Recent Advances in
ANAESTHESIA AND ANALGESIA

R.S. ATKINSON MA MB BChir FFARCS
Consultant Anaesthetist,
Southend Hospital,
Essex, UK

A.P. Adams MB BS PhD FFARCS FFARACS DA
Professor of Anaesthetics in the University of London
at the United Medical and Dental Schools of Guy's
and St Thomas's Hospitals, London;
Honorary Consultant Anaesthetist,
Guy's Hospital, London, UK

Recent Advances in
ANAESTHESIA AND ANALGESIA

EDITED BY
R.S. ATKINSON
AND
A.P. ADAMS

NUMBER SIXTEEN

CHURCHILL LIVINGSTONE
EDINBURGH LONDON MELBOURNE AND NEW YORK 1989

CHURCHILL LIVINGSTONE
Medical Division of Longman Group UK Limited

Distributed in the United States of America by
Churchill Livingstone Inc., 1560 Broadway, New York,
N.Y. 10036, and by associated companies, branches
and representatives throughout the world.

First published 1989

ISBN 0 443 04041 9
ISSN 0309-2305

British Library Cataloguing in Publication Data
Recent advances in anaesthesia and analgesia
No. 16
1. Anesthesia
2. Analgesia
I. Atkinson, R. S. II. Adam, A. P.
617'.96 RD81

Produced by Longman Singapore Publishers Pte Ltd
Printed in Singapore

Preface

In the years which have passed since the publication of Volume 15, the editors have been aware of the enormous cascade of publications in books and journals. The average anaesthetist is busy with a heavy load of clinical work and finds it difficult to keep abreast of developments. The editors have had this very much in mind when choosing topics for the present volume. Some of the chapters review recent advances in clinical methods; others take a new look at long established problems and seek to throw new light on matters still under debate.

Once again the editors have been fortunate to obtain the help of authorities in their respective fields. They have also extended their policy of inviting contributions from outside the British Isles; this time there are two contributions from Australia.

The anaesthetist is always concerned with respiratory physiology and the opportunity is taken to have a new look at the alveolus. What is the future of nitrous oxide in anaesthetic practice? Does recent knowledge of the side effects of this popular agent foreshadow its decline in anaesthetic practice? The subject is reviewed in this volume.

Many more drugs are nowadays given by continuous infusion and this topic is reviewed, as is the subject of sedation in the operating room and the intensive care unit. Both are important to the clinical anaesthetist whether or not he or she practises outside the traditional theatre environment. The increased interest in the use of local analgesic methods also merits a chapter.

Trauma is always with us and presents a challenge to reduce mortality and morbidity. Fluid therapy continues to promote debate. What is the best solution to administer and under what circumstances? There is some overlap between these two subjects which are considered by two separate contributors, each a recognized authority in his subject, but this is considered advantageous in an important field. Craniofacial surgery is of growing surgical interest. The associated problems for the anaesthetist can be formidable, particularly in small children, and deserve a chapter for their consideration.

Volume 15 contained a chapter on morbidity and mortality in anaesthetic practice. The important subject of safety continues to exercise anaesthetists' minds as shown by the confidential enquiries carried out and by the statements on monitoring published by both College and Association. In this volume some space is devoted to monitoring. There is consideration in some depth of both capnography and oximetry, two methods now coming into general use. The monitoring of neuromuscular block is also treated in a separate chapter.

Chronic pain and its management remains of perennial concern. Anaesthetists continue to play a large part in the organization of pain clinics. There is, therefore, a chapter on this subject. The role of aminoglycosides in this context will be new to many anaesthetists, but receives consideration here.

It is hoped that this current volume in the *Recent Advances in Anaesthesia and Analgesia* series will continue to be interesting and informative to examination candidates, to established anaesthetists and to those in remote parts where many current journals are not readily available.

The editors thank the contributors for their hard work and cooperation without which this volume could not be produced. The publishers are also thanked for their considerable courteous help in its production.

Southend and London, 1989   R.S.A.
                                                                                   A.P.A.

Contributors

ANTHONY P. ADAMS MB BS PhD FFARCS FFARACS DA
Professor of Anaesthetics in the University of London at the United Medical and
Dental Schools of Guy's and St Thomas's Hospitals, London, UK

JAYNE GALLAGHER MB BS FFARCS
Sir Jules Thorn Research Senior Registrar, Pain Relief Clinic, Department of
Anaesthetics, Guy's Hospital, London, UK

VALERIE A. GOAT MB ChB FFARCS
Consultant Anaesthetist, Radcliffe Infirmary, Oxford, UK

W. HAMANN MD PhD
Professor of Physiology, The Chinese University of Hong Kong, Shatin, Hong
Kong; Visiting Consultant, Pain Relief Clinic, Department of Anaesthetics, Guy's
Hospital, London, UK

BRIAN A. HILLS ScD (Cantab.)
Professor and Head of Department of Physiology, The University of New
England, Armidale, NSW, Australia

KEN HILLMAN MB BS FFARCS FFARACS
Director of Anaesthetics, Intensive Care and Coronary Care, The Liverpool
Hospital, Sydney, NSW, Australia

K.L. KONG MB BS FFARCS
Lecturer in Anaesthesia, University of Birmingham, Birmingham, UK

A.B. LOACH MA MB BChir FFARCS DA
Consultant Anaesthetist, Nuffield Department of Anaesthetics; Honorary
Clinical Lecturer, University of Oxford, Oxford, UK

A.C. PEARCE MRCP FFARCS
Consultant Anaesthetist, Lewisham and North Southwark Health District, Guy's
Hospital, London, UK

J.W. SEAR MA BSc PhD FFARCS
Clinical Reader in Anaesthetics, Nuffield Department of Anaesthetics,
University of Oxford, John Radcliffe Hospital, Oxford, UK

J.C. STODDART MD BS FFARCS
Consultant in Anaesthesia and Intensive Care, Royal Victoria Infirmary,
Newcastle upon Tyne, UK

D.C. WHITE MB BS FFARCS
Consultant Anaesthetist, Northwick Park Hospital and Clinical Research Centre,
Harrow, Middlesex, UK

SHEILA M. WILLATTS FRCP FCAnaes.
Consultant Anaesthetist, Bristol Royal Infirmary, Bristol, UK

Contents

1. New alveolar models

B.A. Hills

The need to provide ample oxygenation of the patient during anaesthesia requires the integrity of the gas transfer surface and the very delicate architecture of the terminal air spaces to be maintained. Hence it is highly desirable to have a realistic model of those spaces, especially the alveolus, by which to rationalize the effects of clinical procedures or the course of any lung disease. The two primary considerations are *mechanical* in maintaining compliance and *homeostatic* in avoiding oedema; while both can contribute to atelectasis and other forms of reducing the effective surface available for gas transfer.

LUNG MODELS

While there is considerable controversy surrounding the model to use for the alveolus, there is a large measure of agreement in mechanical approaches to the lung as a whole. A fibrous continuum originally described by Orsos[1] and further morphological studies of connective tissue at the microscopic level by Weibel and Bachofen[2] and Weibel and Gil[3] has led Weibel and Bachofen[4] to adopt more of a structural engineering approach. Their model is based upon two networks of force-bearing line elements, one comprising the pleura, interlobar and interlolubar septa while the other is the lattice of alveolar entrance rings on which the alveolar walls are 'draped'. This model is very good for interpreting compliance ($V : P$) curves up to 80% total lung capacity (TLC) in the saline-filled lung and even up to 100% TLC if one of the two parallel networks is composed of both collagen elements and distensible elastic elements.

While these models are excellent at high lung volume where structural forces attributable to parenchymal tissue predominate, problems arise when interpreting the mechanical differences between air-filled and liquid-filled lungs at low volumes relevant to normal ventilation. It then becomes necessary to select an alveolar model and one is effectively assumed whatever mathematical relationship is adopted between lung volume and surface area. Models for whole lung have been well reviewed by Hoppin and Hildebrandt.[5]

INTERFACIAL FACTORS

The basic problem with interpreting volume : pressure ($V : P$) data at low transmural pressures is the predominance of interfacial factors. This is clearly demonstrated by liquid filling excised lungs as originally demonstrated by von Neergaard,[6] who found that the pressure needed to inflate lungs with air was much higher than that with isotonic liquid. In fact, the ratio of transmural pressures needed to return a lung to

1

functional residual capacity (FRC) indicates that interfacial forces contribute between three quarters and seven eighths of total recoil according to data from von Neergaard and from Ardila, Horie and Hildebrandt.[7]

THE 'BUBBLE' MODEL

Von Neergaard offered two possible explanations for his observations. Firstly, he realized that, when a liquid replaces air at a dry surface, the surface energy of the solid — in this case epithelium — is changed. The second explanation he offered for the dramatic change in compliance was that liquid filling would eliminate the interface between air and any aqueous fluid lining the alveolus. Until quite recently[8] only his second interpretation received any attention, and by far the most popular alveolar model today is that of a one-sided bubble. The interfacial contribution to lung recoil that predominates at lower lung volumes is then attributed to the collapsing pressure (ΔP) as related to the surface tension (γ) and radius of curvature (r) by the Laplace equation:

$$\Delta P = 2\gamma/r \qquad (1)$$

Thus the mechanics of the alveolus are most important since not only do alveoli account for at least 60% of lung volume but the curvature of the interface (liquid or solid) is one of the greatest, the lowest values of r giving the highest values for ΔP in equation (1). The simplicity of this expression has indirectly contributed to the popularity of the 'bubble' model but raises the question of how to accommodate such a wide range of alveolar sizes as occur from the hila to the diaphragmatic surface or of curvature within a single alveolus. This raises the major issue of alveolar stability.

ALVEOLAR STABILITY

One of the amazing features of the normal lung is that an area of the order of 90 m^2 can be held apart at the micro level during ventilatory movements. Its remarkable stability has often been compared with that of a foam,[9] but such a mass of *closed* bubbles of different sizes can co-exist for the same surface tension because each can possess a different internal pressure. However, when they are interconnected as occurs in the lung, the smaller ones with a lower value of r in equation (1) would have higher collapsing pressures (ΔP) than larger ones and so air would flow so as to enlarge the larger ones and deflate the smaller ones. The resulting changes in radii then exacerbate the difference, accelerating collapse of the smaller alveoli as ΔP rises hyperbolically.

Advocates of the 'bubble' model then point out that there can be equal recoil (ΔP) in two alveoli of different sizes if they have different surface tensions (γ) each bearing the same ratio to curvature, i.e. if γ/r is in equation (1) is the same for each. Clements et al[10] have demonstrated in vitro how the surfactant known to line the alveolus has the capability of changing the surface tension when placed on the surface of water. Moreover, the surface tension decrease in surface area corresponds to a collapsing bubble, and vice versa for an enlargng bubble, the rates of change ensuring that (γ/r) values reach and maintain a common value *during a single inflation*.

This traditional explanation for alveolar stability is most plausible and appears to remove one of the major shortcomings of the 'bubble' model until it is realized that the continuity of the liquid lining inherently assumed in the model should extend between alveoli either via terminal bronchioles or via the pores of Kohn. If the liquid surface is continuous between adjacent alveoli, it is difficult to postulate different values of surface tension without entering into complex arguments related to the surface viscosity of surfactant.[11]

One further point is that, as soon as a monolayer of surfactant on the smaller bubble is compressed more than the monolayer on the larger bubble, surfactant will be more rapidly derecruited into the aqueous hypophase (liquid lining). Surface tension tends towards an equilibrium value, whether by derecruitment into the hypophase or recruitment from it. Thus, over a longer period than one compression, the same inequality in (γ/r) and, hence, in collapsing pressure would be re-established. Another possibility is that lamellar bodies (active surfactant) might 'pop' to the surface more rapidly in smaller alveoli but, no such *differential* aspect has been demonstrated although the basic mechanism is plausible.[12]

Arguments such as these have cast doubt upon the bubble model but those for and against have all assumed that each alveolus is mechanically independent of its neighbours.

INTERDEPENDENCE

The structural advantages of the back-to-back configuration of alveoli in maintaining spatial integrity of the gas-transfer surface has been emphasized by Mead, Takashima and Leith.[13] This concept of interdependence undoubtedly applies to larger lung units clearly separated by connective tissue but any role at the micro-level is much less obvious. The role of connective tissue in alveolar distensibility and collapsibility has been comprehensively reviewed by Turino and Laurenco.[14] The pertinent question is whether interalveolar forces can impart sufficient stability to accommodate the shortcomings imparted by surfactant as a monolayer on a liquid lining.

This question is answered to some degree by the practical fact that atelectasis occurs at all. Alveolar collapse is easily induced by compromising the surfactant system — either in disease as seen in cases of the respiratory distress syndrome (RDS), or experimentally by detergent rinsing.[15] These basic facts clearly indicate a large degree of *independence* of whatever alveolar model is adopted. However, the importance of surface forces in lung recoil emphasizes the pivotal role of surfactant and need to consider not only alternative alveolar models but each combination of model and mode of action of surfactant.

TRADITIONAL ROLES ATTRIBUTED TO SURFACTANT

Surfactant is a mixture of predominantly phospholipid and protein (4%) produced in its surface-active state by alveolar type II cells as lamellar bodies. These unravel upon secretion onto the alveolar surface forming tubular myelin. The composition of surfactant has been reviewed in much detail in the text edited by Robertson and van Golde,[16] but the predominant and by far the most surface-active component of the phospholipid is Lα-dipalmitoyl phosphatidylocholine — otherwise known as dipalmitoyl lecithin (DPL).

From this point onwards, theories diverge according to the role attributed to surfactant and whether or not there is a continuous hypophase on which it can locate. This issue was first raised by Pattle[17] when reviewing conflicting electron micrographic studies of lung tissue in its normal physiological state. There is no doubt that a continuous liquid lining exists in many pathological states. However, if a continuous liquid lining is a normal physiological state, a mechanism needs to be postulated for control of its thickness but, as Brooks[18] points out, none has been forthcoming.

The traditional theory is that lamellar bodies 'pop to the surface' of the fluid lining (aqueous hypophase) spreading rapidly and greatly reducing surface tension.[12] Its recruitment to the surface is generally considered to be facilitated by some of the proteins present,[16] probably because the soluble proteins can act as carriers for the highly insoluble DPL by forming loose associations in the form of lipoprotein.

When located at the air-aqueous interface, the surfactant is conventionally attributed the following properties:

1. It reduces surface tension (γ) and, hence, the transmural pressure (ΔP) needed to inflate the smallest units of the lung, thereby 'making breathing easy'.

2. It imparts the ability to change surface tension with area, thereby confering alveolar stability for the reasons discussed above.

3. By reducing surface tension, a less negative interstitial pressure is needed in order to prevent alveolar flooding.

Conceptually, oedema can form either by two adjacent bubbles/alveoli tending to collapse and suck fluid into the intervening interstitial space or by the extent of the negative pressure that arises in the liquid lining. Since the Laplace equation predicts a positive pressure (ΔP) on the 'air' side of the interface by the bubble configuration then, if the airways are open to atmosphere taken as the pressure datum, there is a negative pressure ($-\Delta P$) in the aqueous hypophase as discussed later with respect to aveolar flooding.

SHORTCOMINGS OF THE 'BUBBLE' MODEL

When von Neergaard[6] substituted values for ΔP and r into the Laplace equation (Equation 1) for porcine lungs, he obtained γ values not far in excess of the equilibrium surface tension (25 dyne/cm). However, scanning electron micrographs and morphological studies in general leave no doubt that curvature of the alveolar surface is much greater, i.e. much more concave with respect to air at the septal corners. Such studies also show many convex areas — especially where red cells are bulging through the underlying capillaries — indicating a very dynamic state with rapidly changing contours. In some places, the surface can be convex in one plane and concave in the perpendicular plane when, if r_1 and r_2 are the respective radii of curvature, the comprehensive Laplace equation must be used, viz.

$$\Delta P = \gamma(r_1 + r_2) \tag{2}$$

when ΔP can be zero for such a 'saddle' where $r_1 = -r_2$.

If this equation is used for the septal corner,[5] where $r_1 = \infty$ and $r_2 = 10 \ \mu m$, γ must be less than 5 dyne/cm for ΔP not to exceed a physiologically acceptable collapsing pressure of 5 cm H_2O. If one considers mammals such as the bat and the shrew where, even for a perfectly spherical bubble, r cannot exceed 15 μm, Equation (1) gives even lower values[8] for γ. Hence the surface tension needs to be 7 dynes/cm or less for the 'bubble' model to be valid, while many authors[5] consider that it should be 'near zero'.

ALVEOLAR SURFACE TENSION

Many measurements have been made of the surface tension imparted by DPL or by surfactant recovered by lung lavage or solvent extraction from lung tissue. Values range from 'near zero' (less than 2 dynes/cm) to the equilibrium surface tension or just above.[11] However, the vast majority of studies have invoked the Wilhelmy principle illustrated in Figure 1.1 in conjunction with the Langmuir trough as first employed in pulmonary studies by Clements.[19] Surfactant is deposited on an aqueous pool in a spreadable solvent which then evaporates leaving a monolayer or the monolayer is recruited from the hypophase by leaving lung rinsings in the trough.

The Langmuir trough was widely used by physicists and physical chemists at the beginning of this century to study the very interesting phase changes that occur in monolayers, corresponding to gas, liquid and solid forms. They used the largest film compressions possible, representing area changes of 5 : 1 or even 10 : 1, in order to obtain the maximum physical information. When the same 'physical' area changes are used on monolayers of lung surfactant, or pure DPL, it is easy to obtain 'near zero' readings on the transducer used to measure the force (F) by the Wilhelmy method. A

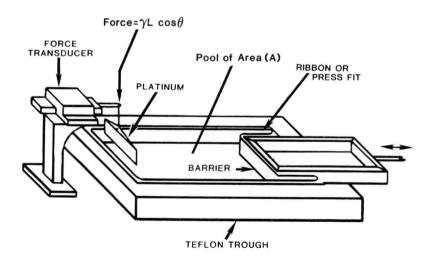

Contact angle θ; wetted perimeter L; surface tension γ

Fig. 1.1 The Langmuir trough long used by physical chemists to study phase changes and other properties of surfactant monolayers by effecting large changes in the areas of monolayers deposited on the surface of a pool. Also demonstrated is the Wilhelmy method very popular among physiologists for measuring the surface tension of the pool as the vertical force (F/L); although this really measures the apparent surface tension ($\gamma.\cos \theta$).

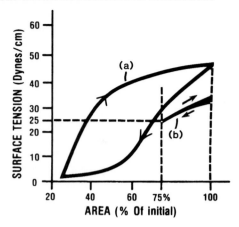

Fig. 1.2   Typical loops for monolayers of DPL on the Langmuir trough: (a) for apparent surface tension measured by the Wilhelmy method (F/L in Fig. 1.1) cycled over area changes of 5:1 commonly used in 'physical' studies; and (b) for true surface tension (γ) cycled over more physiological area changes. (Data from Barrow & Hills (1979b), with permission.)

typical loop for *apparent* surface tension (F/L) versus area (A) is shown in Figure 1.2. Figures such as these that show (F/L) approaching zero — or even negative values — at maximum monolayer compression are much quoted in standard physiological texts,[20] in support of the 'bubble' model. Little mention is made, however, of the fact that the surface tension over much of the cycle is very much higher with the average, approximating the equilibrium value.

CONTROVERSIAL ISSUES

In the foregoing discussion, the term 'apparent surface tension' was used for (F/L) in Figure 1.1 because it equals $\gamma \cos \theta$, and not γ alone. θ is the contact angle, i.e. the angle between the solid–liquid and liquid-air phases at the triple point where all three phases meet and the liquid 'grips' the flag, thus pulling it downwards. The conventional argument is that, for a perfectly clean plate, θ is zero when $\cos \theta$ is unity and (F/L) gives a true reading of γ. Thus Notter and Finkelstein[21] criticize the work of Barrow and Hills[22] who found large contact angles at high compressions when reproducing the loops for F/L, shown in Figure 1.2, on the basis that they were using greasy plates. However the 'grease' is DPL itself, which is readily adsorbed to the plate[11] and, when allowance is made for contact angle, the minimum surface tension is far above zero and certainly too high to be compatible with the 'bubble' model.

While most of the surface-tension data in the physiological literature has been obtained using the Wilhelmy method, methods that avoid contact-angle artefact have recently been pursued. The pulsating bubble method pioneered by Enhorning[23] gives $\gamma : A$ loops with 'near-zero' values at maximum compression but values exceeding 30 dynes/cm at the other end of the cycle. The minimum value can be reduced by larger area changes, but the maximum is then increased, indicating that inertial factors may be accentuating the difference.[11] Similar reasons caused another dynamic method, that conceived by Lord Rayleigh, to be discontinued for use with liquids over ranges where surface energy was so much less than the kinetic energy of the system.[24] The pulsating bubble method has the further disadvantage of departing from the well controlled conditions of the Langmuir trough.

Methods compatible with the Langmuir trough and independent of contact angle are the du Noüy ring, as used on surfactant by Barrow and Hills,[25] and the original method of Langmuir.[26] These studies showed that surface tension could be reduced to a minimum 7 dynes/cm upon a 'physical' compression of 5 : 1.[27]

AREA CHANGES

This 'physical' (5 : 1) compression is needed in order to transform a recruited monolayer into the 'solid' state — the only state of surfactant capable of giving 'near zero' values for the apparent surface tension (F/L). Such compressions are also needed to reduce the true value of γ to 7 dynes/cm, which is about the maximum value that can be used to satisfy conditions for homeostasis as discussed later.

The point that has been conveniently overlooked in much of the traditional literature is how 'physical' compressions of 5 : 1 can be used in *physiological* studies when the barrier of the Langmuir trough is ostensibly used to simulate respiratory area changes. Many relationships between area (A) and lung volume (V) have been proposed, ranging from isometric changes $(A \propto V^{2/3})$ to $A \propto V^{1/3}$ for morphological studies,[28] while Whimster[29] has proposed a 'concertina' model of the alveolus in which area does not change at all. Even when changing lung volume between FRC and TLC, it is difficult to justify an area change of more than 26% while, for normal tidal volume, it is probably 6.3%[11] and certainly unlikely to exceed that 25% limit originally proposed by Pattle.

When DPL films or monolayers of lung surfactant are cycled over these more physiological area changes using measurement methods independent of the contact-angle artefact, the results are shown in Figure 1.2. The major feature is that the surface tension does not fall below 18 dynes/cm, while another interesting ancillary observation is that of negligible surface tension: area hysteresis. Negligible hysteresis avoids one of the major objections to any model based upon the large 'physical' $\gamma : A$ loops (Fig. 1.2) needed to reach near-zero values of surface tension. Surface tension (γ) multiplied by area (A) has the dimensions of work, so that such a large loop represents a very large loss of work. It would be ridiculous for the body to locate a substance at the surface of any bubble lining that would make it work so much harder. Hence the negligible hysteresis recorded over physiological area changes in Figure 1.2 makes much more sense teleologically. In fact, careful examination of the loop when cycled to steady state indicates slight inversion, i.e. the conversion of some other form of energy into work, a possible source being waste metabolic heat.[11] This has interesting clinical implications where there is a delicate balance between the work needed for ventilation and the work that the muscles of the chest wall and diaphragm are capable of providing — such as found in cases of respiratory distress syndrome (RDS) or the weaning of a patient from a ventilator.

So far we have followed the approach of determining the appropriate γ value to use in the Laplace equation (equation (1)), but the reverse approach has been used by Horie and Hildebrandt when the $\gamma : A$ curve derived from $V : P$ data shows little resemblance to any obtained on the Langmuir trough. There are several incogruencies, such as the decrease in surface tension with increasing surface area; this point was raised earlier in discussing the original work of von Neergaard.

STATE OF SURFACTANT IN THE LUNG

Returning to values of surface tension that are so crucial to the 'bubble' model, it is probably fair to state that no one has produced 'near zero' γ without employing non-physiological compressions of the monolayer, not even the apparent surface tension reduced in magnitude by contact-angle artefact. The fact that surface tension rises rapidly upon expansion to values well over 30 dynes/cm (Fig. 1.2) is not discussed in traditional theories.

The counter argument is that, as lamellar bodies rapidly 'pop' to the surface of the aqueous hypophase, surfactant is recruited so rapidly that minimal compressions are then needed to produce a monolayer in the 'solid' phase. However, surfactant such as that contained in lamellar bodies, has a monolayer melting point[30] of about 28.5°C. In other words, it is a surface eutectic mixture of phopholipids, just as solder has a melting point lower than any of its components. Since the whole-surfactant melting point is so much lower than that of DPL (41°C) — the predominant and only component capable of reaching 'near zero' γ for any area change — it is then speculated that respiratory area changes are needed to 'squeeze-out' other components of lung phospholipid,[31,32] elevating the melting point above a human core temperature of 37°C. However, it would require a phenomenal rate of refinement relative to gross recruitment in order to elevate the melting point to 37°C. If lower rates of recruitment are proposed, then de-recruitment of DPL that is facilitated by protein would be too rapid to maintain the solid state of the monolayer and so the debate continues.[11]

Nevertheless, it has been pointed out that, even in the unlikely event of 100% refinement to raise the monolayer melting point to 41°C, lethal core temperatures are several degrees higher, with Schmidt-Nielson[33] quoting 43°C for man and 42–44°C for eutherian mammals with essentially the same surfactant system and up to 46°C for birds. Moreover, 47°C is the point at which the mechanics of excised lungs break down[34]. This temperature is too high to correlate with a monolayer — even of 100% pure condensed DPL — located on an aqueous hypophase.

These arguments are also difficult to explain using another alveolar model in which the refined solid surfactant floating as a raft on the aqueous hypophase is considered to form a solid shell imparting alveolar stability.[35]

Intellectually satisfying as the 'bubble' model may appear, with the convenience of relating lung mechanics to the surface factors that predominate at lower lung volumes, it fails to offer adequate explanations for many pieces of evidence.

ALTERNATE APPROACHES TO SURFACTANT

Hitherto we have discussed surfactant located at the surface of a liquid layer or aqueous hypophase assumed to line the alveoli, where its only role is to reduce and generally modify surface tension. However non-biological surfactants produced for industrial purposes have long been developed for the highly desirable properties that they can impart to solid surfaces, which also have surface energies that can be reduced. For this to occur, however, the surfactant needs to be adsorbed to the surface — a process of reversible physical or chemical attachment usually effected through electrical charges in the polar (water seeking) end of the molecule. Almost all muscosal surfaces in vivo are negative as a result of fixed carboxyl and sulphonyl groups, so the orientation of the choline group is ideal for producing a net force of attraction. Moreover interspersion of cations such as Ca^{2+} in the plane of the phosphate ions can neutralize those ions, leaving the strongly charged quaternary ammonium ions to attach the molecule to the negative surface as a 'pseudocationic' surfactant. This orientates the surfactant with its non-polar fatty-acid chains outwards where they can pack together with those on neighbouring sites to form a thin hydrocarbon exterior. Like all hydrocarbon surfaces, e.g. candle wax or polyethylene, this would be hydrophobic and therefore water repellent. Moreover, lecithin molecules that are locked in position at their polar ends now have a transition temperature[36] for 'chain melting' at 46°C. This corresponds much more closely to the point of breakdown of lung mechanics and could explain the thermal shortcomings of the 'bubble' model described above.

WATER REPELLENCY

In many ways, the fine architecture of the terminal air spaces of the lung resembles that of delicate fabrics where quaternary ammonium surfactants are widely used as 'softeners' to prevent clumping while generally maintaining the spatial integrity of the very fine filaments.[37] Many of the same surfactants are also water repellents[38] and this raises the question whether DPL adsorbed to the epithelial surface could be performing the same function in the alveolus.[8] When adsorbed to cotton carboxylated to simulate the negative charges found in vivo, DPL is a very effective water repellent, inducing a pressure for water penetration well in excess of pulmonary arterial pressure.[39] This has led to an alternative alveolar model depicted in Figure 1.3a where it is compared with the 'bubble' model (Fig. 1.3b).

The major advantage of DPL adsorbed to carboxylated cotton is that it represents a discontinuous liquid lining and therefore one that will not undergo self-accelerating collapse, thus the question of alveolar stability is no longer a problem. At least, this is so until oedema occurs to the point at which the 'corner pools' link up and form a continuous lining but as a *pathological* and not the normal *physiological* state.

Compliance ($V : P$) data can be interpreted on the basis that contact angles change during the respiratory cycle;[40] while a sigh is needed to re-establish compliance by re-establishing edges to the pools from which fluid may have encroached over the intervening 'dry patches'. The water-repellent model is based upon two types of surface, 'wet' and 'dry'. This is supported by experiments in which nebulized water droplets[41] and small fluorocarbon droplets[42] have been found to behave in one of two different ways upon initial contact, either spreading instantly or remaining intact as an adhering bead.

The surface is tensioned by the 'pools' gripping the epithelium to pull it taut over the dry patches — a mechanism for which an equilibrium surface tension of 25 dynes/cm would seem preferable to one that is 'near zero'. An equilibrium surface

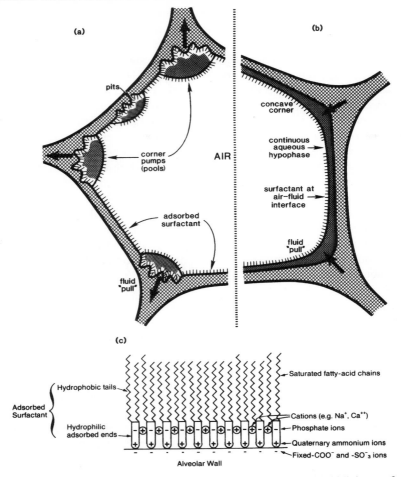

Fig. 1.3 (a) The water-repellent model of the alveolus with a discontinuous liquid lining confined to the 'pits' and 'pools' from which it can 'grip' the dry epithelium at the triple point (Fig. 1.1), tensioning it and storing excess as immersed 'pleats' analogous to soaking wrinkles. With oedema, the 'pools' can assume a convex profile (as shown) when a significant surface tension (e.g. equilibrium) provides a positive force returning fluid to the interstitium. If flooding continues, the 'pools' and 'pits' overflow and fluid 'bursts through' from the pores in the dry patches to form the 'bubble' model (b) but as a pathological state. Water repellency in (a) is imparted by adsorption of surfactant (c) where cations in the plane of the phosphate ions can enhance cohesion of the adsorbate while neutralizing that half of the zwitterion to leave the lecithin as effectively a cationic surfactant characterized by strong adsorption. (Figures from Hills (1988)[11] with permission.)

tension is much more compatible with a very basic observation in lung mechanics — that of holding the lung at low volume after completing several $V:P$ cycles when transmural pressure hardly changes. Interpreted into $\gamma:A$ cycles using the 'bubble' model by Bachofen et al,[43] this implies a constant surface tension of 2–3 dynes/cm, which is totally uncharacteristic of monolayers of lung surfactant on a Langmuir trough (see Fig.1.1). After compression to such a low surface tension, the surfactant is rapidly derecruited into the hypophase[44] until it returns to an equilibrium value, probably facilitated by the protein and Ca^{2+}

It has also been argued[8] that the lowest surface tension is not necessarily the best mechanically because breathing represents an exchange of potential energy between the chest wall and lungs. Since at lower volumes the lungs store most of that energy as surface energy, too low a range of surface tension would limit its ability to store that energy.

There are many other mechanical arguments evaluating the two models,[11] as illustrated in Figure 1.3, that are too lengthy to include in this text but, teleologically, it does not make sense to cover the gas-transfer surface with a liquid layer that adds another barrier to gas diffusion.

Before discussing the other general area of comparison, homeostasis, it is desirable to discuss morphological evidence for what is emerging as the knub of the issue — whether the liquid lining is continuous or not.

MORPHOLOGICAL STUDIES

One would imagine that a few good electron microscopic studies (e.m.s.) would immediately clarify the situation. They certainly leave no doubt that the 'bubble' model applies *after* alveolar flooding but e.m.s. can be selected to support any model for the normal physiological state.

Colacicco[45] claims that the alveolus is normally totally dry and that both liquid and surfactant linings are artefact, surfactant only being released by the Type II cell on flooding. There are certainly many opportunities for introducing artefact in the fixation process and many of the original workers find a continuous liquid lining, while many do not.[17] The difficult question is whether the surface on which no liquid can be seen in really dry or has a liquid layer too thin to detect or is instantly wetted upon advance of any meniscus during respiratory movement. Mathematically, the last two cases would be equivalent to a continuous liquid lining.[46] Electron micrographs can be produced that show droplets standing proud on 'dry' surfaces[47,48] as though such surfaces were hydrophobic. The choice of fixative could influence the outcome, especially now that glutaraldehyde is used almost universally and yet, as Untersee et al[49] point out, aldehydes tend to destroy the hydrophobic surface. Thus a non-wettable surface prior to fixation could appear wettable after fixation.

ALVEOLAR EPITHELIUM

The other approach to the wettability question is to determine whether the alveolar epithelium is lined with hydrophilic or hydrophobic substances. Using various stains, Meban[50] and others were able to demonstrate a continuous layer of acid mucosubstance on the alveolar epithelium, which would therefore appear highly wettable. However, those workers were fixing the tissue via the airways when mucus, known to be secreted from cells lining more proximal air spaces, could have been transported to that surface where it would tend to attach if the surface were hydrophobic. A loose attachment could occur because mucus is an excellent wetting agent for hydrophobic surfaces immersed in water.[51] Hence it could be most significant that Gil & Weibel[52] do not find any mucoid lining to the alveolus when 'fixing from behind', i.e. via the pulmonary vasculature.

Those authors emphasize the need for that fixation route and, when doing so,[28,47] find many interesting features, chief of which are:

1. The liquid lining is present as relatively deep 'pits' and 'pools' separated by areas where no fluid can be seen; although that does not mean that the liquid layer is not present but too thin to visualize.

2. There is a remarkably smooth contour of the alveolar surface, even at points where the interface with air changes from liquid to apparently dry. It is as though the liquid were gripping the epithelium at the edges of the 'pits' and 'pools' pulling it taut. It would only seem possible to impart sufficient tension if the surface tension were well above zero and there were a triple point (see Fig. 1.1) at which to apply its grip. For a triple point to occur, the surface between the 'pools' would need to be dry and not instantly wettable. An analogy has been drawn with a window sash as a model by which the 'pool' can apply an almost constant tension to the whole surface.[11]

3. The epithelium with the 'pools' and 'pits' is crumpled into what Gil et al,[28] appropriately term 'pleats' showing a remarkable transition from the smooth contour of the apparently dry surface and, again, indicating a 'periphery of grip' separating them.

4. The excess epithelium gathered as 'pleats' in the 'pits' and 'pools' strongly resemble soaking wrinkles in cutaneous epithelium, again raising the question of why the whole surface is not wrinkled if there were really a continuous liquid lining. This point is reinforced upon liquid filling the lung when, indeed, the whole alveolar surface does display the same wrinkled contour.[28]

5. Dense osmiophilic boundaries can be seen on both the liquid–air and epithelial surfaces as discussed later.

It has therefore been claimed that the morphology tends to support the model of a discontinuous liquid lining depicted to Figure 1.3a, although Gil[53] disputes this on the basis that no contact angle can be seen with the fluid bulging into the air space. The counter-argument[54] is that there *is* a contact angle in the normal *physiological* state but that it is formed by the epithelium folding under, i.e. into the 'pit' or 'pool' to give their characteristically steep sides rather than the fluid bulging outwards. The latter would only be needed in the *pathological* case to resolve any excess fluid where the contour would now become convex with respect to air as the corner 'pool' becomes a corner 'pump'[39] with a positive pressure for returning oedema fluid to deeper structures, i.e. curvature is in the desired direction and the effect is self-regulating as ΔP in Equation 1 become less positive as r approaches ∞ with resolution of the oedema. Contrary to predictions based upon the 'bubble' model, an equilibrium surface tension would be more effective for this purpose than a 'near zero' value, which, in any case, is difficult to substantiate as discussed above.

Before leaving morphological studies, however, there remains the vital question of whether surfactant is directly adsorbed to alveolar epithelium, which is a cornerstone of the water repellent model (Fig. 1.3c). When substituting tannic acid for much of the glutaraldehyde as the fixative, Ueda et al.[55] have indeed demonstrated a third line equally spaced from the ubiquitous 'tramlines' representing the lipid bilayer of the epithelial membrane. Later studies by Ueda et al.[56] have shown that this might be multilaminar but, whichever it is, it is directly attached to the alveolar surface consistent with adsorption (see Fig. 1.3a). This is compatible with the finding of Cavagna et al.[57] that surfactant is adsorbed to epithelial cells rather than derived from alveolar fluid recovered by lavage; although those authors attributed no functional significance to their observation at the time.

DISJOINING PRESSURE

Attractive as the water repellent model may appear with its 'window-sash' mechanism for tensioning, there would appear one major shortcoming, namely how to restore water repellency after flooding. After all, touching the inside of a tent in the rain starts a drip that runs down the wall recruiting more pores, which then augment the flow. This could explain the exponential rise in alveolar oedema when an elevated vascular driving force is maintained[58] and why, after a critical point, it cannot be reversed even if vascular pressure is returned to normal. This would correspond to the stage at which 'pools' and 'pits' have overflowed to the point where they have linked up and formed a continuous liquid lining, which becomes thicker until the collapsing pressure of the ever decreasing 'bubble' (ΔP increases as r decreases in equation (1) becomes too great for homeostatic forces to cope.

Up to this point, reversal would be aided by an interesting phenomenon by which hydrophobic surfaces covered with water generate a disjoining pressure,[59] which tends to rupture that layer and expose dry surface. This is seen in everyday life by siphoning water out of a Teflon-lined frying pan. When the depth is reduced to 1–1.5 mm, the layer ruptures spontaneously and similar depths have been recorded using adsorbed monolayers of surfactant deposited in vitro from amniotic fluid or by solvent.[60] If the disjoining pressure can rupture a water layer of this thickness, it should be easier to rupture one of alveolar dimensions (150 μm) even if surface tension is lowered.

The phenomena forms the basis of a common industrial use of surfactants as 'de-watering agents' by which the application of one or two drops can cause water held by capillarity in a structural matrix to be immediatley expelled.[8] It would be tempting to speculate something similar occurring when the newborn takes it first breath. This view is supported by the extremely hydrophobic nature of the human amnion,[61] which has been exposed to surfactant in amniotic fluid of only one eleventh the concentration in foetal aspirates.

PULMONARY OEDEMA

The success of using Starling-type forces in explaining fluid balance across the endothelium of many tissues has, in the author's opinion, dominated approaches to fluid balance across pulmonary epithelium. Surfactant is seldom mentioned, if at all, despite the dominance of surface factors in lung mechanics in general. If lymph flow is increased more than about eight fold[62] either by raising pulmonary arterial pressure above 23–25 mm Hg or by reducing oncotic pressure below about 10 mm Hg[63] or various combinations, fluid starts to collect as interstitial oedema. When the increase in lung weight exceeds about 35%[64] there is quite a sudden 'burst through' of fluid onto the alveolar surface which is then difficult to reverse, Staub[65] appropriately comparing this process as an overflowing bathtub. Since the conventional 'bubble' model of the alveolus assumes a liquid lining *before flooding*, transport equations relating hydrostatic forces to the gradient in oncotic pressure[66] require an exceedingly low protein permeability.[67] *Upon Flooding*, however, alveolar cedema is found to have virtually the same composition as lymph and, hence, interstitial fluid,[68] while pulmonary epithelium becomes highly conductive to protein.[69] This is most surprising or 'disconcerting' as Staub[65] describes it since, in terms of Stavermann reflexion coefficients used for quantifying the osmotic effectiveness of protein, it implies a sudden switch from 0 to 1, i.e. from one extreme to the other. This is difficult to believe.

No such sudden switch would be implied, however, if there were no liquid layer before flooding, in which case Starling-type forces would not apply. If it were a simple case of water repellency, then the relevant criterion for alveolar oedema is determined by the relative magnitudes of the interstitial fluid pressure and the critical penetration pressure determined by the surface energy of the dry epithelium. This flow or no-flow situation would explain the sudden onset of alveolar flooding, while the absence of any appreciable oncotic pressure would explain the difficulty in reversing it, i.e. the 'overflowing bathtub' effect. Hence Starling forces would seem inappropriate at the epithelial surface. Moreover the adage that 'water goes wherever protein goes' could be turned around for a purely hydrodynamic system to read 'protein goes wherever water goes'.

NEGATIVE INTERSTITIAL PRESSURE

The absence of any barrier to the diffusion of solutes across the epithelial surface and, hence, absence of any oncotic pressure, means that interstitial fluid has the same hydrostatic pressure as that of fluid on the alveolar surface. If the alveolar fluid has a convex profile with respect to air this will be positive, while it will be negative if it is concave as discussed above in relation to the 'bubble' model. The concept of negative interstitial pressure is highly controversial since it raises such questions concerning the driving force for lymph flow and how pericapillary filtrate derived from a positive pressure source (the vessel) can be reduced to negative pressures. The only answer is that lymph drainage would need to be an active pumping mechanism driven by respiratory movements as expounded by Guyton.[70]

However the mechanism cannot be totally one of pumping since flow rates are highly dependent upon back-pressure (P_2) according to Drake et al.[71] Moreover, if the pumping mechanism is ignored and the unknown upstream pressure is P_1, then the unknown driving force $(P_1 - P_2)$ should be proportional to the lymph flow rate Q, which can be measured. When Drake et al. plotted Q against P_2 to achieve their primary goal of characterizing flow resistance as the gradient, the intercept on the P_2 axis gave P_1. It can be seen from their data that this value is not only *positive* at about $+8$ mmHg but is of just about the magnitude predicted from mean arterio-venous values. It is therefore difficult to see how a negative segment fits into what would otherwise appear a simple gradient of positive pressure.

The experimental evidence in support of a negative interstitial pressure (of about -6 mmHg) has been well reviewed by Guyton et al[72] but ultimately depends upon the validity of an experiment based upon implanting a perforated capsule, as in Guyton's provocative 'ping-pong ball' experiment. The author has confirmed Guyton's negative readings in subcutaneously deposited capsules but was never able to get the capsules totally free of gas, in which case the negative pressure could have been derived from the inherent unsaturation of gases in tissue.[11].

In any case, any negative pressure must be small to be accommodated by Starling-type forces at the epithelium (greater than -7 mmHg) and hence would require surface tension at the septal corners to be 'near zero' — a state very difficult to justify on the basis of the arguments expounded earlier.

CRITIQUE

If the very popular 'bubble' model is very difficult to justify on both mechanical and homeostatic grounds, do any other models offer any better basis for explaining the many facets that need to be considered? Models based upon a totally dry alveolus[45] or floating rafts forming a solid 'shell' of surfactant[35] are convenient for explaining certain aspects but need much more detailed development by their proponents before they can be fully evaluated. The same applies to a model based upon continual alveolar drainage proposed by Hoppin & Heldebandt[5] central to which is the concept of negative interstitial pressure.

The water repellent model is most compatible with the morphology and obviates the need to propose negative interstitial pressure while satisfying many detailed aspects of lung mechanics. However, it has been generally criticized on two fronts, the first being how surfactant can be replenished on the 'dry patches'. This can be answered on the basis that surfactants can diffuse across the solid surfaces to which they are adsorbed[11] while they are present in lymph[73] and hence in the interstitial fluid at the ends of the pores on the surface. The second criticism concerns the good correlation found between the clinical status and the surface tension of fluid recovered from the newborn. This is easily answered[11] on the basis that any substance which is surface active at the fluid-air interface is also surface active at solid surfaces and is thus readily adsorbed. However, as Brooks[18] pointed out, it remains 'unthinkable' to many that the lung surface is not 'totally moistened'.

Hopefully this discussion has made quite clear how intimately the alveolar model is related to the role adopted for surfactant, which cannot be dismissed because surface forces dominate over the normal range of lung volumes.

REFERENCES

1. Orsos F 1936 Die Gerustsysteme der Lunge and deren physiologische and pathologische Bedeutung. I. Normal-anatomische Verhaltnisse. Beitrage Klin Tuberk 87: 568–609
2. Wilson T A, Bachofen H 1982 A model for mechanical structure of alveolar duct. Journal of Applied Physiology 52: 1062–1070
3. Weibel E R, Gil J 1977 Structure-function relationships at the alveolar level. In: West J B (ed) Bioengineering aspects of the lung, Vol. 3 Dekker, New York, p. 1–81
4. Weibel ER, Bachofen H 1979 Structural design of the alveolar septum and fluid exchange. In: Fishman AP, Renkin EM (eds) Pulmonary edema. American Physiological Society, Washington
5. Hoppin F G, Hildebrandt J 1977 Mechanical properties of the lung. In: West J B (ed) Bioengineering aspects of the lung Dekker, New York, pp. 83–162
6. Von Neergaard K 1929 Neue Auggasungen uber einen Grundbegriff der Atammechanik die Retraktionskraft der Lunge, adhangig von der Oberflachenspannung in den Alveolen. Zeitschrift furdie gesamte experimentale Medizinische 66: 373–394
7. Ardila R, Horie T, Hildebrandt J 1974 Macroscopic isotropy of lung expansion. Respiration Physiology 23: 105–115
8. Hills B A 1981 What is the true role of surfactant in the lung? Thorax 36: 1–4
9. Pattle R E 1955 Properties, function and origin of the alveolar lining layer. Nature 175: 1125–1126
10. Clements J A, Hustead R F, Johnson R P, Gribetz I 1961 Pulmonary surface tension and alveolar

stability. Journal of Applied Physiology 16: 444–450
11. Hills B A 1988 The biology of surfactant. Cambridge University Press, Cambridge
12. King R J 1974 The surfactant system of the lung. Federation Proceedings 33: 2238–2247
13. Mead J, Takashima T, Leith D 1970 Stress distribution in lungs: a model of pulmonary elasticity. Journal of Applied Physiology, 28: 596–608
14. Turino G M, Laurenco R V 1972 The connective tissue basis of pulmonary mechanics. In: Mittman C (ed) Pulmonary emphysema and proteolysis. Academic Press, London, pp. 33–50
15. Niemann G, Bredenburg C E 1985 High surface tension pulmonary oedema induced by detergent aerosol. Journal of Applied Physiology 58: 129–136
16. Robertson B, Van Golde L M G 1984 Postscript: surfactant research, current concepts and perspectives for the future. In: Robertson B, Van Golde L M G (eds) Pulmonary Surfactant. Elsevier, Amsterdam, pp. 549–564
17. Pattle R E 1960 Surface tension and lining of the lung alveoli. In: Caro C G (ed) Advances in respiratory physiology. Ch. 3, Williams & Wilkins, Baltimore
18. Brooks R E 1970 Lung surfactant: an alternative hypothesis. American Review of Respiratory Disease 104: 585–586
19. Clements J A 1962. Surface phenomena in relation to pulmonary function. Physiologist 5: 11–28
20. Clements J A, Tierney D F 1965 Alveolar instability associated with altered surface tension. In: Fenn W O, Rahn H (eds) Handbook of physiology: respiration, vol. II American Physiological Society, Washington, pp. 1565–1583
21. Notter R H, Finklestein J N 1984 Pulmonary surfactant: an interdisciplinary approach. Journal of Applied Physiology 57: 1613–1624
22. Barrow R E, Hills B A 1979 Surface tension induced by dipalmitoyl lecithin in vitro under physiological conditions. Journal of Physiology 297: 217–227
23. Enhorning G 1977 Pulsating bubble technique for evaluating pulmonary surfactant. Journal of Applied Physiology 43: 1098–203
24. Champion F C 1939 University Physics Vol. I. General physics. London: Blackie
25. Barrow R E, Hills B A 1979. A critical assessment of the Wilhelmy method in studying lung surfactants. Journal of Physiology 295: 217–227
26. Langmuir I 1916 The constitution and fundamental properties of solids and liquids. Journal of the American Chemical Society 38: 2221–2297
27. Hills B A 1985 Alveolar liquid lining: Langmuir method used to measure surface tension in bovine and canine lung extracts. Journal of Physiology 359: 65–79
28. Gil J, Bachofen H, Gehr P, Weibel E R 1979 Alveolar volume–surface area relation in air- and saline-filled lungs fixed by vascular perfusion. Journal of Applied Physiology 47: 990–1001
29. Whimster W F 1970 The microanatomy of the alveolar duct system. Thorax. 25: 141–149
30. Teubner J K, Gibson R A, McMurchie E J 1983 The influence of water on the phase transition of sheep lung surfactant: a possible mechanism for surfactant phase transitions in vivo. Biochimica et Biophysica Acta, 750: 521–525
31. Watkins J C 1968 The surface properties of pure phospholipids in relation to those of lung extracts. Biochimica et Biophysica Acta 152: 293–306
32. Galdston, M, Shah DO 1967 Surface properties and hysteresis of dipalmitoyllecichin in relation to the alveolar lining layer. Biochimica Biophysica Acta 137: 255–263
33. Schmidt-Nielson K 1979 Animal physiology: adaptation and environment, Cambridge University Press, Cambridge, p. 232
34. Horie T, Ardila R, Hildebrandt J 1974 Static and dynamic properties of excised rat lung in relation to temperature. Journal of Applied Physiology 36: 317–322
35. Bangham A D, Miller N G A, Davies R J, Greenough A, Morley CJ 1984 Introductory remarks about artificial lung expanding compounds (ALEC). Colloids and Surfaces 10: 337–341
36. Chapman D, Williams R M, Ladbrooke B D 1967 Physical studies of phospholipids. VI. Thermotropic and lyotropic mesomorphism of some 1,2-diacyl-phosphatidylcholines (lecithins). Chemistry Physics of Lipids, 1: 445
37. Evans W P 1969 Cationic fabric softeners. Chemistry and Industry 11: 893–903
38. Adamson A W 1967 Physical Chemistry of Surfaces, 2nd edn, Wiley, New York, pp. 352–367
39. Hills B A 1982 Water repellency induced by pulmonary surfactant. Journal of Physiology 325: 175–186
40. Hills B A 1983 Contact-angle hysteresis induced by pulmonary surfactants. Journal of Applied Physiology 54: 420–426
41. Hills BA 1989 Further evidence for a discontinuous liquid lining to the alveolus. Proceedings Australian Physiological & Pharmacological Society 20: 31P
42. Schürch S, Goerke J, Clements J A 1976 Direct determination of surface tension in the lung. Proceedings of the National Academy of Science (USA) 73: 4698–4702
43. Bachofen H, Hildebrandt J, Bachofen M 1970 Pressure-volume curves of air- and liquid-filled

excised lungs — surface tension in situ. Journal of Applied Physiology 29: 422–431
44. Hildebran J N, Goerke J, Clements J A 1979 Pulmonary surface film stability and composition. Journal of Applied Physiology 47: 604–611
45. Colacicco G 1985 Arguments against and alternatives for an extracellular surfactant layer in the alveoli of mammalian lung. Journal of Theoretical Biology 114: 641–656
46. Wilson T A 1981 Effect of alveolar wall shape on alevolar water stability Journal of Applied Physiology 50: 222–224
47. Weibel E R, Bachofen H 1979 Structural design of the alveolar septum and fluid exchange. In: Fishman A P, Renkin E M (eds) Pulmonary edema. American Physiological Society, Washington
48. Kisch B 1958 Electron microscopy of the lungs in acute pulmonary oedema. Experimental Medical Surgery 16: 17–28
49. Untersee P, Gil J, Weibel E R 1971 Visualization of extracellular lining layer of lung alveoli by freeze-etching. Respiration Physiology 13: 171–185
50. Meban C 1978 Surface viscosity of surfactant films from human lungs. Respiration Physiology 33: 219–227
51. Hills B A 1985. Gastric mucosal barrier: stabilization of hydrophobic lining to the stomach by mucus. American Journal of Physiology (Gastrointestinal and Liver Physiology) 244: G561–G568
52. Gil J, Weibel E R 1972 Morphological study of pressure-volume hysteresis in rat lungs fixed by vascular perfusion. Respiration Physiology, 15: 190–213
53. Gil J 1983 Alveolar surface, intra-alveolar fluid pools and respiratory volume changes. Journal of Applied Physiology 54: 321–324
54. Hills B A 1987 Bursting the alveolar bubble. Anaesthesia 42: 467–469
55. Ueda S, Ishii N, Masumoto S, Hayashi K, Okayasu M 1983 Ultrastructural studies on surface lining layer (SLL) of the lung, part II. Journal of the Japanese Medical Society: Biological Interfaces 14: 30–35
56. Ueda S, Kawamura K, Ishii N, Matsumoto S, Hayashi O, Okayasu M, Saito M, Sakurai I 1986 Morphological studies on surface lining layer of the lungs, part IV. Surfactant-like substance in other organs (pleural cavity, vascular lumen and gastric lumen) than lungs. Journal of the Japanese Medical Society: Biological Interfaces 17: 132–156
57. Cavagna G I, Stemmler E J, DuBois A 1967 Alveolar resistance to atelectasis. Journal of Applied Physiology 22: 441–452
58. Drake R E, Smith J H, Gabel J C 1980 Estimation of the filtration coefficient in intact dog lungs. American Journal of Physiology 238 (Heart and Circulation Physiology 7): H430–H438
59. Derjaguin B V, Kusakov M, Lebedeva L 1939 Range of molecular action of surfaces and multi-molecular solvate (adsorbed) layers. Doklady Akademii Nauk USSR 23: 671–673
60. Hills, B A (1984) De-watering capabilities of surfactants in human amniotic fluid. Journal of Physiology 348: 369–381
61. Hills B A, Cotton D B 1986 Release and lubricating properties of amniotic surfactants and the very hydrophobic surfaces of the amnion, chorion and their interface. Obstetrics and Gynecology 68: 550–554
62. Erdmann J A, Vaughan T R, Brigham K L, Woolverton W C, Staub N C 1975 Effect of increased vascular pressure on lung fluid balance in unanesthetized sheep. Circulation Research 37: 271–284.
63. Guyton A C, Lindsey A E 1959 Effect of elevated left atrial pressure and decreased plasma protein concentration on the development of pulmonary oedema. Circulation Research 7: 649–657
64. Iliff I D 1971 Extra-alveolar vessels and oedema development in excised dog lungs. Circulation Research, 28: 524–532
65. Staub N C 1983 Alveolar flooding and clearance. American Review of Respiratory Disease 127: 544–550
66. Staub N C 1984 Pathophysiology of pulmonary edema. In: Staub N C, Taylor A E Edema. Raven, New York, pp. 719–746
67. Egan, E A (1983). Fluid balance in the air-filled space. American Review of Respiratory Disease 127: 537–539
68. Vreim C E, Staub N C 1976 Protein composition of lung fluids in acute alloxan edema in dogs. American Journal Physiology, 230: 376–379
69. Hayward G W (1955). Pulmonary oedema. British Medical Journal 2: 1361–1366
70. Guyton A C 1966 A textbook of medical physiology 3rd. edn. Saunders, Philadephia, p. 550
71. Drake R E, Adcock D K, Scott R L, Gabel J C 1982 Effect of outflow pressure upon lymph flow from dog lungs. Circulation Research 50: 865–869
72. Guyton AC, Barber BJ, Moffatt DS 1978 Theory of interstitial pressures. In: Hargens AR (ed) Tissue fluid pressure and composition. Williams & Wilkins, Baltimore, pp. 11–20
73. Tarpey M M, O'Brodovich H M, Young S L 1983 Role of lymphatics in removal of sheep lung surfactant. Journal of Applied Physiology 54: 984–988

2. A review of nitrous oxide

D. C. White

Nitrous oxide occupies a unique place in the history of anaesthesia and is unique among anaesthetic agents in several ways, which will be described later.

HISTORY

This gas was discovered by Joseph Priestley in 1772 and in a lengthy publication in 1800 describing his researches, facsimile copies of which are now available.[1] Humphry Davy, then 21 years of age, made his famous suggestion that 'it may probably be used with advantage during surgical operations'. This suggestion was not acted upon until 1844 when the American dentist Horace Wells, after seeing a demonstration of the effects of nitrous oxide by Gardner Q. Colton, himself inhaled the gas and had a tooth painlessly extracted. By the middle of January 1845, Wells had 15 successful cases of painless extractions to his credit.[2] At this time, Wells carried out his unsuccessful public demonstration in Boston and he was discredited. The low lipid solubility of nitrous oxide was the cause of his failure and, it may be surmised, of his suicide at the age of 33 years. However, Wells' 15 successful cases justify the claim that nitrous oxide was the first anaesthetic agent to be regularly used. This series of cases antedates the first public demonstration of ether anaesthesia by 21 months.

After a temporary period of eclipse by ether, nitrous oxide was re-introduced and was widely used from 1867 onwards. By 1868, the gas was available in London compressed into metal cylinders and has continued in general use until the present day. In view of the large number of compounds that have been used as anaesthetics and whose use has continued for shorter or longer periods it is remarkable that nitrous oxide continues to be used. Many more patients have been anaesthetized with nitrous oxide then with any other agent and at present, it continues, to be more widely used than any other agent.

It might be concluded from this enormous volume of clinical experience that nitrous oxide is the best agent so far produced. Reasons for thinking otherwise are now being advanced and will be discussed below. It is not yet clear whether these reasons are strong enough to affect our use of nitrous oxide and this review attempts to summarize the present situation.

CHEMISTRY

Nitrous oxide is the only inorganic compound (with the exception of xenon) that has been used to produce general anaesthesia. This is not due to some unusual pharmacological property but is a consequence of its degree of solubility in blood and lipid, together with its chemical stability in the body.

The molecule of nitrous oxide is linear and assymetrical, having the significant resonance structures[3] of:

$$-:\overset{..}{N}:\overset{+}{N}::O: \quad :N:::\overset{+}{N}:\overset{..}{O}:-$$

Although biochemically stable, nitrous oxide is a thermodynamically unstable endothermic compound that supports combustion by decomposing into its elements thus liberating oxygen. A temperature above 450° is required to initiate this reaction:

$$2N_2O \rightarrow 2N_2 + O_2 - 163 \text{ kJ}$$

Because a candle burns more brightly in nitrous oxide than air (an observation made originally by Joseph Priestley) it was believed that nitrous oxide could give up oxygen with beneficial effect in the body and this belief persisted until the classical publication of Courville.[4] This book gave convincing evidence that the lesions in the central nervous system following the administration of nitrous oxide without enough oxygen resulted from hypoxia.

PHYSICAL PROPERTIES

The physical properties of nitrous oxide are as follows:

1. Molecular weight 44
2. Boiling point $-88.5°C$
3. Critical temperture 36.43°C
4. Critical pressure 72.5 bar
5. Specific gravity 1.53 at zero °C (air $=$ 1)
6. Partition coefficients at 37°C
   a. oil/water 3.2
   b. water/gas 0.435
   c. oil/gas 1.4
   d. blood/gas 0.468
7. Velocity of sound in N_2O : 262 m/s (O_2 : 317). The note of a whistle[5] goes down $1\frac{1}{2}$ tones when blown with N_2O instead of O_2.

MANUFACTURE

Several methods of manufacturing nitrous oxide may be employed and these are described by Wynne.[6] The major part of the world's supply of the gas is obtained by heating ammonium nitrate

$$NH_4NO_3 \rightarrow N_2O + 2H_2O + 58.6 \text{ kJ}$$

In older plants this is performed by heating solid ammonium nitrate to a temperature between 245 and 270°C. In more modern plants, an aqueous solution of 83% ammonium nitrate is used. This is available as a by-product of the large scale manufacture of ammonia.

Accurate temperature control of the process is essential because the reaction is exothermic. Above 270°C, impurities increase and above 290°C the reaction becomes explosive. Serious explosions have occurred in nitrous oxide manufacturing plants when the temperature has gone out of control. In the older type of plants using solid ammonium nitrate, the retort in which the exothermic reaction has been initiated by heat has to be externally cooled by water. In newer plants using ammonium nitrate solution, temperature control is obtained by the addition of more solution.

Impurities

Several very toxic substances occur as impurities in nitrous oxide. These include ammonia, carbon monoxide, chlorine and the higher oxides of nitrogen. Scrubbing with permanganate solution, sulphuric acid and water is necessary to remove these impurities and their permitted concentrations in nitrous oxide for medical use are specified and tested for. (European and US standards maximum permissible NO/NO_2 5 ppm in gas). In addition to nitrous oxide, at least seven other oxides of nitrogen are known.[3] Those of importance as contaminants of medical nitrous oxide are nitric oxide and nitrogen dioxide. Nitric oxide combines with air to form the even more toxic nitrogen dioxide, which is an equilibrium mixture $NO_2 \leftrightharpoons N_2O_4$, the point of equilibrium in the mixture depending on temperature.

The higher oxides of nitrogen can be detected by smell at a concentration of about 5 ppm and cause respiratory distress at 100 ppm. An insidious feature of these compounds is that pulmonary damage may not become apparent until the development of pulmonary oedema many hours later. Clinical features of poisoning with the higher oxides of nitrogen are intense cyanosis arising from methaemoglobinaemia, pulmonary oedema and circulatory collapse. A series of papers dealing with all aspects of this subject are to be found in the June issue of the British Journal of Anaesthesia, 1967, Vol. 34.

THE VIRTUES OF NITROUS OXIDE AS AN ANAESTHETIC AGENT

The remarkable longevity of nitrous oxide as an anaesthetic agent has already been noted. The only other agent with a comparable history, diethyl ether, has been little used in the western world since the introduction of halothane in the early 1950s, and its production for anaesthetic use in the UK has recently ceased. It is to be expected, therefore, that nitrous oxide would have considerable virtues as an anaesthetic agent and it is appropriate that these should be considered before discussion of any adverse features. These virtues include:

1. Low blood solubility
2. Minimal adverse effects at clinically used concentrations
3. Advantages when used with other volatile agents
4. Accuracy of administration
5. Non-irritant properties
6. No metabolism
7. Analgesic properties

Low blood solubility

Blood solubility regulates speed of onset and offset of anaesthesia (induction and eduction), the lower the blood solubility the faster these are.[7] With a blood/gas partition coefficient (λ) of 0.46, nitrous oxide is considerably less soluble than any agent in current use, with the exception of cyclopropane. However, two agents currently being developed, sevoflurane[8] and I- 653[9] have comparably low solubilities in blood — 0.6 and 0.42 respectively.

Low blood solubility confers a further advantage in ease of control of anaesthesia. A change of inspired concentration rapidly results in a change of blood concentration so that lightening or deepening of anaesthesia is quickly achieved. Also, the alveolar concentration reflects the inspired concentration quite closely after only a few breaths so that blood levels of nitrous oxide can be estimated from knowledge of the inspired concentration. With agents of greater solubility, this information can only be obtained from the end-tidal (end-respiratory) anaesthetic concentration, measurement of which is not always easy.

Clearly, low blood solubility is a prime asset in an inhalational agent but there is another aspect. Low blood solubility is, in general terms, associated with low fat solubility[10] and this means low anaesthetic potency. Nitrous oxide, having a minimum alveolar concentration (MAC) of 104 is at a disadvantage in this respect and this point is considered later.

Minimal adverse effects
At the concentrations of nitrous oxide that are used in clinical practice (50–70%) the adverse effects are slight.

Respiratory effects
All inhalational agents increase respiratory rate and decrease tidal volume. With most agents this reduces effective ventilation and the $PaCO_2$ rises. This effect may be reduced by surgical stimulation but the overall effect remains one of a decrease in effective ventilation. With nitrous oxide, the increase in respiratory rate is sufficient to compensate for the decreased tidal volume so that, despite the unfavourable change in the ratio of dead space to tidal volume, alveolar ventilation is maintained and $PaCO_2$ does not rise. This remains true even at 1.5 MAC of nitrous oxide when the respiratory rate has been found to be three times the normal value.[11]

Following the classical paper of Whitteridge and Bulbring[12] it has been considered that the tachypnoea associated with inhalational anaesthesia was caused by the increase in the discharge from stretch receptors in the lung that these workers observed. However, the tachypnoea of tricholoroethylene[13] and ether anaesthesia[14] is not abolished by vagotomy, and it seems likely that a central control stimulation is, at least, partly responsible for this effect. Indeed, this possibility was advanced by Whitteridge and Bulbring.

Cardiovascular effects
As with all other anaesthetic agents, the direct action of nitrous oxide on cardiac muscle is depressant.[15] In the normal heart the effect is small and is reduced or entirely obscured by the sympathetic stimulation, which is a feature of the pharmacological actions of nitrous oxide. The interaction between nitrous oxide, other inhalational agents and narcotics will be considered later.

Concentrations of nitrous oxide as low as 40% have been shown to cause increased urinary catecholamines[16] but the sympathetic stimulating effects of the gas are not normally prominent. Perhaps we are so used to the agent being present during general anaesthesia that these effects are not noticed unless sought for. However, if nitrous oxide is used at higher concentrations (which requires the use of a hyperbaric chamber) then the sympathetic stimulating properties of the gas become more apparent. Indeed, in volunteer studies[11] at 1.5 A.T.A. N_2O (i.e. 1.5 MAC — equivalent to 2.5% enflurane) muscle rigidity, catatonic jerking, laboured breathing, sweating and hyperactivity were seen. Subjects became peaceful on reduction of nitrous oxide to 1.1 A.T.A. but it remains one of the unique features of nitrous oxide that it enjoys universal use at subanaesthetic concentrations, although at fully anaesthetizing concentrations and above its effects are so deleterious.

The possibility that nitrous oxide may increase the sensitivity of the heart to exogenous catecholamines does not appear to have been investigated.

Advantages with other inhalational agents

Reduced requirements of potent volatile agents

The provision of 0.5 MAC or more of nitrous oxide reduces the requirement of more potent volatile agent by a proportional amount. In practice, the anaesthetizing effect of a mixture of inhalational agents may be calculated by adding together their fractional MAC values.[7] The reduction by 50% of the amount of enflurane or other agent administered and its substitution by a rapidly acting agent is one of the biggest advantages of the use of nitrous oxide.

Reduced cardiovascular system (CVS) and respiratory depression

Most volatile agents have a fairly uniform depressant action on all vital functions. Because of its sympathetic stimulating action nitrous oxide may, to some extent, antagonize these depressant effects although such an effect is by no means always observed.

In clinical practice, nitrous oxide is usually combined with an approximately equi-MAC concentration of a potent volatile agent, which at low concentrations does not have significant sympathetic blocking action. Under these circumstances, cardiovascular depression is less than if an equal depth of anaesthesia has been maintained by the volatile agent alone. For instance, 70% nitrous oxide plus 1.2% isoflurane resulted in significantly higher arterial pressure and systemic vascular resistance than an equi-MAC concentration of isoflurane alone.[17] If, however, the volatile agent is at a concentration of about 1 MAC or above, the effect of the nitrous oxide will be to produce further depression. Hornbein et al.[18] found that adding 70% nitrous oxide to 0.8% halothane resulted in cardiovascular stimulation but that in the presence of 1.5% halothane the same concentration of nitrous oxide was depressant.

The stimulatory effect of nitrous oxide may also be absent in patients with valvular or coronary heart disease.[19,20] As already described, nitrous oxide does not depress respiration. It might therefore be expected that the addition of nitrous oxide to an anaesthetizing concentration of a volatile agent (with appropriate reduction in concentration of that agent) would result in a lower $PaCO_2$. This is clearly shown for isoflurane in Figure 2.1. Similar effects have been shown for enflurane and nitrous oxide.[21]

Concentration and second gas effects

The administration of, for example, 70% nitrous oxide together with the vapour of an agent such as halothane results in the alveolar concentration of halothane rising more rapidly than would be the case if the halothane were given alone, i.e. the presence of

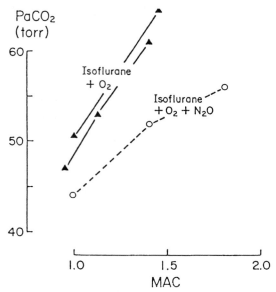

Fig. 2.1 The action of nitrous oxide on the respiratory depressant effect of isoflurane. (Modified from Eger[21].)

the nitrous oxide speeds induction with halothane. This effect has been experimentally demonstrated[22] and two mechanisms are postulated to explain it.

In the first few minutes of breathing a nitrous oxide containing gas mixture the volume of nitrous oxide taken up from the alveolus is large. Any other gases or vapour in the inspired mixture that are not absorbed to the same extent as the nitrous oxide will be concentrated in the alveolar gas mixture. This is the concentration effect. Under normal clinical conditions, the other agent, halothane in this example, would itself be being absorbed at the same time as the nitrous oxide and the concentration effect would be limited to a reduction in the fall of alveolar halothane concentration. However, under experimental conditions designed to show the effect, a small increase in the alveolar concentration of halothane, cyclopropane and ethylene above the inspired concentration has been demonstrated.[23]

The other proposed mechanism is that the volume of gas mixture entering the lungs per breath during induction is larger when a major component of the mixture is nitrous oxide because so much nitrous oxide is absorbed in the first few minutes that more gas than usual passes into the lungs to make good the deficit. This is the second gas effect. If more of the nitrous-oxide-containing gas mixture passes into the lungs then more of its components other then nitrous oxide (e.g. halothane) will enter the alveoli and anaesthetic delivery will be enhanced.

The relative proportions of the part played by these two mechanisms in accelerating induction by an anaesthetic gas mixture of N_2O/other agent/O_2 depends on the blood solubility of the second agent. If this agent is of low solubility (e.g. cyclopropane) then the difference between its inspired and alveolar concentrations will be low and an increase in alveolar ventilation will have little effect in speeding the rate of induction. Elevation of alveolar anaesthetic level by concentration will, however, increase this rate.

If the second agent is of high blood solubility (e.g. diethyl ether) then the limiting factor to rate of induction is delivery of the agent to the alveolus and, in this case, the second gas effect will be responsible for the increased rate of induction when nitrous oxide is added. Administration of carbon dioxide by increasing alveolar ventilation, would have the same effect.

These effects are not, of course, specific to nitrous oxide but, in clinical practice, nitrous oxide is the only gas likely to be used that would result in their occurrence.

Accuracy of administration

Nitrous oxide concentration in gas mixtures can be controlled with accuracy by means of rotameters®. These devices can be accurately calibrated using a stopwatch and a gas volume measuring device such as a spirometer. This is much easier than calibration of a vaporizer — a procedure that ultimately relies on the making up of volumetric standards.

The electronic control of gas mixtures (N_2O and O_2) is also easier and more precise than that of vaporization of volatile agents. Digital flowmeters[24] and various forms of mass flow controllers have been described.[25]

Non-irritant properties

Nitrous oxide is conspicuously non-irritant compared with other inhalational agents. It has no more than a slightly sweet smell, which not everyone can detect. This is a considerable advantage, not only for gaseous induction of anaesthesia, but also during maintenance. This is apparent to anyone regularly using isoflurane for anaesthesia with unpremedicated outpatients.

No metabolism

Since 1964 it has been appreciated that metabolic breakdown of inhalational anaesthetics occurs and it has also become apparent that reactive intermediate compounds, free radicals and inorganic fluoride are the substances chiefly responsible for organ toxicity (liver or kidney) after anaesthesia.

There are considerable technical difficulties in studying in vivo metabolism of nitrous oxide. No suitable radioactive isotopes of nitrogen exist to permit radiolabelling, and the large amoung of various nitrogen compounds present in the body hinder other techniques. Two small loci of nitrous oxide metabolism have been identified. One is the reduction of the gas to nitrogen by bacteria present in the gut. By extrapolation from in vitro observations this has been estimated to amount to 0.004% of the quantity of nitrous oxide taken into the body.[26,27] It has been shown that during this reduction of nitrous oxide, free radical intermediates may be formed.[28] These compounds are potentially harmful but there is no evidence at all of any toxic effects resulting from their temporary presence in the gut at such low concentrations. Bacteria in the gut may themselves synthesize nitrous oxide.

The other identified metabolic process is the interaction between nitrous oxide and vitamin B_{12}, which is described later. The amount of gas taking part in this reaction is too small to be of any significance. Interestingly, the reduction of nitrous oxide by intestinal bacteria may result, at least in part, from the same chemical reactions as in the body since these organisms synthesize B_{12}.

No metabolism of nitrous oxide in the liver has been detected and it can be concluded that, with the probable exception of xenon, nitrous oxide is the least metabolized of any anaesthetic agent.

Analgesic properties

From the first observations of Davy it has been known that nitrous oxide, inhaled at subanaesthetic concentrations, has an analgesic action.[1] The analgesic effect of breathing 20% nitrous oxide has been found to be equivalent to that produced by 15 mg of morphine subcutaneously.[29]

It is unclear why some inhalation agents have an analgesic effect at subanaesthetic concentrations and others do not.[30] However, in the case of nitrous oxide (but not other agents), there is evidence that the analgesic effect, or at least part of it, is brought about by an interaction with the opiate receptor-endorphin system. The chief evidence in support of this view is the partial but significant reversal of nitrous oxide analgesia by naloxone observed in numerous animal studies.[31] This has been confirmed in the human subject.[32] Depletion of endogenous opiate stores may play a part in the acute tolerance to nitrous oxide observed in experimental animals[33] and in humans.[34]

It has always been assumed that the possession of analgesic action was a desirable feature for an inhalational agent and many anaesthetists consider that the administration of opiates is necessary, or at least desirable, during anaesthesia and indeed reduces MAC for several inhalational agents.[35] However, naloxone neither reverses anaesthesia nor increases MAC and, in the case of nitrous oxide, although analgesia is partially reversed, the ED50 for nitrous oxide as assessed by loss of righting reflex in mice (=MAC) is unaffected by naloxone.[36] It therefore appears that anaesthesia is separable from analgesia in this case.

Not only does naloxone not affect anaesthesia produced by inhalational agents, it also does not affect the analgesia produced by such agents other than nitrous oxide.[37,38] This affords further evidence for the existence of other non-opiate pain-control systems as proposed by Watkins & Mayer[39] and others. It also suggests that the opiate receptor-endorphin system is not directly involved in the mechanism of general anaesthesia.

ADVERSE FEATURES OF NITROUS OXIDE

Nitrous oxide has been subjected to closer scrutiny than any other anaesthetic agent in attempt to detect adverse features; in particular, the interaction with vitamin B_{12}, since it can affect DNA synthesis and has the potential for multifarious effects throughout the body. Nevertheless, it seems possible in the present state of knowledge to divide this aspect of research into nitrous oxide into two parts. Firstly, areas in which harmful effects have been clearly demonstrated to a greater or lesser degree:

1. Diffusion into closed spaces
2. Adverse circulatory effects of nitrous oxide
3. Oxidation of B_{12} causing abnormalities in
   a. blood
   b. nervous system

Secondly, areas in which harmful effects have been sought and not (to date) been found or found only to an insignificant or dubious degree:

1. Leucocyte function (cell mediated immune responses)
2. Wound healing
3. Teratogenicity, carcinogenicity, mutagenicity
   a. Laboratory studies
   b. Epidemiological studies
4. Malignant hyperpyrexia
5. Postoperative nausea and vomiting

DIFFUSION OF NITROUS OXIDE INTO CLOSED SPACES

Diffusion is the process of intermingling of molecules that takes place when differing gases (or liquids) are in contact. The process results from the random movement of molecules that occurs in gases and liquids (Brownian movement). The factors regulating the rate of diffusion are: concentration (partial pressure) gradient; molecular size; when passage of gas through liquid films is involved — solubility of the gas in the liquid.

Fick's Law states that the rate of diffusion is proportional to the concentration or partial pressure gradient. Graham's Law states that the rate of diffusion at identical partial pressures through porous plates and some membranes is inversely proportional to the square root of the molecular weight. Differences in gas density, therefore, have only small effects on rate of diffusion. Finally, where gas transfer across blood or water films is involved, the rate of diffusion is proportional to the solubility of the gas in the liquid. This is the major factor regulating diffusion rates of gases into, or out of, spaces within the body as can be seen from Table 2.1 (From Nunn,[40] with permission). The body is normally in equilibrium with atmospheric nitrogen and gas present in any enclosed spaces within the body will contain approximately this concentration of nitrogen. If, however, the subject breathes a nitrogen-free gas mixture containing 60–70% nitrous oxide from a system allowing no rebreathing, then it can be seen from Table 2.1 that nitrous oxide will diffuse into such spaces 25 times as fast as nitrogen can diffuse out. If the space is compliant, e.g. the gut, there will be a volume increase. If the space has rigid walls and is non-compliant, e.g. the middle ear, there will be a rise in pressure. Some cavities, e.g. the pneumothorax, fall between these two clearly defined cases in that there is both a volume increase and an increase in pressure. Such increases may take place at the expense of other tissues normally occupying the space, namely the lungs and mediastinal structures in the case of the pneumothorax.

If the administration of nitrous oxide via a non-rebreathing system is continued long enough all the nitrogen will diffuse out of the space and the pressure and/or volume, having risen to a peak, will return to normal. The nitrogen will have been replaced by nitrous oxide. Also, when the nitrous oxide is withdrawn and air breathing is

Table 2.1   Some physical properties of N_2O related to O_2 and N_2

Gas	Density relative to oxygen	Water solubility relative to oxygen	Diffusing capacity* relative to oxygen
Oxygen	1.00	1.00	1.00
Nitrogen	0.88	0.515	0.55
Nitrous oxide	1.37	16.3	14.0

*Diffusing capacity of a gas is the rate of its transfer divided by the tension gradient across the interface.

resumed, the process goes into reverse and a subatmospheric pressure may be present for a while in any cavity until there has been time for nitrogen to diffuse back. This low pressure phase has been studied only in the case of the middle ear (see below).

The sites within the body in which air filled cavities are normally present (e.g. the middle ear) or where air has been accidentally introduced (e.g. pneumothorax) or deliberately (e.g. air encephalogram) in which increases of volume and/or pressure have been described following the administration of nitrous oxide are as follows:

1. Compliant
   a. Stomach & Gut
   b. Pneumothorax
   c. Pneumoperitoneum
   d. Surgical emphysema
   e. Air embolus
2. Non-compliant
   a. Middle ear
   b. Nasal sinuses
   c. Intercranial
      i. subdural
      ii. cisternal
   d. Vitreous cavity

Individual sites will be considered below.

Stomach and gut

Under normal conditions, the volume of gas in the gut is not large and increase in its volume due to nitrous oxide is not important but when intestinal obstruction is present the volume of gas may be much greater and its expansion by nitrous oxide could cause problems. Assuming that no nitrogen is absorbed, the theoretical increase in volume that could result from breathing 66% nitrous oxide is 200%.

Figure 2.2a shows the increase in volume that can be expected in a fully compliant space from breathing nitrous oxide assuming that no nitrogen diffuses out from the space while the nitrous oxide diffuses in.

Figure 2.2b shows the increase in volume found by Eger & Saidman[41] in loops of small intestine (si), colon (c) and stomach (s) in dogs in which halothane/oxygen anaesthesia was changed to 70–80% nitrous oxide. It can be seen that the volume change is not of rapid onset but nevertheless it can be considered undesirable, particularly in the case of small babies.

The effects of nitrous oxide on postoperative bowel motility have been investigated.[42] It was found that any excess of the gas was absorbed long before peristalsis was reestablished. The use of nitrous oxide does not delay the return of gastronintestinal function in patients undergoing bowel surgery.

Pneumothorax

The risk of accumulation of nitrous oxide in pneumothorax cavities producing tension pneumothorax has long been recognized[43] and a similar risk applies when sub-pleural blebs or lung cysts are present. Such cavities may be non-communicating or

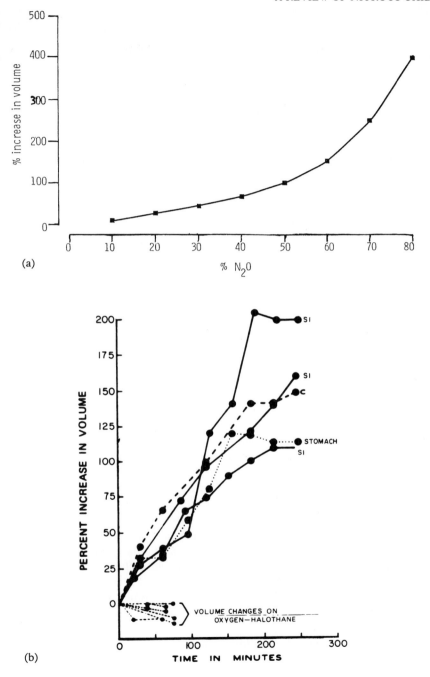

Fig. 2.2 (a) Volume change of compliant space on breathing N_2O (assuming no N_2O diffusing out). (b) Volume change of gut during nitrous oxide anaesthesia. (From Eger & Saidman[41] with permission.)

communicate only by a very narrow orifice, which becomes valvular when there is a volume increase in the cavity. The volume increase in pneumothoraces when nitrous oxide is breathed is rapid. It was found experimentally that, in dogs breathing 68–78% N_2O, the volume of a pneumothorax doubled in 10 minutes and tripled in 30 minutes.[41]

Pneumoperitoneum
The gas most commonly introduced into the peritoneal cavity is carbon dioxide for laparoscopy. Nitrous oxide will diffuse into the gas in the peritoneal cavity but both gases have similar diffusing capacities; the procedure is usually of short duration and the cavity is vented at the end. However, if air is introduced to accustom the abdomen to a proposed large increase in its contents, e.g. the reduction of a large scrotal hernia, then difficulties may arise on breathing high concentrations of nitrous oxide.

Surgical emphysema
Air in subcutaneous tissue will be expanded by nitrous diffusing in. Problems have not been reported from this cause, perhaps because even extensive surgical emphysema is not life threatening.

Air embolus
It was predicted[44] that nitrous oxide would enter and enlarge venous air emboli such as may occur during neurosurgery and also open heart surgery. It was found by Munson & Merrick[45] that this did occur to the extent theoretically predictable. Tuman et al[46] experimentally observed that nitrous oxide increased the size of coronary air embolism. Stopping the administration of nitrous oxide should produce a rapid decrease in the size of such bubbles.

Middle ear and nasal sinuses
The skull cavities are normally vented via the Eustachian tube or various ostia. These may be blocked by inflammatory or other lesions and pressure changes following nitrous oxide administration may be expected. The nasal sinuses remain to be investigated but, in the case of the middle ear, effects have been observed attributable to both raised pressure during nitrous administration and sub-atmospheric pressure after its removal. These effects include rupture of the ear drum, graft displacement, stapes displacement, haematotympanum and temporary or permanent hearing loss. Low pressure in the middle ear after nitrous oxide is particularly common in children probably because the Eustachian tube is compliant and collapses when middle-ear pressure is subatmospheric, thus preventing equilibration of pressures. In one series of 22 children[47] all developed negative pressures, which in some cases lasted more than 24 hours. Rise of pressure during anaesthesia occurs more rapidly in children if positive pressure is used.[48]

Clearly, a case can be made for avoiding the use of nitrous oxide in middle-ear surgery.

Pneumoencephalos
The presence of air pockets anywhere within the skull raises the possibility of harmful pressure changes if nitrous oxide is administered (tension pneumoencephalos). This is

most clearly seen if there is an enclosed space within the brain together with an intact cranial vault. These conditions are present if air is introduced into the ventricles as previously performed for radiological investigation but also from intermittent drainage or aspiration of cerebrospinal fluid (CSF) from the ventricle during surgery via a shunt or ventriculostomy.[49,50] It was advocated that nitrous oxide should be the gas introduced into the ventricle for encephalography. However, if this gas is used the rapid removal of the gas by diffusion at the end of the procedure may cause the ventricle to be compressed with serious consequences.[51]

A supratentorial gas pocket may develop during posterior fossa surgery with the patient sitting.[53] It is suggested[53] that such pockets develop during the operation and are in equilibrium with blood nitrous oxide. Also, the fall in pressure in nitrous-oxide-containing gass spaces within the skull in the immediate postoperative period may be beneficial in lowering intercranial pressure.

The eye
Following surgery for retinal detachment, ophthalmic surgeons may inject a gas bubble into the vitreous cavity to tamponade the retina in place. It is desirable that this bubble remains in place for several days and for this purpose sulphur hexafluoride (SF_6) has been used. It has very low solubility so that it is very slowly absorbed. A bubble of 40% SF_6 and 60% air maintains a constant volume for several days, but if nitrous oxide is given a considerable rise in intraocular pressure can occur. The subject was examined by computer simulation.[54] Their recommendations are that nitrous oxide should be discontinued 15 minutes before injection of the gas bubble. However, the pressure rise is not great if nitrous oxide is withdrawn at the same time as the gas is injected.

Air bubbles may be present in the eye for some time after trauma or surgery, thus care in the use of nitrous oxide may be necessary.

ADVERSE CIRCULATORY EFFECTS OF NITROUS OXIDE

In animals, nitrous oxide significantly reduces the pulmonary vasoconstructive response to hypoxia[55] but it is unclear to what extent these findings can be transferred to the clinical situation.

In the normal patient, pulmonary artery pressures and pulmonary vascular resistance are not significantly affected by nitrous oxide,[56] but when pulmonary hypertension is present nitrous oxide causes a marked increase in mean pulmonary artery pressure and pulmonary vascular resistance[57] and its use may be inadvisable. Several authors have described cases in which infants and small children with pulmonary hypertension have suffered adverse effects when given nitrous oxide. It is hard to be certain that these effects were specific to nitrous oxide since other workers have failed to find increases in pulmonary artery pressure and vascular resistance in infants with pulmonary hypertension given 50% nitrous oxide.[58]

The sympathomimetic stimulant action of nitrous oxide on the heart that normally exceeds its direct depressant effect has already been described. The administration of drugs that tend to block sympathetic stimulation, such as narcotics, may reveal the underlying depressant action. For this reason, the addition of nitrous oxide to high dose narcotic anaesthesia (to reduce the risk of awareness) has been found to cause depression of cardiac function, which is not seen when either drug is given alone. This effect is only of importance when cardiac performance is compromised by cardiac disease. This complex subject is discussed by Meretoga et al[59]

It is safe to conclude that in conditions where there is strong sympathetic stimulation, such as hypovolaemia, nitrous oxide is cardiodepressant[60] and in more complex situations its cardiac effects are not always predictable because of an uncertain balance between its direct depressant and indirect stimulant actions.

INTERACTION BETWEEN NITROUS OXIDE AND VITAMIN B_{12}

The introduction, after 1952, of long-term intermittent positive — pressure ventilation as a therapy for patients either with respiratory difficulty or requiring pharmacological paralysis for conditions such as tetanus, facilitated the use of nitrous oxide for long-term sedation. Several workers described cases in which nitrous oxide had been used continuously for several days and in which granulocytopaenia occurred, but it was unclear which of the many drugs these patients were receiving was responsible. The connection was first made by Lassen et al[61] and was quickly confirmed. On administration of nitrous oxide, even at low concentration, leucopaenia will occur after about 3 days, developing into agranulocytosis in 5–7 days.[63] If the pa-

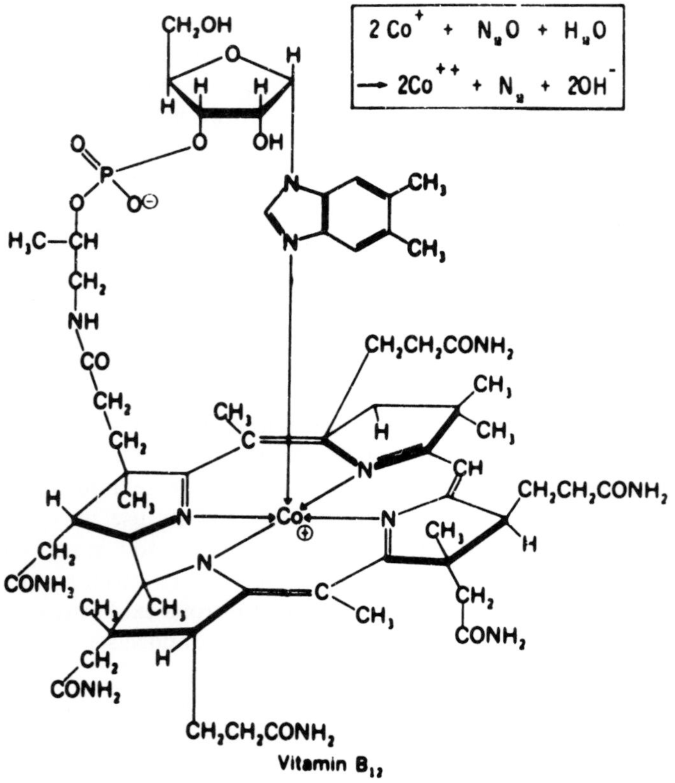

$$2Co^{+} + N_2O + H_2O$$
$$\longrightarrow 2Co^{++} + N_2 + 2OH^{-}$$

Vitamin B_{12}

Fig. 2.3 Molecular structure of vitamin B_{12}.

tient does not succumb, recovery of the bone marrow occurs within 4 days of withdrawal of the nitrous oxide. Treatment with vitamin B_{12} was found to have no effect.

In 1968, a paper was published in a chemical journal[63] describing the interaction between nitrous oxide and vitamin B_{12}. The clinical significance of this was not appreciated for 10 years. In 1978, Amess et al[64] established that giving nitrous oxide for 24 hours affected DNA synthesis as measured by the deoxyuridine suppression test (described below). Shortly after this[65] it was shown that the selective inactivation of vitamin B_{12} inhibited the action of methionine synthase.

It is now necessary to briefly describe the metabolic pathway affected by this inhibition. Vitamin B_{12} is a cobalamin, its molecular structure is shown in Figure 2.3. The function of the cobalt can be compared with that of the iron in haemoglobin and, as can be seen, the tetrapyrolle ring structure in both molecules is similar. Furthermore, the oxidation of Co by N_2O is analogous to the oxidation of Fe by chemical oxidizing agents to form metIhaemoglobin. In the case of Co the nitrous oxide converts the monovalent CobIalamin to the bivalent CobIIalamin, in which form it can no longer function as a methyl carrier.

Vitamin B_{12} is a co-factor in two enzyme reactions. These are methionine synthase and methyl malonase coA mutase. The interaction between B_{12} and N_2O does not affect the second of these reactions.

Methionine is a sulphur-containing essential amino acid. It is available from food and by metabolism of homocysteine, another sulphur-containing amino acid also available from the diet. Folates, also of dietary origin, are necessary for this conversion.

The enzyme methionine synthase, together with B_{12}, transfers a methyl group from methyl-tetrahydrofolate to convert homocysteine to methionine. At the same time, by losing its methyl group, methyl-tetrahydrofolate becomes tetrahydrofolate. This is shown in Figure 2.4. Following this transmethylation, the two products take part in several reactions (shown in Figure 2.4), which result in the formation of deoxythymidine from deoxyuridine. Deoxythymidine is an essential component of DNA. Inhibition of DNA synthesis is thought to be the cause of the haematological and fetotoxic effects of nitrous oxide (described below). The neurological effects (also described below) may result from the depletion of s-adenosyl methionine (SAM), see Figure 2.4.

Abnormalities in this metabolic pathway are detected by several tests, the commonest of which are given below, arranged in order of sensitivity:

1. measurement of methionine synthase activity in tissues e.g. liver, brain, a biopsy is needed

2. deoxyuridine (dU) suppression test

3. detection of megaloblastic changes by microscopy of bone marrow; this test was devised by Matz to assess folate metabolism, i.e. the production of 5,10 methylne tetrahydrofolate from methyltetrahydrofolate as shown in Figure 2.4.

The dU suppression test involves the short-term tissue culture of a small sample of bone marrow and is based on the observation of Killman from autoradiographic evidence that pre-inoculation of normal bone marrow with deoxyuridine reduces the incorporation of tritiated thymidine into DNA. With normal bone marrow cells, in the synthesis of DNA, 90% of the deoxythymidine incorporated into DNA comes from

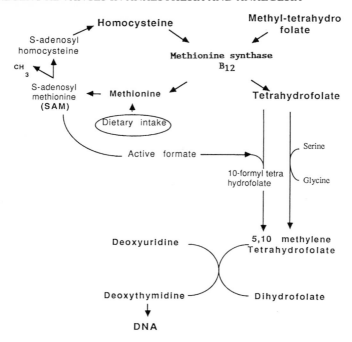

Fig. 2.4 Metabolic pathway of B_{12}/methionine synthase.

the metabolism of deoxyuridine and less than 10% from additional radiolabelled thymidine added to the reaction mixture. In B_{12} deficiency and other abnormalities of folate metabolism, the folate substrate needed for deoxythmidine synthesis is deficient and this results in increased uptake of thymidine from the added radiolabelled thymidine. If the bone marrow being tested is deficient in folate then the amount of thymidine incorporated into the DNA may rise from less than 10% to as much as 60%. The presence of deoxyuridine can be said to suppress the uptake of thymidine — hence the name of the test.

Duration of exposure

The duration of exposure to nitrous oxide required to produce significant bone marrow depression is clearly important. Before giving data on this subject it should be mentioned that, although nitrous oxide impairs DNA synthesis in experimental animals, man is the only species in which megaloblastic changes are seen. For this reason, animal work on the subject uses the dU suppression test as a measure of impaired DNA synthesis.

In rats, the shortest exposure to nitrous oxide (50%) to give an abnormal dU suppression test was 1 h, with maximum effect seen at 6 h and maintained with daily exposures for 15 days with return to normality 24 h after withdrawal of nitrous oxide.[66]

The earliest sign of abnormality caused by nitrous oxide is found by assay of methionine synthase activity, usually in the liver. In the rat, the inactivation of the enzyme by 50% N_2O is rapid, having a half-time of 5.4 min.[67] In man, the time course is slower, 46 min[67] or 2 h.[68] These measurements were made on hepatic tissue obtained by biopsy. No inactivation of methionine synthase activity in human placenta was found following nitrous oxide administration of up to 30 min for caesarean section.[69] Presumably, the duration of exposure was inadequate.

Intermittent exposure to N_2O, such as Entonox during physiotherapy, has been found to produce a megaloblastic bone marrow.[70]

The inhaled concentration of nitrous oxide required to inactivate methionine synthase has been studied in the mouse only and found to have an ED50 of 10%.[71]

Prevention or reversal of B_{12}–nitrous oxide interaction

It is clearly important to discover to what extent the biochemical lesions produced by nitrous oxide can be prevented or reversed by restoring the levels of deficient metabolites. The substance that has been most studied in this respect is folinic acid (5-formyl tetrahydrofolate (THF), leucovorin, citrovorum factor). This compound is freely available and is used in chemotherapy as an antidote to folic acid antagonists such as methotrexate. It is converted to 5:10 methylene THF (see Figure 2.4) and so restores the metabolic pathway leading to DNA synthesis.[72]

It was found that two parenteral doses of 30 mg of folinic acid prevented the development of an abnormal dU suppression test and megaloblastic changes in the bone marrow in 4 out of 5 patients ventilated for 24 h with 50% nitrous oxide.[73] Smaller doses were ineffective. Kano et al[74] found that, in patients subjected to nitrous oxide anaesthesia for up to 11 h, the abnormal dU suppression test was corrected almost to normal within 1 h of giving 15 mg of folinic acid. Similar findings were reported by Nunn et al[75]

Neurological effects of vitamin B_{12}–N_2O interaction

In addition to impairment of DNA synthesis, a clinical feature of vitamin B_{12} deficiency is an inability to synthesize myelin causing a neuropathy that usually develops insidiously in peripheral nerves and progresses to involve the posterior and lateral columns of the spinal cord. A neuropathy of this type occurring in 15 patients was described by Layzer[76.] Thirteen of these patients inhaled nitrous oxide intermittently for 'recreational' purposes. In unscavenged dental surgeries nitrous oxide levels may be considerably higher than in operating theatres and in a survey of over 30 000 dentists and their assistants Brodsky et al[77] found an incidence of less than 2% of neurological symptoms that might have been resulted from neuropathy.

The cases recorded by Layzer[76] showed no macrocytosis; however, bone marror was not examined. Sweeney et al[78] examined both blood and marrow of 21 dentists exposed to nitrous oxide in their surgeries. In 3 cases, an abnormal dU suppression test was found, the full blood count was normal with no macrocytosis but in 2 of the cases a slight increase in hypersegmented neutrophils was seen. No neurological abnormalities were found in this group of subjects. The lowest weekly concentration at which definite haematological abnormality was found was 1800 ppm. These dentists carried a personal sampling device from which a measurement of the individual weekly dose of nitrous oxide could be made and a correlation between the dose and the appearance of an abnormal dU suppression test was found.

It can be concluded that neuropathy is unlikely to be a complication of the clinical use of nitrous oxide in normal subjects. Study of this aspect of nitrous oxide toxicity is complicated by wide differences in species susceptibility. Rats appear immune but monkeys develop neurological signs in a few days of breathing 15% N_2O. The neurological damage in monkeys can be greatly reduced by supplementation of the diet by 2 g of methionine daily.[79]

MEASUREMENT OF INDIVIDUAL EXPOSURE TO NITROUS OXIDE

Several sampling devices have been described, to be carried by the individual, which accumulate a sample of the gas breathed by the carrier. In the work of Davenport et al[80], a small evacuated canister that drew gas in via a capillary tube from a sampling point close to the nares was carried. Head space analysis of urine samples has also been advocated.[81] Nitrous oxide is measured by gas chromatography or infra-red spectrophotometry.

EFFECT OF NITROUS OXIDE ON CELL-MEDIATED IMMUNE RESPONSES

The evidence on the effects of nitrous oxide on chemotaxis and phagocytosis is not entirely consistent. Nunn & O'Morain[82] and Moudgil et al[83] found that nitrous oxide applied in vitro depressed neutrophil chemotaxis. Hill et al[84] found increased chemotaxis in volunteers who breathed 60% N_2O for 1 hour. Although motility may be impaired by nitrous oxide, phagocytosis is not.[85] It seems likely that the metabolic responses to surgery are more important in this area than the effects of nitrous oxide.

Wound healing
Because of possible effects on leucocyte function and cell reproduction, a study on the effects of nitrous oxide on the strength of healing incisions was carried out on rats.[86] The results were negative.

MUTAGENIC, CARCINOGENIC OR TERATOGENIC EFFECTS OF NITROUS OXIDE

The very extensive use of nitrous oxide has already been referred to. A National Institute of Health estimate of 24.5 million anaesthetics involving nitrous oxide per year in the USA is quoted by Baden et al[87] Because of this, evidence of even a very low level of mutagenicity or carcinogenicity has potential importance but has not been found to date. The subject is reviewed by Baden[88] and further experiments by the same workers[87] failed to show carcinogenic potential of nitrous oxide in mice.

As to teratogenicity or other effects on the reproductive process the picture is less clear. In small rodents (rats, mice and hamsters) nitrous oxide produces increased fetal resorption and growth retardation and congenital abnormalities — particularly of the skeleton. To produce these effects, exposure to high concentrations (e.g. 75%) of nitrous oxide for more than 12 h/d are required. In the rat the ninth day of pregnancy appears the optimum time for teratogenesis on exposure. The work of Lane et al[88,89] and Mazze et al[90] confirm that these effects on the reproductive process are specific to nitrous oxide and are not found with other anaesthetic agents. Evidence that the teratogenic effect of nitrous oxide is connected with an effect on vitamin B_{12} is provided by Keeling et al[91], who found that pretreatment with folinic acid partially reduced the teratogenic effects of exposure of rats to 75% nitrous oxide for 24 h on the ninth day of pregnancy.

Extrapolation of these findings (which are by no means constant) from rodent to man is hardly possible. However, several studies have sought fetal malformations following anaesthetics with nitrous oxide given during pregnancy.[92] Their conclusions have been uniformly negative.

There have been a large number of epidemiological surveys attempting to discover adverse reproductive effects among people exposed to nitrous oxide (and other anaesthetics) in trace concentrations at their work. This extensive subject is reviewed by Baden. To summarize, the only agreed positive finding is an increase in the rate of spontaneous abortion among exposed personnel. This increase is not great and a causal relationship to nitrous oxide cannot be shown, indeed other factors seem more likely.

The highest level of occupational exposure to nitrous oxide is found among workers in dental surgeries where as much as 1000 ppm may occur.[7] In a large study of dentists and their assistants, exposure to nitrous oxide alone taken as a measure of dose using hours per week spent in rooms in which nitrous oxide was used[93] established a dose-dependent relationship with incidence of abortion (maximum 105%) and a small increase in the wives of dentists (52%). From these data a small, non-dose dependent increase in congenital anomalies was also found among children of female workers. This study remains the strongest evidence for teratogenic effects of nitrous oxide in the human and its conclusions are not generally accepted.[88]

No effect on human spermatozoa was found in anesthesiologists working in well-scavenged operating rooms[94] and no effect of nitrous oxide on in vitro fertilization success rates was found by Rosen et al.[95] Oocyte retrieval was carried out under either isoflurane or isoflurane and nitrous oxide anaesthesia.

Malignant hyperpyrexia
It is generally considered that nitrous oxide is, at most, a weak triggering agent of malignant hyperpyrexia and many authorities consider it a safe agent to use in susceptible patients.[96] However, there is at least 1 case recorded in which nitrous oxide undoubtedly triggered the condition[97] and it seems best to avoid its use if it is suspected that the patient is susceptible.

NITROUS OXIDE AND POSTOPERATIVE VOMITING

It is generally accepted that the use of those agents that have sympathomimetic effects, such as cyclopropane or trichloroethylene, results in more postoperative nausea or vomiting than the use of agents that lack such effects. For this reason and the effects in the middle ear already described, it has been suspected that nitrous oxide might produce postoperative nausea and vomiting. Published work on the subject shows inconsistency and great variation of incidence.

In 1982 Buffington[98] examined 6 798 isoflurane anaesthetics and found that if the concentration of nitrous oxide used exceeded 40% then the incidence of vomiting was signficantly increased. Alexander et al[99] and Melnick & Johnson[100] both found that the use of nitrous oxide greatly increased the incidence but in a well-conducted trial involving 780 patients Muir et al[101] could find no association and this finding was supported by Kortilla et al[102] who surveyed 110 patients having abdominal hysterectomy and also by Gunawardene & White,[103] and Senegupta & Plantevin.[104] The suggestion that middle-ear pressure changes were associated with postoperative vomiting was examined by Montgomery et al[105] in 60 paediatric dental patients 27% of whom vomited. Of these, 48 patients developed subatmospheric pressure in one or both ears postoperatively but there was no association between this factor and vomiting.

Surveying this field does not lead to firm conclusions but the consensus of opinion goes in favour of nitrous oxide. There is also the suspicion that other factors, such as the use of fentanyl, play a larger part than the use of nitrous oxide in affecting the incidence of postoperative nausea and vomiting.

CUFFS AND BALLOONS

Endotracheal tube cuffs and balloons on Swan-Ganz catherers are permeable to gases and when in situ and filled with air are subject to pressure and/or volume changes in the same way as other gas filled cavities. More than 30 papers have been published on this subject, which has the merits of being easy to investigate and lending itself readily to both laboratory and theoretical investigation. However, there are often discrepancies between the in vivo and extracorporeal findings.[106]

The subject is clearly a complex one and many variables determine the change and rate of change of volume or pressure in the cuff or balloon. These variables include the permeability, elasticity and contents of the cuff, its initial volume and pressure, the inspired nitrous oxide concentration, temperature, etc. It is therefore not surprising that very different changes in pressure and volume with time are reported by various observers.

Although sore throat is a common after effect of intubation, serious problems do not commonly occur as a result of cuff pressure after routine anaesthesia. However, it is clearly undesirable to subject the tracheal mucosa to unnecessary pressure, thus care must be taken to inflate to no more than sealing pressure and to remember that pressure may go on rising for 3 hours and to make adjustment accordingly. Suggestions to minimize pressure changes in cuffs include inflating with the respired gas mixture, with N_2O and perhaps best of all, with water or saline. Several constant-pressure inflating devices have also been described. A detailed theoretical and experimental approach to the subject is given by Chandler[107] and an equation predicting cuff pressure changes under defined conditions is derived.

CONCLUSIONS

Until the discovery of its interaction with vitamin B_{12}, the least favourable feature of nitrous oxide was its lack of potency (MAC 104). Since no more than at most 80% (at 1 a.t.a.) could be given without risk of hypoxia, use of the agent alone could not guarantee anaesthesia. Nevertheless, its advantages as described, outweighed its disadvantages, which were fairly well understood and could be contained.

It now appears that all patients anaesthetized with nitrous oxide suffer a biochemical lesion, which can be detected after 1–2 hours and will lead, if continued for more than about 24 hours, to serious bone marrow changes owing to reduction in synthesis of DNA the double helical structure of which carries the genes and is the major component of the cell nucleus. In the adult, the bone marrow is the most rapidly dividing tissue so it is perhaps not surprising that it is the tissue most affected by this lesion.

The possible effects of interference with DNA synthesis are protean, but to date, with the exception of bone marrow effects after days of administration and neurological effects after months (or years) of administration, very little hard evidence of harm to the human subject has emerged. Nevertheless it is now being said that nitrous oxide should no longer be used; indeed it is true that if it were a new agent it might not gain the approval of the various official regulatory bodies. The suitability of nitrous oxide for very sick patients (for which it was formerly considered optimum) as well as those deficient in vitamin B_{12} or on anti-folate therapy, is open to question.

Work is now in progress to demonstrate the safety of nitrous oxide both for intermittent exposure.[108] and prolonged anaesthesia[109] but even in the absence of further evidence it is likely that the use of nitrous oxide will decline. This may be due as much to interest and enthusiasm for new techniques and their supposed advantages as to positive evidence of harm from the old. Such new techniques may themselves have defects but if they are as reticent in appearing as those of nitrous oxide many years may elapse before they are discovered.

REFERENCES

1. Davy H 1800 Researches, chemical and philosophical chiefly concerning nitrous oxide: a facsimile reproduction. Butterworths, London
2. Duncum B 1947 The development of inhalation anaesthesia. Oxford University Press, Oxford
3. Kleinberg J, Agersinger W J, Griswold E 1960 Inorganic chemistry, Heath, Boston
4. Courville C B 1939 Untoward effects of nitrous oxide anaesthesia. California Press Publishing Association, California
5. Wright B M 1977 Whistle discriminator for oxygen and nitrous oxide. Lancet 2: 1008
6. Wynne J M 1985 Physics, chemistry and manufacture of nitrous oxide. In: Eger E I II (ed) Nitrous oxide. Elsevier, New York
7. Eger E I II 1974 Anesthetic uptake and action. Williams & Wilkins, Baltimore
8. Holaday D A 1983 Sevoflurane: An experimental anesthetic. In: Brown B R (ed) New vistas in anesthesia. Davis Philadelphia
9. Eger E I II 1987 Partition coefficients for I-653 in human blood, saline and olive oil. Anesthesia Analgesia 66: 971–973
10. White D C 1985 Appraisal of inhalation anaesthetic agents. In: Kaufman L (ed) Anaesthesia Review 3, Churchill Livingstone, Edinburgh
11. Hornbein T F, Eger E I II, Winter P M, Smith G, Wetstone D, Smith K H 1982 The minimum alveolar concentration of nitrous oxide in man. Anesthesia Anaglesia 61: 553–556
12. Whitteridge D, Bulbring E 1944. Changes in activity of pulmonary receptors in anaesthesia and their influence on respiratory behaviour. Journal of Pharmocological & Experimental Therapeutics 81: 340–359
13. Ngai, S H, Katz R L, Farhie S E 1965 Respiratory effects of tricholorethylene, halothane and methoxyflurane in the cat. Journal of Pharmocological and Experimental Therapeutics 148: 123–130
14. Muallem M, Larson C P Jr, Eger E I II 1969 The effects of diethyl ether on $PaCO_2$ in dogs with and without vagal, somatic and sympathetic block. Anesthesiology 30: 185–191
15. Motomura S, Kissin I, Aultman D F, Reves J 1984 Effects of fentanyl and nitrous oxide on contractility of blood perfused papillary muscle of the dog. Anesthesia Analgesia 63: 47–50
16. Eisele J H, Smith N T 1972 Cardiovascular effects of 40% nitrous oxide in man. Anesthesia Analgesia 51: 956–963
17. Dolan W M, Stevens W C, Eger E I II, Cromwell T H, Halsey M J, Shakespear T F, Miller R D 1974 The cardiovascular and respiratory effects of isoflurane — nitrous oxidre anaesthesia. Canadian Anaesthetists' Society Journal 21: 557–568
18. Horbein T F, Martin E W, Bonica E J, Freund F G, Parmentier P 1969 Nitrous oxide effects on the circulatory and ventilatory responses to halothane. Anesthesiology 31: 250–260
19. Stoelting R K, Reis R R, Longnecker D E 1972 Haemodynamic responses to nitrous oxide —

halothane and halthane in valvular heart disease. Anesthesiology 37: 430–435

20. Moffitt E A, Sellina D H, Garry R J, Raymond M J, Matloff J M, Bussell J A 1983 Nitrous oxide added to halothane reduces coronary flow and myocardial oxygen consumption in patients with coronary disease. Canadian Anaesthetists' Society Journal 30: 5–9

21. Lam A M, Clement J L, Chung E C, Knill R L 1982 Respiratory effects of nitrous oxide during enflurane anesthesia in humans. Anesthesiology 56: 298–303

22. Epstein RM, Rackow H, Salanitre E, Wolf GL 1964 Influence of the concentration effect on the uptake of anesthetic mixtures: the second gas effect. Anesthesiology 25: 364–371

23. Stoelting R K, Eger E I II 1969 An additional explanation for the second gas effect: a concentrating effect. Anesthesiology 30: 273–277

24. Boaden R W, Hutton P 1986 The digital control of anaesthetic gas flow. Anaesthesia 41: 413–418

25. Baker W C, Pouchot J F 1983 The measurement of gas flow, parts 1 and 2. Journal of the Air Pollution Association 33: 66- 72 & 156–162

26. Hong K, Trudell J R, O'Neill J R, Cohen E N 1980 Biotransformation of nitrous oxide. Anesthesiology 53: 354–355

27. Hong K, Trudell J R, O'Neill J R, Cohen E N 1980 Metabolism of nitrous oxide by human and rat intestinal contents. Anesthesiology 52: 16–19

28. Bosterling B, Trudell J R, Hong K, Cohen E N 1980 Formation of free radical intermediates during nitrous oxide metabolism by human intestinal contents. Biochemical Pharmacology 29: 3037–3038

29. Chapman W P, Arrowood J G, Beecher H K 1943 The analgesic effect of low concentrations of nitrous oxide compared in man with morphine sulphate. Journal of Clinical Investigation 22: 871–875

30. Dundee J W, Moore J 1960 Alterations in response to somatic pain associated with anaesthesia, IV: the effects of sub-anaesthetic concentrations of inhalation agents. British Journal of Anaesthesia 32: 453–459

31. Finck A D 1985 Nitrous oxide analgesia. In: Eger E I II (ed) Nitrous oxide. Elsevier, New York

32. Yang J C, Clark W C, Ngai S H 1980 Antagonism of nitrous oxide analgesia by naloxone in man. Anesthesiology 52: 414–417

33. Rupreht J, Ukponwanoe M, Dworacek B, Admiraal P V, Dzolgic M R 1984 Enkephalase prevented tolerance to nitrous oxide analgesia in rats. Acta Analgesia Scandinavica 28: 617–620

34. Rupreht J, Dworacek B, Bonke B, Dzolgiv M R, van Eindhoven J H, de Vlieger M 1985 Tolerance to nitrous oxide in volunteers. Acta Anaesthesiologica Scandinavica 29: 635–638

35. White D C 1987 Narcotics in general anaesthesia. In Kaufman L (ed) Anaesthesia Review 4. Churchill Livingstone, Edinburgh, pp. 166–179

36. Smith R A, Wilson M, Miller K W 1978 Naloxone has no effect on nitrous oxide anaesthesia. Anesthesiology 49: 6–8

37. Smith E H, Rees J M H 1981 The effects of naloxone on the analgesic activities of general anaesthetics. Experientia 37: 289–290

38. Lawrence D, Livingstone A 1981 Opiate-like analgesic activity in general anaesthetics. British Journal of Pharmacology 73: 435–442

39. Watkins L R, Mayer D L 1982 Organization of endogenous opiate and non-opiate pain control systems. Science 216: 1185–1192

40. Nunn J F 1987 Clinical aspects of the interaction between nitrous oxide and vitamin B_{12}. British Journal of Anaesthesia 59: 3–13

41. Eger E I II, Saidman L J 1965 Hazards of bowel obstruction and pneumothorax. Anesthesiology 26: 61–72

42. Giuffre M, Gross J B 1986 The effects of nitrous oxide on postoperative bowel motility. Anesthesiology 65: 699–700

43. Hunter A R 1955 Problems of anaesthesia in artificial pneumothorax. Proceedings of the Royal Society of Medicine 48: 765–766

44. Nunn J F 1959 Controlled respiration in neurosurgical anaesthesia. Anaesthesia 14: 413–414

45. Munson E S, Merrick H C 1966 Effect of nitrous oxide on venous air embolism. Anesthesiology 27: 783–787

46. Tuman K J, McCarthy R J, Overfield B S, Ivankovich A D 1987 Effects of nitrous oxide during ventricular and coronary air embolism in swine. Anesthesia Analgesia 66: S180

47. Blackstock D Gettes M A 1986 Negative pressure in the middle ear in children after nitrous oxide anaesthesia. Canadian Association Journal 33: 32–35

48. Casey W F, Drake-Lee A B 1982 Nitrous oxide and middle-ear pressure: a study of induction methods in children. Anaesthesia 37: 896–900

49. Artru A A 1982 Nitrous oxide plays a direct role in the development of tension pneumocephalus intraoperatively. Anesthesiology 57: 59–61

50. Drummond J C 1984 Tension pneumocephalos and intermittent drainage of ventricular C.S.F.

Anesthesiology 60: 609–610
51. Collan R, Iivanainen M 1969 Cardiac arrest caused by rapid elimination of nitrous oxide from cerebral ventricles after encephalography. Canadian Anaesthetists' Society Journal 16: 519–524
52. Macgillivray R S 1982 Pneumocephalus as a complication of posterior fossa surgery in the sitting position. Anaesthesia 37: 722–725
53. Skahen S, Shapiro H M, Drummond J C, Todd M M, Zelman v 1986 Nitrous oxide withdrawal reduces intercranial pressure in the presence of pneumoencephalus. Anesthesiology 65: 192–195
54. Stinson T W, Donlon J V 1982 Interaction of intraocular air and sulfur hexafluoride with nitrous oxide. A computer simulation. Anesthesiology 56: 385–388
55. Sykes M K, Hurtig J B, Tait A R, Chakrabarti M K 1977 Reduction of hypoxic pulmonary vasoconstriction in the dog during administration of nitrous oxide. British Journal of Anaesthesia 49: 301–307
56. Price H L, Cooperman L H, Warden J C, Morris J J, Smith T C 1969 Pulmonary haemodynamics during general anaesthesia in man. Anesthesiology 30: 629–636
57. Schulte-Sasse U, Hess W, Tarnow J 1982 Pulmonary vascular responses to nitrous oxide in patients with normal and high pulmonary vascular resistance. Anesthesiology 57: 9–13
58. Hickey P R, Hansen D D, Strafford M, Thompson J E, Jones R E, Mayer J E 1986 Pulmonary and systemic haemodynamic effects of nitrous oxide in infants with normal and elevated pulmonary vascular resistance. Anesthesiology 65: 374–378
59. Meretoga O H, Takkunen O, Heikkila, Wegelius U 1985 Haemodynamic response to nitrous oxide during high dose fentanyl pancuronium anaesthesia. Acta Anaesthesiologica Scandinavica 29: 137–141
60. Weiskopf R B, Bogetz M S 1985 Cardiovascular action of nitrous oxide or halothane in hypovolemic swine. Anesthesiology 63: 509–510
61. Lassen H C A, Henriksen E, Neukircb F, Kristensen H S 1956 Treatment of tetanus: severe bone marrow depression after prolonged nitrous oxide anaesthesia. Lancet 1: 527–530
62. Wilson P, Martin F I R, Last P M 1956 Bone marrow depression in tetanus. Lancet 2: 442
63. Banks R G, Henderson R J, Pratt J M 1986 Reactions of gases in solution III: some reactions of nitrous oxide with transition- metal complexes. Journal of the Chemical Society (A) 3: 2886–2890
64. Amess J A L, Burman J F, Rees G M, Nancekievell D G, Mollin D L 1975 Megaloblastic hemopoiesis in patients receiving nitrous oxide. Lancet 2: 339–340
65. Deacon R, Lumb M, Perry J, Chanarin I, Minty B, Halsey M J, Nunn J F 1978 Selective inactivation of vitamin B_{12} in rats by nitrous oxide. Lancet 2: 1023–1024
66. Deacon R, Lumb M, Perry J, Chanarin I, Minty B, Halsey M, Nunn JF 1980 Inactivation of methionine synthase by nitrous oxide. European Journal of Biochemistry 104: 419
67. Royston B D, Nunn J F, Weinbren H K, Royston D, Cormack R S 1988 Rate of inactivation of human and rodent hepatic methionine synthase by nitrous oxide. Anesthesiology 68: 213–216
68. Koblin D D, Waskell L, Watson J E, Stokstad E L, Eger E I II 1982 Nitrous oxide inactivates methionine synthetase in human liver. Anesthesia Analgesia 61: 75–78
69. Landon M J, Toothill V J 1986 Effect of nitrous oxide on placental methionine synthase activity. British Journal of Anaesthesia 58: 524–527
70. Nunn J F, Sharer N M, Gorchein A, Jones J A, Wickramsinghe S N 1982 Megaloblastic haemopoiesis after multiple short-term exposure to nitrous oxide. Lancet 1: 1379–1381
71. Koblin D D, Watson J E Deady J E, Stokstad E L, Eger E I II 1981 Inactivation of methionine synthetase by nitrous oxide in mice. Anesthesiology 54: 318–324
72. Herbert V, 1985 Biology of disease: megaloblastic anaemias. Laboratory Investigation 52: 3–19
73. Amos R J, Amess J A, Nancekievill D G, Rees G M 1954 Prevention of nitrous oxide-induced megaloblastic changes in bone marrow using folinic acid. British Journal of Anaesthesia 56: 103–107
74. Kano Y, Sakamoto S, Sakuraya K, Kubota T, Taguchi H, Miura Y, Takaku F 1984 Effects of leucovorin and methylcobalamin with N_2O anaesthesia. Journal of Laboratory and Clinical Medicine 104: 711–717
75. Nunn J F, Chanarin I, Tanner A G, Owen F R 1986 Megaloblastic bone marrow changes after repeated nitrous oxide anaesthesia: reversal with folinic acid. British Journal of Anaesthesia 58: 1469–1470
76. Layzer R B 1978 Myeloneuropathy after prolonged exposure to nitrous oxide. Lancet 2: 1227–1238
77. Brodsky J B, Cohen E N, Brown B W Jr., Wu M L, Whitcher C E 1981 Exposure to nitrous oxide and neurologic disease among dental professionals. Anesthesia Analgesia 60: 297–301
78. Sweeney B, Bingham R M, Amos R J, Petty A C, Cole P V 1985 Toxicity of bone marrow in dentists exposed to nitrous oxide. British Medical Journal 291: 567–569
79. Scott J M, Dinn J J, Wilson P, Weir D S 1981 Pathogenesis of subacute combined degeneration: a result of methyl group deficiency. Lancet 1: 334–340

80. Davenport H T, Halsey M J, Wardley-Smith B, Wright B M 1976 Measurement and reduction of occupational exposure to inhaled anaesthetics. British Medical Journal 2: 1219–1221
81. Sonander H, Stenquist O, Nilsson K 1985 Nitrous oxide exposure during routine anaesthetic work. Acta Anaesthesiologica Scandinavica 29: 203–208
82. Nunn J F, O'Morain C 1982 Nitrous oxide decreases motility of human neutrophils in vitro. Anesthesiology 56: 45–48
83. Moudgil GC, Forrest JB, Gordon J 1984 The effect of volatile anaesthetics and nitrous oxide on human leukocyte chemotaxis in vitro. Canadian Anaesthetists' Society Journal 31: 631–637
84. Hill GE, English JB, Stanley TH, Kawamura R, Loeser EA, Hill HR. 1978 Nitrous oxide and neutrophil chemotaxis in man, British Journal of Anaesthesia. 50: 555–558
85. Welch W D, Zaccari J 1982 Effect of halothane and N_2O on the oxidative activity of human neutrophils. Anesthesiology 57: 172–176
86. Algie T G, Seth A, Barbenel J C, Galloway D J, Gray W M, Spence A A 1985 Nitrous oxide and wound healing. British Journal of Anaesthesia 57: 621–623
87. Baden J M, Kundomal Y R, Luttropp M E, Mazze R I, Kosek J C 1986 Carcinogen bioassay of nitrous oxide in mice. Anesthesiology 64: 747–750
88. Lane G A, Nahrwold M L, Tait A R, Taylor-Busch M, Cohen P J 1980 Anesthetics as teratogens: Nitrous oxide is fetotoxic, xenon is not. Science 210: 899–901
88. Baden J M 1985 Mutagenicity, carcinogenicity and teratogenicity of nitrous oxide. In: Eger E I II (ed) Nitrous Oxide. Elsevier, New York
89. Lane G A, DuBoulay P M, Tait A R, Taylor-Busch M, Cohen P J 1981 Nitrous oxide is teratogenic: halothane is not. Anesthesiology 55: A252
90. Mazze R I, Fujinaga M, Rice S A, Harris S B, Baden J M 1986 Reproductive and teratogenic effects of nitrous oxide, halothane, isoflurane and enflurane in Sprague-Dawley rats. Anesthesiology 64: 339–344
91. Keeling P H, Roche D A, Nunn J F, Monk S J, Lumb M J, Halsey M J 1986 Folinic acid protection against nitrous oxide teratogenicity in the rat. British Journal of Anaesthesia 58: 528–534
92. Konieczko K, Chapple JC, Nunn JF. 1987 Fetotoxic potential of general anaesthesia in relation to pregnancy. British Journal of Anaesthesia 59: 449–454
93. Cohen E N, Brown B W, Wu M L et al 1980 Occupational disease in dentistry and chronic exposure to trace anaesthetic gases. Journal of the American Dental Association 101: 21–31
94. Wynobek A J, Brodsky J, Gordon L, Moore DH, Watchmaker G, Cohen E N 1981 Sperm studies in anesthesiologists. Anesthesiology 55: 527–532
95. Rosen M A, Roizen M F, Eger E I II, Glass R H, Martin M, Dandekar P V, Dailey P A, Litt L 1987 The effect of nitrous oxide on in vitro fertilization success rates. Anesthesiology 67: 42–44
96. Gronert G A 1980 Malignant hyperthermia. Anesthesiology 53: 395–423
97. Ellis F R, Clarke I M, Appleyard T N, Dinsdale R C 1974 Malignant hyperpyrexia induced by nitrous oxide and treated with dexamethasone. British Medical Journal 4: 270–271
98. Buffington C W 1982 Reflex actions during isoflurane anaesthesia. Canadian Anaesthetists' Society Journal 29: s35–s43
99. Alexander G D, Skapski J N, Brown E M 1984 The role of nitrous oxide in postoperative nausea and vomiting. Anesthesia Analgesia 63: 175
100. Melnick B M, Johnson L S 1987 Effects of eliminating nitrous oxide in outpatient anesthesia. Anesthesiology 67: 982–984
101. Muir J J, Warner M A, Offord K P, Buck C F, Harper J V, Kunkel S E 1987 Role of nitrous oxide and other factors in postoperative nausea and vomiting: a randomized and blinded prospective study. Anesthesiology 66: 513–518
102. Kortilla K, Hovorka J, Erkola O 1987 Nitrous oxide does not increase the incidence of nausea and vomiting after isoflurane anaesthesia. Anesthesia Analgesia 66: 761–765
103. Gunawardene R D, White D C 1988 Propofol and emesis. Anaesthesia 43 (suppl.) 65–67
104. Sengupta P, Plantevin D M 1988 Nitrous oxide and day case laparoscopy: effects on nausea, vomiting and return to normal activity. British Journal of Anaesthesia 60: 570–573
105. Montgomery C J, Vaghadia H, Blackstock D 1988 Negative middle-ear pressure and postoperative vomiting in pediatric outpatients. Anesthesiology 68: 288–291
106. du Boulay P M, Nahrwold M L 1982 In vivo response of air- filled balloon-tipped catheters to nitrous oxide. Anesthesiology 57: 530–532
107. Chandler M 1986 Pressure changes in tracheal tube cuffs. Anaesthesia 41: 287–293
108. Reagan J O, Gerson J I, Davey F R, Oates R P, Morris M S 1987 Intermittent low-dose N_2O does not cause metaloblastic anemia. Anesthesia Analgesia 66: S146
109. Tyson G, Bishop M J, Bashein G, Cullen B F 1987 Prolonged anaesthesia with nitrous oxide: Is it hazardous? Anesthesia Analgesia 66, S182

3. Drugs by infusion: their use during intravenous anaesthesia and intensive care

J.W. Sear

During anaesthesia or in the intensive care unit, there is often need to maintain therapeutic drug concentrations for long periods of time. Under these circumstances, use of continuous infusions rather than repeated intravenous incremental doses of a drug may be preferable; as with the latter there will be oscillation of the plasma drug concentration between subtherapeutic trough values and peak concentrations associated with toxic or adverse side-effects.

In order to administer drugs by infusion rationally, the anaesthetist must understand the disposition and metabolism of the individual drugs concerned — otherwise therapeutic nihilism may ensue. This review will consider the ways that drugs are handled by the body; those factors which may result in alterations in the duration or intensity of drug effect; and the relationships, where known, between drug infusion rate, drug concentration and drug effect for several individual groups of drugs.

When drugs are given by the intravenous route, their distribution within the body as well as their elimination are the net result of the various physiological and pharmacological processes governing these two separate, yet dependent, events. Drug behaviour may be described by either physiologically based or mathematically based models. In the former, which are also termed 'perfusion models', drug disposition is related to the various drug tissue: plasma coefficients, tissue mass and tissue or organ blood flow. Tissues with similar partition coefficients and blood flow per unit mass may then be combined together into 'compartments'. It will be understandable, therefore, that a compartment does not have fixed anatomical boundaries nor does it necessarily comprise only one type of tissue. Such models have limitations because they necessarily incorporate several assumptions, such as average organ mass, average organ blood flow, and so on. In this way, they ignore those alterations in blood flow occurring in the presence of concurrent disease states, or through other concurrently administered therapeutic agents.

In mathematically based models, descriptions of drug behaviour are based on knowledge of the dose of drug administered, and the plasma (blood) concentration/time profile. For most drugs, this profile after a single intravenous dose is a curvilinear function. Mathematically, it can be described by a polyexponential equation. Two or more separate phases are recognized in the decline of the plasma drug concentration and these represent drug distribution within the body and drug elimination. The drug concentration (C_p) at any time 't' may then be calculated from the various terms of the polyexponential equation:

$$C_{p.t} = \text{sum of } A_i(n) \, e^{-ki(n)t}$$

where $A_i(n)$ are the equation constants, and $ki(n)$ the rate constants of the different exponential terms.

Most drugs are eliminated by first order rate processes, thus implying that a *constant fraction* of drug within the body is eliminated per unit time. Although the rate constants define the decline in the plasma drug concentration, the concept more frequently used is that of the 'half-life', i.e. the time necessary for the plasma drug concentration to fall by 50%. After 4 or 5 half-lives, the plasma drug concentration will have declined to about 6% of its original value.

Based on these rate constants and their associated half-lives, it is possible to construct mathematical models describing the body's handling of a drug. For further explanation of those concepts, the reader is referred to any of the reviews listed at the end of this chapter.

By relating plasma drug concentrations to the total administered dose, various volumes of drug distribution can be calculated (V_1, V_2, Vdss) — where V_1 is the volume of the central kinetic compartment; V_2 that of the peripheral compartment(s); and Vdss (the overall apparent volume of distribution at steady state) the sum of V_1 and V_2. For many drugs, especially those with a high liposolubility, Vdss will be large and in excess of total body mass. The calculation of Vdss assumes the steady-state partitioning of drug between plasma and all tissues of the body to be unity. This is a necessary assumption, as only plasma drug concentrations can be measured.

The third characteristic of a drug's kinetic profile is clearance (Cl), that is the volume of blood or plasma from which drug is completely removed per unit time. Clearance is independent of drug concentration, although it is related to both the elimination rate constant (k_{el}) and the volume of distribution (Vd):

$$Cl = K_{el} \cdot Vd$$

Clearance may also be expressed in terms of an individual's organ's ability to remove drug, based on determination of the 'extraction ratio' (see later). For any organ or tissue, drug clearance will be influenced by:

Table 3.1   Effect of increased hepatic blood flow (HBF) and enzyme activity on the disposition of high and low extraction compounds

	Low extraction drugs (<0.3)	High extraction drugs (<0.7)
Effect of increased HBF:		
Systemic clearance	unchanged	increased
Oral clearance	unchanged	unchanged
Bioavailability	unchanged	increased
Half-life	unchanged	decreased
Intensity of effect	unchanged	may be decreased
Duration of effect	unchanged	shortened
Effect of increased enzyme activity:		
Systemic clearance	increased	unchanged
Oral clearance	increased	increased
Bioavailability	unchanged	decreased
Half-life	decreased	unchanged
Intensity of effect	may be shortened	unchanged
Duration of effect	may be shortened	unchanged

1. Blood flow
2. Intrinsic ability of the organ to extract that drug
3. Plasma drug binding

Hepatic clearance (the main route of drug elimination) is the product of hepatic blood flow and the extraction ratio.

If the hepatic extraction ratio (ER) is high (>0.7), drug clearance will be highly dependent on liver blood flow; changes in liver enzyme activity having only a minimal effect on drug clearance. In contrast, for drugs with a low ER (<0.3) only a fraction of the available drug is removed per unit time. Thus, excess drug is available for clearance. Changes in liver blood flow will have little effect on drug clearance, while changes in liver enzyme activity or an increase in the free (or unbound) drug fraction will result in a large increase in drug clearance (Table 3.1)

KINETICS OF INTRAVENOUS INFUSIONS

When a continuous infusion of drug is maintained for long periods of time, plasma drug concentrations increase in a curvilinear fashion until steady-state levels are achieved. At that point, the rate of drug administration must exactly equal the rate of drug removal from the body. The relationship between infusion rate and steady state concentration may be given by:

$$C_{ss} = K_{01}/Cl$$

where C_{ss} is the steady-state drug concentration; K_{01} is the infusion rate; and Cl is the clearance. The time to achieve steady-state concentrations will vary from drug to drug. However, it is independent of the infusion rate, the latter only governing the ultimate concentration reached. In general, drug concentrations within 10% of the final true steady state concentration will be reached by infusions of duration greater than 3 times the drug elimination half-life. However, this assumes the infused drug to be pharmocologically inert, having no dynamic effects that may themselves influence drug distribution and elimination. For most of the intravenous anaesthetic agents, their administration is accompanied by changes in cardiac output and regional blood flow, such that steady-state concentrations are achieved sooner than otherwise predicted.

As defined earlier, the three basic kinetic parameters (half-life, volume of distribution and clearance) are inter-related:

$$T_{1/2\,el} = 0.693 \cdot Vd/Cl$$

Thus, if a drug has a large Vd, there will be a long elimination half-life, and it will take a long period of time to reach steady state concentrations when administered by a single, fixed rate infusion. More rapid steady state concentrations can be achieved by use of complex infusion schemes:

1. Combination of a loading dose followed by a single constant rate infusion. The size of the loading dose may be based on either the initial volume of drug distribution (V_1), the Vdss or the apparent volume of distribution during the elimination phase ($V\beta$). In general, the dose administered is calculated as the product of desired target concentration and Vd. If the dose is based on V_1, subtherapeutic concentrations (below C_{ss}) will persist for some period of time; while if Vdss or $V\beta$ are used, initial drug con-

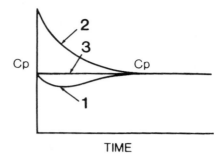

Fig. 3.1   Plasma concentration against time curve after two different loading doses prior to a continuous infusion. For curve 1, the loading dose was determined based on the initial volume of distribution (V_1); for curve 2, on the apparent volume of distribution at steady state (Vdss). Curve 3 represents the target steady-state plasma drug concentration.

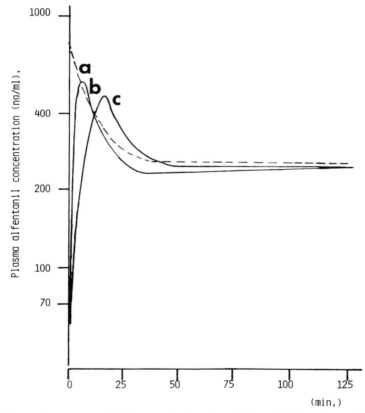

Fig. 3.2   Plasma drug concentration/time profiles for three different infusion schemes for administration of a loading dose of alfentanil (100 μg/kg) followed by an infusion of 1 μg/kg.min^{-1}: (a) 100 μg/kg bolus following by the alfentanil infusion (1 μg/kg.min^{-1}); (b) Rapid loading infusion (20 ug/kg.min^{-1} for 5 minutes) followed by infusion (1 μg/kg.min^{-1}); (c) Rapid loading infusion (6.67 μg/kg.min^{-1} for 16 min) followed by infusion (1 μg/kg.min^{-1}).

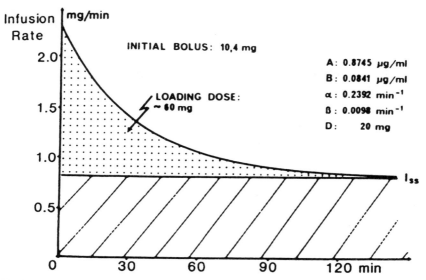

Fig. 3.3 BET (Bolus-elimination-transfer) infusion scheme for etomidate, with data to achieve a constant plasma drug concentration of 0.5 μg/ml. This consists of an initial bolus dose (10.4 mg), a constant rate infusion to replace drug lost by elimination (metabolic clearance) i.e. 0.8 mg/min, and an exponentially declining infusion rate to compensate for drug transfer to the peripheral tissues (loading dose approximately 60 mg over 170 min). The bolus dose and infusion rates for the BET scheme have been based on kinetics derived following administration of a single dose of 20 mg etomidate (D). From this kinetic study, the parameters A, B, a, and b are the ordinate constants and hybrid rate constants of the bi-expoential equation that describes the decline in the plasma etomidate concentration.

centrations will exceed the desired target levels (Fig. 3.1). For drugs with a narrow therapeutic range, supra-therapeutic concentrations may result in toxic or other untoward side-effects.

2. Double infusion regimens, based on the principles described by Wagner.[1] Two differing rate infusions are used: the first (a rapid infusion) fills up the body distribution volumes, while the second (a slower maintenance rate) is at the rate needed to maintain the target concentration, and is therefore related to the clearance of the drug. The concentration/time profile for this technique initially undershoots the target concentration and then overshoots — the magnitude of the overshoot may be limited by extending the duration of the rapid infusion phase (Fig. 3.2)

3. Combination of a single bolus dose, and more than one consecutive constant rate infusion(s). This approach was originally proposed by Kruger-Thiemer[2] and then developed by many others. It has been adapted for the administration of several groups of drugs used in anaesthetic practice (e.g. propofol, etomidate and midazolam, and alfentanil). Such a scheme may be broken down into three separate components — the bolus dose (X) to achieve the target concentration (X = $V_1 . C_{ss}$); a maintenance infusion to replace drug lost by metabolism or excretion ($Q_1 = Cl . C_{ss}$); and thirdly an exponentially declining infusion (Q_2) (or a series of stepwise declining rate infusions) to compensate for drug transfer from the blood and central kinetic compartment to the peripheral tissues (Fig. 3.3):

$$Q_2 = V_1 . C_{ss} . K_{12}e^{-k12t}$$

4. A fourth and novel approach to the attainment of constant plasma drug concentrations without recourse to complex computerization was described by Riddell and colleagues.[3] An exponentially decreasing drug delivery rate is achieved by removing solution from a container at a constant rate, while replacing with solvent at the same rate. Riddell described its use for infusions of lignocaine; but more recently, McMurray and colleagues have used the same method for infusion of methohexitone for the maintenance of anaesthesia.[4]

NON-LINEAR KINETICS

So far, the distribution and elimination of intravenous drugs has been discussed in terms of first-order rate reactions. However, there are limitations to the application of this methodology to all drugs. For example, there are few studies investigating the linearity of kinetic parameters over a wide dose input range[5]. In addition, many biophysiological processes incorporate transport mechanisms utilizing either carrier proteins or enzyme systems for drug metabolism. Both of these processes are saturable and, under such circumstances, the rates of reaction may not be first-order, but constant and independent of the substrate concentration (i.e. zero-order).

In clinical practice, zero-order processes are uncommon as the capacity of most carrier transport systems and enzyme pathways are in excess of therapeutically effective drug (substrate) concentrations. Those reactions that do occur often involve drugs that are predominantly eliminated by hepatic metabolism. Increasing drug doses will result in higher plasma drug concentrations, longer elimination half-lives, and proportionately greater 'area under the curve' (i.e. decreased clearance). Enzyme saturation can occur with ethanol, salicylates, theophylline and phenytoin and, in the case of the intravenous agents, thiopentone if given by repeated doses or continuous infusion such that the plasma drug concentration exceeds 40–50 μg/ml. Surgical anaesthesia with thiopentone is seen at concentrations between 39 and 42 μg/ml in the absence of nitrous oxide,[6] and 15–20 μg/ml with nitrous oxide.[7]

Each of these approaches assumes a stable plasma drug concentration to be associated with a steady dynamic effect.

PLASMA DRUG CONCENTRATIONS AND DRUG EFFECTS

Few, if any, of the intravenous anaesthetic agents have narrow therapeutic ranges with precise concentrations being associated with desired dynamic effects in all patients. In addition, there are many factors that will influence drug kinetics and therefore alter the drug concentration achieved by a given infusion.

An area of recent controversy and interest has therefore been the relative merits of fixed-rate infusion regimens as compared with infusion rates varied to achieve clinically adequate anaesthesia. It seems logical to vary the infusion rate of an hypnotic or opioid according to the systemic arterial pressure or somatic response, as has been the traditional practice for the volatile agents.

Ausums and his colleagues in Leiden therefore conducted several studies using the opioid alfentanil aimed at demonstrating the need for differing drug concentrations for different surgical events.[8] The infusion of alfentanil supplemented 67% nitrous oxide in oxygen anaesthesia; the initial rate being 50 μg/kg.h^{-1} This rate was then adjusted up or down in 25 μg/kg.h^{-1} steps between 25 and 150 μg/kg.h^{-1} according to clinical response. In addition, bolus doses (7–14 μg/kg) were used to rapidly suppress any acute response indicating inadequate anaesthesia. Blood samples were collected every 10 minutes until the first patient response, and then at 2, 5 and 15 minutes thereafter. Thus, they were able to define (using logistical analysis) plasma drug concentrations associated with a known probability of non-response to a given surgical stimulus. For intubation, the Cp_{50} concentration of alfentanil (concentration at which there is a 50% chance of a response) was 475 ng/ml (95% limits: 418–532 ng/ml), while for skin incision, the Cp_{50} was 279 ng/ml (95% limits 238–320). During surgery, the Cp_{50} was 270 ng/ml for breast surgery, 309 ng/ml for lower abdominal surgery and 412 ng/ml for upper abdominal surgery. Recovery of consciousness with spontaneous breathing was seen at concentrations of alfentanil *below* 200 ng/ml. This concentration may have significant dynamic effects on ventilatory function,[9,10] as it represents the Cp_{50} value (i.e. at 200 ng/ml, 50% of patients can be predicted to require naloxone). If we extrapolate from Ausum's findings, the concentration of alfentanil at which no patient would require naloxone (for inadequate ventilation) would be about 120 ng/ml. Thus, not only is there need for different drug concentrations for different surgical procedures, but also different concentrations are required at different times during any single operation.

COMPUTERIZED CONTROL OF ANAESTHETIC DELIVERY

The administration of drugs by infusion may be achieved either by gravity infusion sets or by more sophisticated delivery systems (e.g. volumetric pumps or syringe pumps),which may be controlled in various manners. Control systems for anaesthetic delivery may be classified into one of two main groupings: open loop systems and closed loop systems.

Open-loop systems

These are pre-programmed systems (such as constant rate infusions, the dilutional strategies of McMurray and colleagues,[4] or Wagner's two-stage infusion regimen[1]). These do not require a priori a computer for drug delivery. The predetermined infusion criteria will be based on mean kinetic data for a defined population — usually either volunteers or healthy (ASA) I surgical patients. Further refinements of the infusion regimens may be achieved by derivation of true population kinetic parameters using non-linear regression programmes such as ELSFIT or NONMEM. Because of the dynamic as well as the kinetic differences between patients, a given threshold plasma drug concentration will vary between individuals. Thus, using fixed infusion regimens (often inappropriately dependent on patient weight), some patients will receive more and some less than is clinically necessary. Hence the concepts of MAC (for inhalational agents) or MIR (minimum infusion rate) offer only guidelines as to actual dosage requirements.[11,12,13]

The open-loop system may be further refined by incorporation of a feedforward control. Examples of this include systems to compensate for changes in cardiac output and alveolar ventilation during pulsed halothane anaesthesia.[14] As yet, this approach has not been applied to intravenous infusions during anaesthesia.

Closed-loop systems

Closed-loop control for administration of intravenous anaesthetic (hypnotic) and potent analgesic drugs is difficult to achieve as the control variables (depth of anaesthesia or analgesia) are hard to define and measure. With inhalational anaesthetic agents, control may be readily achieved by defining the set-point in terms of a given end-tidal vapour concentration, which, by implication, represents a given partial pressure of anaesthetic. At present, there are no facilities to monitor intravenous anaesthetic concentrations *on line*.

Recent studies have attempted to use the physiological effects of intravenous anaesthetics as the control variables. For example, such end-points might include the e.e.g. (or one of its derivatives), lower oesophageal contractility, or the reflex evoked e.m.g[15,16,17] None of these indices appear suitable alone for the satisfactory control of intravenous drug delivery but a combination of end-points might often improve results. Thus, Schils et al[18] used the combination of blood pressure and spectral edge frequency to control halothane delivery;[18] while Jordan and colleagues have monitored blood pressure, heart rate and CO_2 production as the control parameters when infusing fentanyl to supplement 60% nitrous oxide in oxygen.[19]

Another example of closed-loop control involves infusion of sodium nitroprusside (SNP), or isoflurane from a servo-controlled vaporizer, for the induction and maintenance of arterial hypotension. Millard and colleagues adapted a self-tuning adaptive control programme and, by using an infusion of sodium nitroprusside as an addition to a basal 1% halothane anaesthetic, achieved mean arterial pressures of 50–55 mmHg.[20] Low et al reported good control ($\pm$ 5mmHg) in 7 out of 14 patients, and moderate control ($\pm$ 10mmHg) in another 3 patients. Control was inadequate in the remaining 4 patients owing to marked oscillation of the blood pressure.[21] Furthermore, Westenskow et al have observed increasing dose requirements for nitroprusside when used in an experimental animal model to maintain hypotension.[22] This was thought to reflect the progressive change in sensitivity to SNP with time owing to an increased release of both renin and angiotension. Thus, improved control has been obtained with similar feedback systems when animals or patients have been pre-treated with beta-adrenoceptor blocking agents such as propranolol, or the alpha$_2$-adrenoceptor agonist, clonidine.[23]

Of the other physiological variables, the magnitude of muscle contraction is probably the easiest to measure, and feedback systems for control of neuromuscular blockade have been described.[24-26] There are, however, few data investigating the efficiency of such systems. In a clinical comparison of computer-controlled versus manually-controlled infusions of vecuronium to achieve the common end-point of blockade of 90% twitch height, Asbury et al found the variability of paralysis to be 21% with computer control as against 187% with manual control. In addition to the improved control, drug dosage was also reduced.[27]

FACTORS AFFECTING KINETICS OF DRUGS BY INFUSION

For a single bolus of a drug, alterations in kinetics result in changes in the concentration/time profile — with an accompanying prolongation or shortening of the duration of effect, coupled with possible changes in the magnitude of this effect. For drugs given by infusion, changes in kinetics will primarily alter steady state drug concentrations (C_{ss}) and, in turn, the magnitude of dynamic responses. Changes in the

C_{ss} for a given infusion rate may reflect alterations in the hepatic extraction ratio, in plasma protein binding, in liver blood flow, or changes in the excretion rate of drugs eliminated unchanged through the kidneys.

Extraction ratio

When blood passes through any tissue or organ, drug removal may take place. The extraction ratio (ER) may be defined as:

$$ER = C_{in} - C_{out}/C_{in}$$

For drugs metabolized in the liver, hepatic clearance (Cl_H) is the product of Q and ER, where Q equals hepatic blood flow. Thus hepatic clearance depends on both flow to the organ and the ability of the liver to extract drug from it. The ER must reflect the activity of the liver's drug metabolizing enzyme system (the microsomal mixed function oxygenases — MFOs). The intrinsic ability of these enzymes to metabolize drug may also be expressed as the 'intrinsic clearance' (Cl_{int}); this represents the maximal ability of the liver to remove drug and is independent of organ blood flow.

Plasma protein and tissue binding

In the body, an equilibrium exists between drug bound to plasma and other tissue binding proteins, and the free or unbound drug. The extent of this binding will affect both drug distribution and elimination.

Changes in drug binding, through either drug–drug interactions or disease processes may significantly alter the volume of distribution of a drug. Similarly, changes in binding may influence drug distribution within the intravascular space, with changes in the whole blood: plasma drug ratio. For example, both liver disease and protein losing renal nephroses may cause a decrease in the plasma albumin concentration, and therefore reduced protein binding. Another important group of binding proteins are the acute-phase reactant proteins (especially alpha$_1$ acid glycoprotein), which are signficantly increased in concentration in chronic inflammatory diseases (such as rheumatoid arthritis, glomerulonephritis, Crohn's disease), malignancy, surgery, trauma, renal transplantation, and myocardial infarction.

In general, alterations in protein binding (and therefore in the percentage free fraction) are only important for drugs with high binding (>95%). Since, for a drug given by infusion, C_{ss} equals rate of infusion/clearance, alterations in protein binding will influence total drug concentrations in different ways depending on the ER. For drugs with a low ER, any increase in the free fraction will be reflected by an increase in the volume of drug distribution and a fall in the total drug C_{ss}. Because clearance is dependent on the free fraction, the free drug concentration will remain unaltered.

However, for a drug with a high ER, the rate of clearance is independent of the extent of protein binding. Thus, with the increase in free fraction, there will be a similar fall in the plasma total drug concentration owing to the increased volume of distribution; but *with continued administration* and with an *unaltered* clearance, the total drug C_{ss} will in time return to its previous value, while there will be an associated increased free fraction. This may result in increased pharmacological effects from a given drug infusion rate, and possible toxicity.

Liver blood flow

This can be altered in three ways, namely physiological interventions, pharmacological agents and pathological processes.

Physiological interventions

Those altering cardiac output will alter liver blood flow, and therefore the clearance of flow dependent drugs (e.g. methohexitone, propofol, ketamine, lignocaine, etc.). Such factors include hypocapnia secondary to excessive ventilation (decrease in cardiac output caused by the raised intrathoracic pressure), hypercapnia causing splanchnic vasoconstriction secondary to increased sympathetic activity, hypoxia (perhaps), and volume depletion.

Pharmacological agents

Several drugs administered to the peri-operative patient will alter the distribution and clearance of intravenous agents. These include alpha- and beta-adrenoceptor agonists and antagonists, histamine H_2-receptor antagonists, calcium-channel blocking drugs, and anti-arrhythmic drugs (lignocaine, amiodarone).

Beta-adrenoceptor antagonists. These reduce total liver blood flow leading to a decrease in the clearance of the flow-dependent drugs. Propranolol has also been demonstrated to impair the clearance of antipyrine — a capacity-limited drug. This latter property is related to the liposolubility of the different blocking agents.

Histamine H_2-receptor antagonists. These drugs (particularly cimetidine) decrease the clearance of several flow-limited drugs (e.g. lignocaine, propranolol, chlormethiazole, fentanyl, midazolam); these effects being the result of a reduction in hepatic blood flow. However, Mojaverian et al failed to demonstrate such an effect on the clearance of morphine in the presence of cimetidine.[28]. Increases in the C_{ss} of diazepam (a capacity-limited drug) have also been observed when co-administered with cimetidine. This latter effect appears to be mediated through binding of cimetidine to the terminal oxidase (cytochrome P_{450}) of the mixed-function oxidase system. Ranitidine, famotidine and nizatidine do not share these same properties.

Calcium channel blocking drugs. These drugs act by two separate mechanisms, either to increase liver blood flow by splanchnic vasodilation (verapamil, nifedipine) or to decrease it secondary to an inhibition of hepatic enzyme activity (verapamil, diltiazem). Thus, diltiazem has been shown to increase the C_{ss} of digoxin and decrease antipyrine clearance (capacity-limited clearance drugs), while verapamil and nifedipine increase liver blood flow and hence the clearance of drugs such as ICG.

Other drugs of interest include amiodarone, which inhibits oxidative drug metabolism (in the rat) by decreasing hepatic microsomal cytochrome P_{450} content. Any effects of this drug will be long-lasting as it has an apparent elimination half-life of between 40 and 100 days. Lignocaine may cause either increased or decreased drug clearance — at low dosage rates (60 μg/kg/.min^{-1}) the drug acts as vasodilator; at higher doses (50–200 mg) it depresses the myocardium.

Pathological processes

As may be expected, drug disposition will be altered in disease states where there is hepatic or renal impairment, or both.

Severe liver disease decreases total effective hepatic blood flow (through both intra- and extra-hepatic shunting) and decreases hepatocyte function (Table 3.2). This will

Table 3.2 Predominant pathophysiological changes in various types of liver disease (Adapted from Blaschke TF (1977): *Clinical Pharmacokinetics 2*, 32–44 with permission from the author and publishers.)

Disease	Total liver blood flow	Liver cell mass	Liver cell function
Cirrhosis			
Mild	↓	↔ or ↑	↔
Severe	↓	↓	↓
Acute inflammatory liver disease			
Viral hepatitis	↔ or ↑	↔ or ↓	↓
Alcoholic hepatitis	↔ or ↓	↑, ↔ or ↓	↓

normally result in increases in C_{ss} for drugs given by infusion. However, accompanying changes in plasma protein binding for xenobiotics having a low free fraction may lead to increases in the volume of total drug distribution and hence a decrease in the total drug concentration.[29]

Acute renal failure, as well as chronic renal insufficiency, will also alter plasma protein binding; in addition, cellular metabolism and drug metabolite elimination. In uraemia, the plasma-protein binding of basic drugs is largely unaltered, but there will be a significant decrease in the binding (mainly to albumin) of acidic drugs. As a result, distribution volumes are increased, and may be accompanied by increases in total drug clearance. Free drug clearance remains unchanged.

There are few data on the influence of renal disease of the disposition of intravenous anaesthetic drugs by infusion. Ball et al demonstrated an increase in morphine-like activity (probably morphine and cross-reacting morphine-6-glucuronide) when morphine was infused in ITU patients with renal failure.[30] Similar increases in active metabolite concentrations have been reported by Szeto et al and colleagues when pethidine administration was studied in patients with chronic pain and impaired renal function.[31]

Other pathological processes that may alter drug disposition include severe cardiac disease and perhaps chronic hypoxic pulmonary disease.

INFUSIONS OF SPECIFIC GROUPS OF DRUGS

Within anaesthesia and intensive care, the physician has a number of clinical situations where maintenance of a steady blood or tissue drug concentration is important for the efficacy of treatment. Some examples have already been highlighted, but the three basic components of anaesthesia (hypnosis, analgesia and muscle relaxation) provide further illustrations of present day applications and knowledge.

Hypnotics

The current rationale for anaesthetic techniques using continuous infusions of hypnotic agents stems from three main considerations:

1. Concern over the organ-toxic effects of volatile anaesthetic agents in the anaesthetized patient.

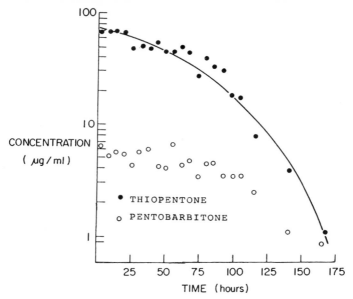

Fig. 3.4 Post-infusion plasma concentrations of thiopentone and pentobarbitone in a single patient[32] who had received a very large dose (502 mg/kg) over 42 h. The solid line represents the predicted values for thiopentone using the V_{max} and K_m estimates. The pentobarbitone is a metabolite.

2. Concern over the effects of chronic exposure to trace concentrations of anaesthetic gases or vapours on the health of operating room personnel.

3. The introduction of intravenous drugs with more appropriate kinetic profiles (viz. onset of sleep within one arm–brain circulation time; predictable and short duration of action followed by rapid inactivation of the drug by hepatic or plasma metabolism; non-cumulative; inactive, non-toxic metabolites; absence of toxicity or allergenicity towards the solvent; minimal cardiorespiratory effects).

Although the archetypal drug, thiopentone, remains the standard by which other induction agents are judged, its properties are less than ideal when given by continuous infusion (e.g. cumulation of drug, with prolongation of recovery). This results from two separate mechanism: firstly, a change in the kinetics from a first order to a zero-order reaction when plasma drug concentrations exceed 40–50 μg/ml; and secondly, from the formation of a pharmacologically active metabolite, pentobarbitone (Fig. 3.4).[32] This latter barbiturate has a longer elimination half-life (20–52 h) when compared with that of thiopentone (10–12 h) under first-order kinetic conditions. However, many authors have successfully employed infusions of thiopentone (at rates between 150 and 300 μg/kg.min^{-1}), either alone or as a supplement to 67% nitrous oxide in oxygen for the provision of anaesthesia.[7,33]

Other hypnotics with more desirable kinetic profiles include methohexitone, di-isopropyl phenol, ketamine and midazolam. The kinetics of these agents when given by continuous infusion are shown in Table 3.3, together with the range of infusion rates (and associated therapeutic plasma drug concentrations) when used to supplement either 67% nitrous oxide or infusions of opioids for the provision of clinical anaesthesia. Data for etomidate by infusion are included for completeness — although

Table 3.3 Dynamic and kinetic properties of hypnotic agents given by continuous intravenous infusion

	$T^{1/2}$ (min)	Vd (l)	Cl_p (ml/min)	Infusion rates for anaesthesia (+ N_2O or opioids) (μg/kg.min^{-1})	Concentration during anaesthesia (μg/ml)
Thiopentone	210–690	90–210	150–300	150–300	15–25
Methohexitone	90–240	80–280	820–840	60–120	2–10 (?)
Midazolam	120–150	90–130	250–500	0.125–0.25	0.3–0.4
Etomidate	70–280	140–340	880–1600	10–30	0.5–0.6
Propofol	180–720	400–1800	1300–1900	50–200	1.5–3.0
Ketamine	90–170	200	930–1230	40–60	0.5–1.8

the effects of this drug on steroid biosynthesis in the adrenal cortex render its use unacceptable for the maintenance of anaesthesia.[34]

What advantages do the intravenous agents show over the volatile agents? The cardiovascular effects of continuous infusions of hypnotic agents when used to supplement 67% nitrous oxide in oxygen have been studied by Prys-Roberts and his colleagues. In a review comparing the effects of infusions of methohexitone and propofol to supplement 67% nitrous oxide in oxygen with the three main volatile agents at equipotent concentrations (1 MAC or 1 MIR), there was less cardiovascular depression when assessed in terms of the mean arterial blood pressure or cardiac output.[35] Few arrhythmias were observed with the hypnotic agents. However, at 2 MIR, both methohexitone and Althesin caused less depression of arterial pressure and cardiac output than has been described for propofol, although the latter is, in turn, less depressant than halothane or enflurane. Propofol, nitrous oxide, anaesthesia in the absence of surgical stimulation results in a resetting of the baroreceptor reflex set-point without any depression of sensitivity.[36] This is in contrast to infusion anaesthesia with Althesin or methohexitone where significant depression of reflex activity has been observed.[37] Thus, when infusions of propofol or methohexitone were administered to supplement nitrous oxide anaesthesia for patients undergoing body surface surgery, higher heart rates for comparable mean arterial blood pressures were found in the methohexitone group.[38]

Besides depression of these general cardiovascular indices, infusions of etomidate, thiopentone, Althesin and propofol all produce dose-related reductions in total hepatic blood flow.[39] (P. Foëx, J. Diedericks & J. W. Sear, unpublished). Similar decreases in liver blood flow have been found during use of the volatile agents.[40] Infusions of ketamine have generally been associated with cardiovascular stimulation. However, recent studies show a similar dose-related, although smaller magnitude decreases in mean arterial pressure and systemic vascular resistance, but with no change in cardiac output.[41] Thus, during ketamine anaesthesia there was no significant alteration of total liver blood flow.

Despite these changes in liver blood flow, infusions of the hypnotic agents (with the possible exceptions of thiopentone, methohexitone and ketamine) cause only minimal disturbance on the plasma activities of routinely measured liver function tests.

The combinations of midazolam with either fentanyl or alfentanil have been used to supplement both nitrous oxide- and oxygen-enriched air for anaesthesia. Plasma midazolam concentrations of about 400 ng/ml were found to be needed to achieve hypnosis, while the combination with fentanyl resulted in satisfactory analgesia with good cardiovascular control. However, these techniques have the disadvantage of postoperative drowsiness and a frequent need for naloxone to overcome respiratory depression at extubation. Further studies with the shorter-acting opioid alfentanil and a reduced target midazolam concentration (300 ng/ml) have led to improved recovery without loss of cardiovascular stability.[42]

Multiple increments or infusions of propofol have no effect on the normal neuroendocrine response to surgery and trauma[43,44] — in contrast to the prolonged inhibition of cortisol and aldosterone secretion following infusions of etomidate.[34] Other endocrine effects of intravenous agents by infusion have been described.[45] Midazolam (90 μg/kg.h^{-1}) caused an obtunding of the normal increase in plasma cortisol concentrations in patients undergoing minor body surface surgery; in contrast to the effects in patients receiving etomidate where plasma ACTH levels were not increased. Moreover, midazolam did not affect the increase in cortisol following an exogenous injection of ACTH (Synacthen®). However, these data are at variance with our own data following single induction doses of midazolam[46] and with those of Nilsson et al,[42] where an infusion of 25 μg/kg.h^{-1} supplemented by alfentanil was employed. One explanation may be that these latter studies were both in patients undergoing lower abdominal surgery rather than body surface operations. In other studies in the dog, midazolam by infusion was associated with obtunding of the postoperative increase in adrenaline.[48]

Little work has been conducted comparing the respiratory effects of inhalational and intravenous infusion anaesthesia, although respiratory depression appears to be less marked with the latter agents. Unlike the inhalational agents, intravenous infusions do not appear to inhibit pulmonary vasoconstrictor mechanisms in response to hypoxia.[48]

Few systematic studies have evaluated dose requirements of hypnotic agents in the critically ill patient. In a classical paper,[49] Ramsay et al described the use of Althesin by infusion for sedation in the ITU — the rates needed to achieve a sedated but rousable patient varying between 0.01 and 0.23 ml/kg.h^{-1}. Similarly wide inter-individual variations in dose requirements have been reported for thiopentone by infusion for the control of intra-cranial pressure, and infusions of propofol or midazolam for sedation in a general intensive care unit.[44,50]

OPIOIDS BY INFUSION

Infusions of opioids alone may provide anaesthesia.[51] Among the advantages claimed, are greater cardiovascular stability as compared with intermittent bolus doses, and a reduction in the metabolic response to surgery and trauma. However, to counterbalance these positive aspects is the severe respiratory depression encountered postoperatively.

The diposition kinetics are shown in Table 3.4, the therapeutic plasma concentration range and the minimum effective analgesic concentration for several opioids. The latter two parameters vary according to an individual patient's sensitivity, the type of surgery, and the presence of adjunctive drugs such as nitrous oxide or volatile agents. For drugs such as pethidine, fentanyl, alfentanil and sufentanil, where there is rapid equilibration between the plasma and the drug's central site of action, a close

Table 3.4   Dynamic and kinetic properties of some of the commonly used opioids

	$T^{1/2}$ (min)	Vd (litres)	Cl_p (ml/min)	Therapeutic range (ng/ml)	MEAC* (ng/ml)
Morphine	150–210	100–150	400–950	15–100	15–25
Pethidine	180–240	250–300	700–1200	300–1500	300–650
Fentanyl	120–300	200–350	400–800	2–25	1–3
Alfentanil	90–200	40–60	150–350	50–500	100–350
Sufentanil	120–300	120–180	700–1100	0.3–2	Unknown

*MEAC = minimum effective analgesic concentration.

relationship exists between the blood concentration and the intensity of effect.

Initial reports using continuous infusions of fentanyl for anaesthesia appeared in the late 1970s and early 1980s.[52,53] By use of a continuous infusion technique the dose can be more easily titrated to effect, therefore the amount of drug administered can be reduced and recovery times improved. As a simple formula, infusion regimens for fentanyl aim for a concentration of about 18–20 ng/ml when the drug is used as a sole agent for cardiac surgery (loading dose of 50–75 μg/kg, and a maintenance rate of 0.3–0.5 μg/kg.min^{-1}). When used as part of a balanced anaesthetic technique for major abdominal surgery, steady state fentanyl concentrations of about 5 ng/ml are needed (10 μg/kg loading dose and 2 μg/min); while for out-patient surgery, fentanyl concentrations between 2 and 4 ng/ml are appropriate.

Although Ausums and colleagues have demonstrated the rationale for different concentrations of the opioid alfentanil according to the nature of the surgical stimulus,[8] this approach requires considerable technological support that is outside the easy access of most clinical anaesthetists. Thus, several authors have adopted use of fixed infusion regimens with supplementation of the basal rate either by bolus doses of the opioid or volatile agents at times of clinically inadequate anaesthesia or haemodynamic instability. It is therefore relevant to review the currently available data.

In a preliminary study, Andrews et al reported the analgesic effects of an infusion of fentanyl 3 μg/kg.h^{-1} as supplement of 67% nitrous oxide, and compared it with 20 μg/kg.h^{-1} alfentanil.[9] Patients were ventilated to normocapnia, and volatile supplementation (halothane <0.5%) was only added if the heart rate or arterial pressure increased by more than 15% in response to surgical stimulation. At the completion of surgery, the infusions were continued for a further hour to provide postoperative pain relief.

During surgery, halothane was needed in 3 out of 8 patients receiving fentanyl and in all 8 patients receiving alfentanil. One hour after the end of anaesthesia, and with the infusion of the opioid continued, there was a 28% (mean) decrease in minute ventilation in both groups. The slopes of the CO_2 ventilatory response curves were 35% of the awake value in the fentanyl group and 48% in the alfentanil patients (plasma fentanyl and alfentanil concentrations were 3.0 ng/ml and 121.8 ng/ml; with calculated clearances of 16.7 and 2.7 ml/kg.min^{-1} respectively). After a further hour, when the respective plasma drug concentrations were 1.71 and 20.8 ng/ml, the slopes of the CO_2 response curves were 53.9% and 69% of baseline.

One proposed advantage of an infusion technique was the likely reduction in total opioid dose given per unit time when compared with multiple intermittent administrations. Studies by White have compared the use of variable rate infusion with incremental dosage techniques, and shown a 40% reduction in opioid dose, improved intra-operative conditions (lower incidence of purposeful movements, cardiovascular changes or respiratory depression) and decreased times to awakening.[54] However, the incidence of common postoperative side-effects was unchanged.

Other authors have investigated both fixed and variable rate infusions of alfentanil and sufentanil to supplement nitrous oxide in oxygen; and compared them with either fentanyl by infusion or volatile supplementation. Using higher intra-operative alfentanil infusion regimens (50 and 100 μg/kg.h^{-1}), O'Connor et al found improved operating conditions and no significant postoperative depression;[10] our own data (unpublished) and those of Raeder et al, van Beem et al, and Zuurmond et al would concur with O'Connor's findings[55-57] In a study of fentanyl and alfentanil by either bolus dosing or continuous variable rate infusion to supplement 67% nitrous oxide in the spontaneously breathing patient, Coe et al found alfentanil to be associated with a lower incidence of chest wall rigidity and ventilatory depression, although there was a higher incidence of mild bradycardia and hypotension[58] More rapid recovery was observed after alfentanil.

Phitayakorn and colleagues investigated infusions of fentanyl and sufentanil for out-patient anaesthesia.[60] Sufentanil has a faster onset of action and a shorter elimination half-life, hence recovery should be more rapid than after fentanyl. However, at clinically equivalent infusion rates (3.9 μg/min fentanyl versus 0.53 μg/min sufentanil — a potency ratio of approximately 7:1), there were no differences in recovery — although more patients in the fentanyl group reported postoperative pain necessitating further analgesic drugs. The incidence of nausea was significantly lower after sufentanil (20% compared with 52%). Taken together, these side-effects may dictate an important role for sufentanil in ambulatory practice.

Within the ITU, we have demonstrated a wide range of infusion rates of alfentanil (0.6–8.4 mg/h: median 1.73 mg/h) needed to provide adequate analgesia to supplement midazolam sedation.[60] Thus, in this environment there is clear indication that titration of dose to effect is of more value than the adoption of empirical regimens.

Other opioids administered by infusion include morphine, papaveretum and pethidine. The first two drugs have a greater role in providing analgesia in the recovery period and in the ITU rather than in the operating theatre, where the sedative and euphoric side-effects may be disadvantageous to rapid patient recovery. For postoperative analgesia, infusions of pethidine of the order of 0.4–0.5 mg/min may be needed after major intra-abdominal surgery. A recent paper from Ray and Drummond described a successful infusion regimen for morphine based on infusing morphine 1 mg/kg body weight over the initial 24-h recover period.[61] However, both drugs have important, pharmacologically active metabolites (morphine 6-glucuronide and nor-pethidine), which may accumulate within the body in patients with impaired renal function[62-64]

NEUROMUSCULAR BLOCKING DRUGS BY INFUSION

Infusions of suxamethonium (60–90 μg/kg./min^1) provide an easy way of achieving a constant degree of muscle paralysis. However, the characteristics of the neuromuscular blockade often change from an initial depolarizing block (phase I) to a second type of blockade showing the monitoring characteristics (fade of the train-of-four or tetanic stimulus) of the non-depolarizing relaxants (phase II). The onset of phase II is usually heralded by tachyphylaxis and is accelerated by the concurrent use of inhalational agents. In many patients, the spontaneous recovery from phase II blockade is slow, although it can be reversed by the normal anticholinesterase agents. It is then followed by a decrease in suxamethonium requirement. However, use of these agents must first depend on the clear establishment of phase II blockade, and it has been usual clinical practice to observe a waiting period of at least 10–20 min to allow plasma suxamethonium levels to decline.

The problems of these different types of phase block are not seen with either vecuronium or atracurium. Because of the short half-lives of these relaxants, maintenace of a twitch height of 5–10% awake value will require regular bolus dosing every 20–30 minutes. Thus, provision of a constant rate infusion will allow a constant level of paralysis — provided drug accumulation does not occur with time. The ideal neuromuscular blocking drug for continuous infusion will, therefore, have several specific properties, such as duration of action not limited by metabolism or excretion, and a rapid attainment of true equilibrium distribution — so providing a rapid 'on' phase.

Established older neuromuscular blocking drugs (e.g. tubocurarine, pancuronium) are thought to act by a separate 'effect compartment' or 'biophase', which is kinetically separate from the central compartment and has the property that drug cannot be eliminated from it directly by chemical or enzymic degradation. This may result in drug cumulation during long-term administration. Thus the development of newer drugs that are either not dependent on a single route of elimination (vecuronium) or that can be continuously degraded in vivo in all body compartments (atracurium) offer considerable advantages.

The kinetics of atracurium in healthy patients show an elimination half-life of about 20 min (range 17–21), clearance of 5.5 ml/kg.min^{-1} (range 5.1–6.1), and volume of distribution of 0.16 l/kg (range 0.15–0.18); the kinetics of vecuronium show an half-life of 62 min (range 24–92), clearance of 4.6 ml/kg.min^{-1} (range 3.6–6.7) and volume of distribution of 0.26 l/kg (0.21–0.31). Most of the other relaxants have elimination half-lives in excess of 2–3 h.

There has been some discussion as to whether spontaneous reversal of neuromuscular blockade is prolonged after infusions of vecuronium and atracurium. Noeldge and colleagues reported a two-fold increase in the time to recovery from 25–75% twitch height after infusions of vecuronium;[65] whereas this has not been subsequently substantiated.[66] Furthermore, d'Hollander and colleagues showed no prolongation of recovery in healthy patients receiving atracurium by infusion during balanced anaesthesia.[67] Similar results have been demonstrated by Wait and colleagues in Oxford (unpublished data)[69] using a servo-controlled infusion regimen to maintain twitch height to 5% awake value. The averaged rates of infusion needed to maintain 90–95% blockade when administered during nitrous oxide-fentanyl anaesthesia are 5–8 μg/kg.min^{-1} atracurium and 0.9–1.7 μkg.min^{-1} vecuronium, and the corresponding plasma drug concentrations (EC$_{95}$) are 10.0 and 0.2 μg/ml respectively.

The rates of infusion, or intermittent dosing rate of atracurium is not significantly altered by either renal failure or liver failure. However, the metabolites of atracurium (laudanosine and the quaternary mono-acetylated alcohol) are stable to Hofmann hydrolysis and may therefore accumulate in the compromised patient. Laudanosine causes convulsions in the dog at plasma concentrations in excess of 17 μg/ml. However, others have demonstrated that maximum laudonosine concentrations after infusion of atracurium to patients with renal and/or hepatic failure are of the order of 2–5 μg/ml, with an absence of clinical signs of convulsive activity or e.e.g. changes[68–70]

While the kinetics and dynamics of atracurium are largely unaltered in renal failure,[69,71] there are data to suggest a prolongation of both properties of vecuronium in this group of patients.[72–75] However, this is not supported by other studies.[73,78,79] The kinetics and dynamics of vecuronium (0.1 mg/kg) have been shown to be unaffected by hepatocellular disease.[80,81] However, at higher doses ($>$0.15 mg/kg),[79,80] a prolonged dynamic effect and reduced drug clearance have been demonstrated. This may be accentuated in patients receiving the drug by continuous infusion.

Newer drugs for neuromuscular blockade include the short-acting agent mivacurium (BW B1090U), and the longer duration agent doxacurium (BW A938U). Mivacurium has an elimination half-life of about 17 minutes, a clearance of 55 ml/kg.min^{-1} and a duration of action to spontaneous recovery to 95% twitch height following an intubating dose, 0.25 mg/kg (3 $\times$ ED$_{95}$), of 30 minutes. It is rapidly broken down by plasma cholinesterase. These properties suggest the drug may have a significant future in administration by continuous infusion. In an open, non-randomized comparison of infusions of mivacurium and atracurium, recovery (25%–75% twitch height) was slower after atracurium; the recovery after mivacurium being about 6 minutes. The mean infusion rate to maintain 90% blockade during non-volatile anaesthesia was 7.5–8.0 μg/kg.min^{-1} (range 3.0–14.1); as with other non-depolarizing agents, potent inhalational agents augment neuromuscular blockade. Thus during isoflurane anaesthesia, rates of the order of 5 μg/kg.min^{-1} (range 1.6–8.7) were needed.[81]

CONCLUSIONS

Administration of intravenous drugs by continuous infusion represents an attempt by the anaesthetist to control the wide oscillations in dynamic drug effects seen following intermittent dosing. This advance in clinical care has arisen hand-in-hand with improvements in the technology of drug delivery (syringe and volumetric pumps, pressurized infusors), a clearer understanding of the relationships between drug kinetics and drug effect, and the ability to monitor these effects and control their magnitude by appropriate feedback mechanisms. Further progress will depend on the pharmaceutical development of drugs with those ideal profiles already outlined. Whether the anaesthetist in the twenty first century will see the replacement of anaesthetic gas Rotameters® and vaporizers by a bank of syringe pumps (each with or without a computer to modulate input according to dynamic effects) must remain to be answered by further laboratory and clinical study.

ACKNOWLEDGEMENTS

The author thanks Dr H. Schwilden and Georg Thieme Verlag, also Dr D.R. Stanski: and J.P. Lippincott for permission to reproduce figures.

REFERENCES

1. Wagner J G 1974 A safe method for rapidly achieving plasma concentration plateaus. Clinical Pharmacology and Therapeutics 16: 691–700
2. Kruger-Thiemer E 1968 Continuous intravenous infusion and multicompartment accumulation. European Journal of Pharmacology 4: 217–324
3. Riddell J G, McAllister C B, Wilkinson G R, Wood A J J, Roden D M 1984 A new method for constant plasma drug concentrations: application to lidocaine. Annals of Internal Medicine 100: 25–28
4. McMurray T J, Robinson F P, Dundee J W, Riddell J G, McClean E. 1986. A new method for producing constant plasma drug levels: application to methohexitone. British Journal of Anaesthesia 57: 1085–1090
5. Murphy M R, Hug C C Jr, McClain D 1983 Dose-independent pharmacokinetics of fentanyl. Anesthesiology 59: 537–540
6. Becker K E 1978 Plasma levels of thiopental necessary for anesthesia. Anesthesiology 49: 192–196
7. Crankshaw D P, Edwards N E, Blackman G L, Boyd M D, Chan H N J, Morgan D J 1985 Evaluation of infusion regimens for thiopentone as a primary anaesthetic agent. European Journal of Clinical Pharmacology 28: 543–552
8. Ausums M E, Hug C C Jr, Stanski D R, Burm A G L 1986 Plasma concentrations of alfentanil required to supplement nitrous oxide anesthesia for general surgery. Anesthesiology 65: 362–373
9. Andrews C J H, Sinclair M, Prys-Roberts C, Dye A 1983 Ventilatory effects during and after continuous infusion of fentanyl or alfentanil. British Journal of Anaesthesia 55 (suppl. 2): 211s–216s
10. O'Connor M, Escarpa E, Prys-Roberts C 1983 Ventilatory depression during and after infusion of alfentanil in man. British Journal of Anaesthesia 55 (suppl. 2): 217s–222s
11. Sear J W, Prys-Roberts C 1979 Dose-related haemodynamic effects of continuous infusions of Althesin in man. British Journal of Anaesthesia 51: 867–873
12. Sear J W, Phillips K C, Andrews C J H, Prys-Roberts C 1983 Dose-response relationships for infusions of Althesin or methohexitone. Anaesthesia 38: 931–936
13. Sear J W, Prys-Roberts C, Phillips K C 1984 Age influences the minimum infusion rate (ED_{50}) for continuous infusions of Althesin and methohexitone. European Journal of Anaesthesiology 1: 319–325
14. Chilcoat R T, Lunn J N, Mapleson W W 1984 Computer assistance in the control of depth of anaesthesia. British Journal of Anaesthesia 56: 1417–1432
15. Schwilden H, Schuttler J, Stoeckel H 1987 Closed-loop feed-back control of methohexital anesthesia by quantitative e.e.g. analysis in humans. Anesthesiology 67: 341–347
16. Evans J M, Davies W L, Wise C C 1984 Lower oesophageal contractility: a new monitor of anaesthesia. Lancet *i*: 1151–1154
17. Hakansson C H, Malcus B 1969 A reflex-controlled automatic anaesthesia device for animal use. Physics in Medicine and Biology 14: 559–562
18. Schils G F, Sasse F J, Rideout V C 1983 Automated control of halothane administration — computer model and animal studies. Anesthesiology 59: A 169
19. Jordan W S, Jaklitsch R R, Heining M P D 1986 Computer applications in intravenous anaesthetic administration. International Journal of Clinical Monitoring and Computing 3: 269–278
20. Millard P K, Hutton P, Pereira E, Prys-Roberts C 1987 On using a self-tuning controller for blood pressure regulation during surgery in man. Computers in Biology and Medicine 17: 1–18
21. Low J M, Millard R K, Curnow J S H, Prys-Roberts C 1983 Closed loop maintenance of deliberate hypotension using sodium nitroprusside infusion during middle ear surgery. British Journal of Anaesthesia 55: 1157p
22. Westenskow D R, Meline L J, Pace N L, Bodily M N 1984 Sodium nitroprusside induced hypotension with computer adjustment for varying drug sensitivity. Anesthesia and Analgesia 63: 281
23. Woodcock T E, Millard R K, Dixon J, Prys-Roberts C 1988 Clonidine premedication for isoflurane-induced hypotension: sympathoadrenal responses and a computer-controlled assessment of the vapour requirement. British Journal of Anaesthesia 60: 388–394
24. Jaklitsch R R, Westenskow D R, Pace N L 1985 Neuromuscular block monitor based on the integrated electromyogram. Journal of Clinical Monitoring 1: 79
25. Wait C M, Goat V A, Blogg C E 1987 Feedback control of neuromuscular blockade: a simple system for infusion of atracurium. anesthesia 42: 1212–1217
26. Webster N R, Cohen A T 1987 Closed-loop administration of atracurium. Steady-state neuromuscular blockade during surgery using a computer controlled closed loop atracurium infusion. Anaesthesia 42: 1212–1217

27. Asbury A J, Brown B H, Linkens D A 1980 Control of neuromuscular blockade by external feedback mechanisms. British Journal of Anaesthesia 52: 633p

28. Mojaverian P, Fedder I L, Vlasses P H, Rotmensch H H, Rocci M L, Swanson B N, Ferguson P K 1982 Cimetidine does not alter morphine disposition in man. British Journal of Clinical Pharmocology 14: 809–813

29. Sear J W, Prys Roberts C 1979 Plasma alphaxalone concentrations during continuous infusion of Althesin. British Journal of Anaesthesia 51: 861–865

30. Ball M, McQuay H J, Moore R A, Allen M C, Fisher A, Sear J W 1985 Renal failure and the use of morphine in intensive care. Lancet i: 784–786

31. Szeto H H, Inturrisi C E, Houde R, Saal S, Cheigh J, Reidenberg M M 1977 Accumulation of normeperidine, an active metabolite of meperidine in patients with renal failure or cancer. Annals of Internal Medicine 86: 738–741

32. Stanski D R, Mihm F G, Rosenthal M H, Kalman S M 1980 Pharmocokinetics of high-dose thiopental used in cerebral resuscitation. Anesthesiology 53: 169–171

33. White P F 1986 Continuous infusions of thiopental, methohexital or etomidate as adjuvants to nitrous oxide for outpatient anesthesia. Anesthesia and Analgesia 63: 282

34. Moore R A, Allen M C, Wood P J, Rees L H, Sear J W 1985 Perioperative endocrine effects of etomidate. Anesthesia 40: 124–130

35. Prys-Roberts C. 1982. Cardiovascular effects of continuous intravenous anaesthesia compared with inhalational anaesthesia. Acta Anaesthesiologica Scandinavica 26 (suppl. 75): 10–17

36. Cullen P M, Turtle M, Prys-Roberts C, Way W L, Dye J 1987 Effect of propofol anesthesia on baroreflex activity in humans. Anesthesia and Analgesia. 66: 1115–1120

37. Carter J A, Clarke T N S, Prys-Roberts C, Spelina K R 1986 Restoration of baroreflex control of heart rate during recovery from anesthesia. British Journal of Anaesthesia 58: 415–421

38. Doze V A, Westphal L M, White P F 1986 Comparison of propofol with methohexital for out-patient anesthesia. Anesthesia and Analgesia 65: 1189–1195

39. Thomson I A, Fitch W, Hughes R L, Campbell D, Watson R. 1986. Effect of certain iv. anaesthetics on liver blood flow and hepatic oxygen consumption in the greyhound. British Journal of Anaesthesia 58: 69–80

40. Chelly J E, Hysing E S, Abernethy D R, Doursout M-F, Merin R G 1986 Effect of inhalational anesthetics on verapamil pharmacokinetics in dogs. Anesthesiology 65: 266–271

41. Thomson I A, Fitch W, Campbell D, Watson R 1988 Effects of Ketamine on liver blood flow and hepatic oxygen consumption. Studies in the anaesthetised greyhound. Acta Anaesthesiologica Scandinavica 32: 10–14

42. Nilsson A, Persson M P, Hartvig P, Wide L 1988 Effect of total intravenous anaesthesia with midazolam/alfentanil on the adrenocortical and hyperglycaemic response to abdominal surgery. Acta Anaesthesiologica Scandinavica 32: 379–382

43. Kay N H, Uppington J, Sear J W, Allen M C 1985 An emulsion formulation of ICI 35868 (propofol) for induction and maintenance of anaesthesia. British Journal of Anaesthesia 57: 736–742

44. Newman L H, McDonald J C, Wallace P G M, Ledingham I McA 1987 Propofol infusion for sedation in intensive care. Anaesthesia 42: 929–937

45. Crozier T A, Beck D, Schlaeger M, Wuttke W, Kettler D 1987 Endocrinological changes following etomidate, midazolam or methohexital for minor surgery. Anesthesiology 66: 628–635

46. Dawson D, Sear J W 1986 Influence of induction of anaesthesia with midazolam on the neuroendocrine response to surgery. Anaesthesia 41: 268–271

47. Glisson S N, Haddad W, Kubak M A, Hieber M F 1983 Midazolam action on catecholamine, cortisol and renin responses to surgical stress in dogs. Anesthesiology 59: A239

48. Bjertnaes L J 1982 Intravenous versus inhalation anesthesia — pulmonary effects. Acta Anaesthesiologica Scandinavica 26 (suppl 75): 18–24

49. Ramsay M A E, Savege T M, Simpson B R J, Goodwin R 1974 Controlled sedation with alphaxalone-alphadolone. British Medical Journal ii: 656–659

50. Shapiro J M, Westphal L M, White P F, Sladen R N, Rosenthal M H 1986 Midazolam infusion for sedation in the intensive care unit: effect on adrenal function. Anesthesiology 64: 394–398

51. Lowenstein E, Hallowell P, Levine F H, Daggett W M, Austen W G, Laver M B. Cardiovascular response to large doses of intravenous morphine in man. New England Journal of Medicine 281: 1389–1393

52. McQuay H J, Moore R A, Paterson G M C, Adams A P 1979 Plasma fentanyl concentrations and clinical observations during and after operation. British Journal of Anaesthesia 51: 543–549

53. Hengstmann J H, Stoeckel H, Schuttler J 1980 Infusion model for fentanyl based on pharmacokinetic analysis. British Journal of Anaesthesia 52: 1021–1025

54. White P F 1983 Use of continuous infusion versus intermittent bolus administration of fentanyl or ketamine during outpatient anesthesia. Anesthesiology 59: 294–300

55. Raeder J C, Hole A 1986 Alfentanil anaesthesia in gall-bladder surgery. Acta Anesthesiologica Scandinavica 30: 35–40
56. van Beem H B H, Meulman H, van Peer A 1987 Clinical experience with a fixed rate of alfentanil infusion. European Journal of Anaesthesiology (suppl. 1): 31–34
57. Zuurmond W W A, van Leeuwen L 1986 Alfentanil v. isoflurane for outpatient arthroscopy. Acta Anaesthesiologica Scandinavica 30: 329–331
58. Coe V, Shafer A, White P F 1983 Techniques for administering alfentanil during outpatient anesthesia — a comparison with fentanyl. Anesthesiology 59: A 347
59. Phitayakorn P, Melnick B M, Vicinie A F 1987 Comparison of continuous sufentanil and fentanyl infusions for outpatient anaesthesia. Canadian Journal of Anaesthesia 34: 242–245
60. Sinclair M, Sear J W, Summerfield R J, Fisher A 1988 Alfentanil infusions in the intensive therapy unit. Intensive Care Medicine 14: 55–59
61. Ray D C, Drummond G B 1988 Continuous intravenous morphine for pain relief after abdominal surgery. Annals of the Royal College of Surgeons of England 70: 317–321
62. Osborne R J, Joel S P, Slevin M L 1986 Morphine intoxication in renal failure: the role of morphine-6-glucuronide. British Medical Journal 292: 1548–1549
63. Sear J W, Hand C W, Moore R A, McQuay H J 1989 Studies on morphine disposition: influence of renal failure on the kinetics of morphine and its metabolites. British Journal of Anaesthesia 62: 28–32
64. Armstrong P J, Bersten A 1986 Normeperidine toxicity. Anesthesia and Analgesia 65: 536–538
65. Noeldge G, Hinksen H, Buzello W 1984 Comparison between the continuous infusion of vecuronium and the intermittent administration of pancuronium and vecuronium. British Journal of Anaesthesia 56: 473–478
66. Gramstad L, Lilleaasen P 1985 Neuromuscular blocking effects of atracurium, vecuronium and pancuronium during bolus and infusion administration. British Journal of Anaesthesia 57: 1052–1059
67. d'Hollander A A, Luyckx C, Barvais L, de Ville A 1983 Clinical evaluation of atracurium besylate requirement for a stable muscle relaxation during surgery: lack of age-related effects Anesthesiology 59: 237–240
68. Yate P M, Flynn P J, Arnold R W, Weatherley B C, Simmonds R J, Dopson T 1987 Clinical experience and plasma laudanosine concentrations during infusion of atracurium in the intensive therapy unit. British Journal of Anaesthesia 59: 211–217
69. Ward S, Boheimer N, Weatherley B C, Simmonds R J, Dopson T A 1987 Pharmacokinetics of atracurium and its metabolites in patients with normal renal function and in patients with renal failure. British Journal of Anaesthesia 59: 697–706
70. Parker C J R, Jones J E, Hunter J M 1988 Disposition of infusions of atracurium and its metabolite, laudanosine, in patients in renal and respiratory failure in an ITU. British Journal of Anaesthesia 61: 531–540
71. Hunter J M, Jones R S, Utting J E 1984 Comparison of vecuronium, atracurium and tubocurarine in normal patients and in patients with no renal function. British Journal of Anaesthesia 56: 941–952
72. Bevan D R, Donati F, Gyasi H, Williams A 1984 Cumulation of vecuronium in renal failure. Anesthesiology 61: A296
73. Gramstad L 1987 Atracurium, vecuronium and pancuronium in end-stage renal failure. Dose-response properties and interactions with azathiopine. British Journal of Anaesthesia 59: 995–1003
74. LePage J Y, Molinge M, Cozian A, Pinaud M, Blanloeil Y, Souron R 1987 Vecuronium and atracurium in patients with end-stage renal failure: A comparative study. British Journal of Anaesthesia 59: 1004–1010
75. Lynam D P, Cronnelly R, Castagnoli K P, Canfell P C, Caldwell J, Arden J, Miller R D 1988 The pharmacodynamics and pharmacokinetics of vecuronium in patients anesthetized with isoflurane with normal renal function or with renal failure. Anesthesiology 69: 227–231
76. Vanacker B F, Van de Walle J 1986 The neuromuscular blocking action of vecuronium in normal patients and in patients with no renal function and interaction vecuronium-tobramyacin in renal transplant patients. Acta Anaesthesiologica Belgica 37: 95–100
77. Fahey M R, Morris R B, Miller R D, Nguyen T L, Upton R A 1981 Pharmacokinetics of ORG NC45 (Norcuron) in patients with and without renal failure. British Journal of Anaesthesia 53: 1049–1053
78. Arden J R, Cannon J C, Lynam D P, Castagnoli K P, Canfell P C, Miller R D 1987 Vecuronium pharmacokinetics and pharmacodynamics in hepatocellular disease. Anesthesia and Analgeisa 66 (2S): S3
79. Hunter J M, Parker C J R, Bell C F, Jones R S, Utting J E 1985 The use of different doses of vecuronium in patients with liver dysfunction. British Journal of Anaesthesia 57: 758–764
80. Lebrault C, Berger J L, D'Hollander A A, Gomeni R, Henzel D, Duvalidestin P 1985

Pharmacokinetics and pharmacodynamics of vecuronium in patients with cirrhosis. Anesthesiology 62: 601–605

81. Powers D, Weber S, Brandom B W, Byers R, Simpson K, Sarner J, Woelfel S K, Cook D R, McNulty B S, Foster V J 1987 BW B1090U infusion requirements in adults during isoflurane or narcotic anesthesia. Anesthesiology 67: A 359

FURTHER READING

Greenblatt DJ, and Koch-Weser J 1975 Clinical pharmacokinetics. New England Journal of Medicine 293: 702–705 and 964–970

Hug CC Jnr. 1978 Pharmacokinetics of drugs administered intravenously. Anesthesia and Analgesia: Current Researches (Cleveland) 57: 704–723

Hull C J 1979 Pharmacokinetics and pharmacodynamics. British Journal of Anaesthesia 51: 579–594

Morgan M 1983 Total intravenous anaesthesia. Anaesthesia 38 (suppl.): 1–9

Sear JW 1983 General kinetic and dynamic principles, and their application to continuous infusion anaesthesia. Anaesthesia 38 (suppl.): 10–25

Sear J W 1984 Pharmacokinetic and pharmacodynamic aspects of continuous infusion anaesthesia — concept of minimum infusion rate as an index of equipotency for intravenous agents. Clinics in Anaesthesiology 2: 223–242

Stanski DR 1987 The role of pharmacokinetics in anaesthesia: application to intravenous infusions. Anaesthesia and Intensive Care 15: 7–14

4. New views on local analgesia

A. Loach

In the past decade, three factors have brought about a re-appraisal of regional techniques. Firstly, the suggestion by Scott[1] of using a local block in combination with light general anaesthesia ('controllable sedation'), to overcome both the patient's reluctance to stay awake during surgery and the surgeon's distrust of an incomplete block, has had considerable impact. Secondly, the realization has grown that excellent postoperative pain relief can be provided easily and quickly with a suitable local block. Finally, surgical developments have created new indications for regional analgesia.

CONTROLLABLE SEDATION

The addition of a sequence of light general anaesthesia to regional analgesia frees the anaesthetist from the imperative of providing a perfect block every time. In practice, this means that blocks can be used much more often, to minimize the requirement for general anaesthesia and to provide postoperative pain relief. Thus experience can be acquired (and with it, confidence) as imperfect blocks are mapped and reasons sought for failures. Then, when there is a strong indication for local analgesia, the required block can be performed accurately and confidently.

The regional block may form a small contribution to the anaesthetic as a whole, as in the addition of an intercostal block during cholecystectomy, or it may form the major part, for instance with a brachial plexus block accompanied by sedation for surgery of the arm. The beauty of the arrangement is its flexibility. Many agents may be used for sedation during regional analgesia but recently interest has centred on the use of midazolam or propofol given as increments or as an infusion.

Fanard et al[2] compared the two drugs when sedating patients who were undergoing orthopaedic procedures under extradural block. He found that there was a greater variation of dose required with midazolam but with better sedation, while those patients who received propofol recovered more quickly.

When such sedatives are used it is preferable to establish the local block first when the patient's co-operation may be needed and then the degree of sedation caused by systemic absorption of local analgesic can be assessed before adding any further drug. This is especially true in the elderly, who are easily sedated by local analgesics and often do not wish for more drowsiness. When benzodiazepines are used, they should be given in small aliquots until a suitable level of sedation is induced: too large a dose produces a state of restlessness and confusion, which may render surgery impossible and control can only be regained by proceeding to general anaesthesia. An infusion of propofol may be used to produce any degree of sedation from drowsiness to general anaesthesia with a very rapid recovery time. While infusion rates of 6–12 mg/kg.h^{-1} are necessary for general anaesthesia, Fanard et al[2] found that an infusion of only 1.74

mg/kg.h^{-1} provided adequate sedation. This interesting drug might form the perfect complement to regional analgesia.

POSTOPERATIVE PAIN RELIEF

Not until relatively recently have doctors concerned themselves with postoperative pain, which has been viewed as an inevitable result of surgery but one which quickly improves with time. It is nevertheless real to patients, and the knowledge that the pain will go away is not an analgesic. Many contemporary techniques of light general anaesthesia with short recovery times may serve only to postpone the pain of surgery unless a deliberate effort is made to provide lasting postoperative analgesia.

Edmonds-Seal et al[3] demonstrated that 40% of patients undergoing surgery of the limbs could enjoy a pain-free interval of 8 hours or more when simple nerve blocks were used. In a study of 929 patients, McQuay, Carroll and Moore[4] compared postoperative analgesic requirements between groups of patients to determine the effect of opiate premedication and local nerve blocks. When neither opiate premedication nor local block were used, the median time to the first request for postoperative analgesia was less than 2 hours; opiate premedication increased the time to more than 5 hours; local analgesic block produced a further significant increase to 8 hours and opiate premedication used with a local analgesic block extended the time to more than 9 hours. This paper is supported by an editorial by Wall[5] which suggests that the blocking of painful afferents may confer more benefit than the control of pain alone: that the avoidance of widespread central nervous system activation that results from painful stimuli improves the patient's recovery.

For peripheral surgery, in particular, the time-honoured prescription of an intramuscular opiate, is an opportunity missed. A suitable regional block can provide focal analgesia without the nausea, vomiting and respiratory depression that accompany parenteral opioids.

NEW SURGICAL TECHNIQUES

The most important new surgical techniques demanding regional analgesia are those based on microsurgical repair of limb injuries. The magnification afforded by the operating microscope and the use of finer suture materials make possible the repair of vessels and nerves down to the size of those found in the digit of a child. In turn, this makes possible reconstructive repair of severe injuries of the limbs and for the upper limb in particular, the replantation of severed parts — even, on occasion, the limb itself. Success rates for replantation in excess of 80% are being claimed in American centres carrying out this work and the microsurgical techniques necessary are now a required skill for orthopaedic surgeons training in the UK.

Regional analgesia is required for microvascular surgery because the accompanying sympathetic blockade maintains a blood supply to precarious replanted parts and flaps. The block is continued postoperatively, often for days, to provide adequate pain relief (which will avoid pain-induced vasoconstriction) and further sympathetic blockade. This has led to the development of catheter techniques to maintain long-lasting blocks.

Further techniques with strong indications for regional analgesia include the creation of a fistula for dialysis in patients with end-stage renal failure and muscle biopsy for investigation of a cryptic myopathy. Some 2000 patients a year are entering a dialysis programme and each will require an arteriovenous fistula in the forearm. Pain relief for these patients, who may be relatively unfit for general anaesthesia, is best provided by a regional block. The accompanying vasodilatation renders the surgery technically easier.

A muscle biopsy, generally taken from quadriceps femoris, is required to establish a diagnosis of myopathy or dystrophy and, occasionally, to investigate the susceptibility of a patient to malignant hyperthermia (MH). General anaesthesia in these patients carries obvious risk from cardiomyopathy, poor respiratory function or, in the case of MH, of inducing the disease. Yet surgeons are reluctant to use local infiltration for the procedure because it is often ineffective or the specimen is spoiled by the introduction of artefacts. Bupivacaine injected into muscle is directly toxic and causes rapid cellular degeneration[6] thus reducing the value of any specimen taken. An elegant solution to this problem is suggested by Gielen and Viering[7] who used the inguinal paravascular technique of Winnie et al[8] to provide regional analgesia distant from the site of biopsy. They further found that the amide local analgesics, prilocaine and bupivacaine, used in this way did not provoke hyperthermic crises in 22 patients subsequently considered to be susceptible to malignant hyperthermia.

ANTITHROMBOTIC EFFECTS OF LOCAL ANALGESICS

While much work has emphasized the reduction in incidence of venous thrombosis and pulmonary embolism associated with spinal and extradural analgesia, interest has been growing in the systemic antithrombotic effects of regional analgesic drugs. Cooke et al[9] first reported the use of intravenous lignocaine in prevention of deep vein thrombosis after hip surgery: a protective effect that was a specific quality of the agent rather than the route of injection as in spinal or extradural application. Using an intravenous infusion of lignocaine for 6 days after hip surgery, Cooke et al found that the incidence of deep vein thrombosis (DVT) in the trial group was 14% compared with an incidence of 78% in the control group, and that the difference between the groups began to diminish after the infusion was discontinued. Luostarinen et al[10] found that lignocaine in particular had an anti-thrombotic effect. In their study, a laser was used to cause microvascular injury in the everted cheek pouch of hamsters, which was moistened either with saline, tocainide or lignocaine. In the animals pre-treated with saline the laser injury resulted in irreversible thrombus formation and permanent standstill of the microcirculation. When pretreated with lignocaine, inhibition of thrombus formation occurred in all cases. They ascribed these anti-thrombotic effects to reduced adhesion between blood cells and also between blood cells and the vessel walls.

Borg & Modig[11] studied the effects of lignocaine, bupivacaine and tocainide on platelet aggregation in vitro. Platelet aggregation was induced in a fresh sample of plasma by the addition of ADP or collagen and the aggregation quantified by the change in light transmission of the sample. In the presence of lignocaine, platelet aggregation did not occur and similar, but smaller, effects were noted with tocainide and bupivacaine. The effect was both dose-related and also time-related. Borg and Modig were at paints to refute extrapolation of these observations to a clinical situation since the plasma concentrations used were greater than those likely to be met clinically. However, they may be too modest: the clear clinical benefit found by Cooke et al[9] may be explained by smaller concentrations of drug acting for much longer than the time limit of the laboratory investigation. The infusion rate of lignocaine used by Cooke (2 mg/min) gave maximum blood levels of 4.0 μg/ml, which are comparable to the levels that might be reached with, for example, a brachial plexus block (vide infra).

The remainder of this chapter is concerned with the development of specific nerve blocks. Actual techniques are difficult to describe and are best learned at a 'hands-on' course such as those organized by the European Society of Regional Anaesthesia (see Appendix, p. 79).

LOCAL ANALGESIA OF THE UPPER LIMB

In the upper limb, regional analgesia may be used for elective procedures on the hand, forearm and elbow and also for accident and emergency work and for day surgery. Because the nerves of supply to the arm are geographically grouped closely together in the brachial plexus, a single injection can provide anaglesia of the whole limb, consequently distal blocks in the arm are less useful. By contrast, the innervation of the leg is derived from three major trunks and proximal blocks are of limited use, while distal blocks have more to offer. In the arm, blocks at the elbow and wrist can be used to make good missing elements from a brachial plexus block. Of the three common approaches to the brachial plexus, axillary, supraclavicular and interscalene, the axillary approach commonly misses the musculocutaneous nerve or the radial nerve while the interscalene approach tends to miss the ulnar nerve.

Pharmacokinetics of brachial plexus block

When local analgesic is injected around a nerve trunk, it will soak into the trunk on an advancing front (Fig. 4.1). Transmission in fibres in the periphery of the trunk will first be blocked and those in the centre of the trunk last. Further, transmission in peripherally placed fibres will be blocked over a longer length of fibre than will be the case for central fibres. Thus analgesia will appear first and last longest in the territory that is supplied by peripheral fibres. If the pool of local analgesic is too small, perhaps because the injection was not accurate enough or too dilute, the fibres in the centre of the trunk will escape blockade.

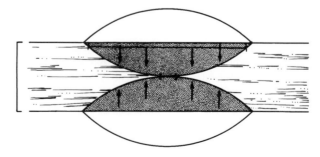

Fig. 4.1   Pharmacokinetics of nerve block. A pool of local analgesic surrounding a nerve trunk will penetrate the trunk on an advancing front. Block of peripheral fibres will occur first followed by more central fibres later. The length of nerve fibre blocked will be greater for peripheral fibres than for central fibres.

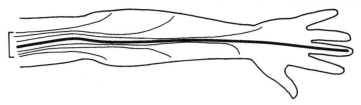

Fig. 4.2 Arrangement of fibres in a nerve trunk. The central fibres are those supplying the most distal part of the limb.

The trunks are arranged so that the central fibres are those with the longest run supplying the extremities of the limb (Fig. 4.2) while shorter fibres are arranged more peripherally as their area of supply is more proximal. After the initial arrangement of nerve fibres into nerve trunks in the brachial plexus there is little crossing of fibres. (For this reason repair of nerve trunks achieves good matching of fascicles and a good functional result whilst repair of the proximal brachial plexus is prejudiced by the difficulty in matching fascicles.) This arrangement also explains why loss of motor power in the upper arm occurs before loss of sensation in the hand, even though motor fibres are larger and more resistant to block. Winnie et al[12] took this argument further. If we consider a trunk of the brachial plexus in cross-section and focus on a peripheral bundle of fibres, which Winnie called a 'mantle bundle', this bundle contains outer motor fibres and inner sensory fibres corresponding to all the early branches of the brachial plexus being motor branches. Similarly, a central bundle ('core bundle') has the same arrangement; with the peripheral fibres being motor and supplying the muscles of the forearm, and the most central fibres carrying sensation from the hand. The onset of block in the arm is as follows: loss of motor power to the shoulder and upper arm; loss of sensation in the upper arm; loss of motor power of the forearm; and loss of sensation to the hand. Commonly, on withdrawing the needle from a supraclavicular block in particular, diminution of power at the shoulder has already begun.

Approaches to the brachial plexus

The axillary approach
Although many approaches to the brachial plexus have been described, only the axillary, the supraclavicular and the interscalene are in common use. The axillary approach is gaining prominence as the best approach for use with accident and emergency or day surgery patients because of its freedom from complications and for long-term blocks it is the approach most suited to catheter techniques. However, the axillary approach is not so consistently successful as the supraclavicular approach and is slower in onset. The success rate of 80–90% reported by Selander[13] is typical. The block is performed with the patient's arm abducted and externally rotated and with the hand positioned behind the head in the sunbathing position. The axillary vessels are then easily palpable. After raising a skin bleb of local analgesic, the needle should be directed medially along the line of the axillary artery until the neurovascular sheath is entered with a 'pop'. Accurate injection is often marked by visible distention of the neurovascular sheath as a linear prominence across the axilla, while the development of a mound subcutaneously is less promising.

In obese patients, the chief landmark of the axillary artery may simply be impalpable. Other common reasons for lack of success are injecting too deeply and the use of an inadequate volume of solution. Bryce-Smith[14] stressed how superficial the neurovascular bundle is in the axilla where it lies subcutaneously. The volume of solution required was studied by Vester-Anderson et al[5] who found that 50 ml was superior to 40 ml of 1% mepivacaine and that 60 ml gave no improvement.

Other manoeuvres will improve the likelihood of success. Peripheral axial streaming of injected solution was radiologically demonstrated by Ang, Lassale and Goldfarb,[16] and this should be prevented using either a tourniquet or by manual compression to ensure that the solution encircles the artery to reach the radial nerve posteriorly. Proximal spread of the solution can be encouraged by reducing the degree of abduction at the shoulder prior to injection. In full abduction, the head of the humerus compresses the sheath posteriorly, again restricting access to the posterior elements of the brachial plexus.[17]

This block depends upon the concept of a tightly fitting fascial sheath, which binds together the brachial plexus, axillary artery and vein, and holds injected local analgesic solution in contact with the nerve trunks long enough for transmission block to occur. Such a sheath is well represented in illustrated textbooks.[18,19] However, there is an apparent inconsistency between the concept of a tightly enclosing fascial sheath and the large volumes already reported that are required to fill it. The answer seems to lie with more recent work by Vester-Andersen et al,[20] who studied the morphology of the sheath by injecting gelatine in cadavers. After allowing the gelatine to set they performed a total dissection of the axilla. The sheath was found not to be tubular as supposed but to possess a tongue inferiorly, which extended down the thoracic wall (Fig. 4.3), presumably to permit a free range of movement at the shoulder. It would then require an increased volume of solution to fill such a space. Furthermore, it was

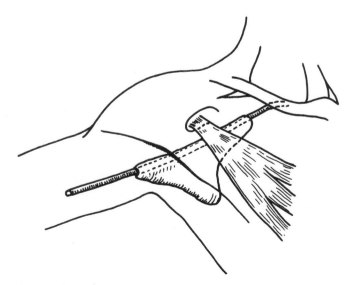

Fig. 4.3   The morphology of the axillary sheath. The sheath is not a tubular structure investing the axillary vessels but has an extension inferiorly down the thoracic wall. From Vester-Andersen et al (1986) with permission.

noted that while the median and ulnar nerves were in direct contact with the injected gelatine at all cross-sections of the sheath, the musculocutaneous, radial and axillary nerves showed no direct contact in several cross-sections, thus explaining the observed difficulty of blocking these nerves by the axillary route.

Thompson and Rorie[21] suggested that patchy axillary blocks may be caused by fibrous septa within the axillary sheath that might loculate injected local analgesic and limit its spread to the plexus. These workers argued that it was necessary to make separate injections for each of the three major branches of the plexus despite common experience that a single injection will give an adequate block in most cases. However, in a further anatomical study, Partridge, Katz and Benirschke[22] found only incomplete feeble fibrous septa and no effective partitioning of the axillary sheath. They also found that the sheath was not, as earlier depicted, a tough fibrous tube but was made up of numerous thin layers closely applied, which could be easily stripped by injection. When dye was injected it spread without difficulty to radial, ulnar and median nerves in every case. When attempting to place needles in the axillary sheath in 5 cases, a 'pop' was felt at a layer superficial to the sheath; that is, the needle was directed towards but not at that point in the sheath. These workers argued that a single injection is all that is required to produce a block and that multiple injections increase the likelihood of neural damage.

Catheter techniques. The duration of a block may be increased by using a higher dose of local analgesic, by adding adrenaline to the solution or by using a catheter and supplementary injections. Long-term brachial plexus blocks are useful for the management of pain after the repair of serious injuries to the hand and arm, regrettably common industrial injuries, and for sympathetic vasoconstrictor blockade. Such blocks have also been used to provide analgesia during continuous passive movement of a painful limb.

The axillary approach is especially suitable for catheter techniques because no great angulation of the catheter is required as it leaves the needle to enter the perivascular space. Selander[23] reported the use of a catheter over a needle that allowed repeated injections for a prolonged block. Plancarte et al[24] used a 17-gauge Tuohy needle to introduce a 22-gauge epidural catheter. The needle was rotated gently as it was advanced to ease its passage and 6 ml of 1.5% lignocaine was injected to distend the sheath before inserting the catheter. Repeated injections were given as necessary for up to 72 hours. Gaumann, Lennon and Wedel[25] used a very similar technique but attempted to thread the catheter as far proximally as possible in order to obtain the benefits of a more proximal block without the complications of a supraclavicular approach. Catheters were inserted a mean distance of 12 cm from the skin and the block was continued for up to 11 days. In 2 patients who had undergone replantation procedures, the catheter was re-inserted after its initial removal had been followed by deterioration in limb blood flow. In both of these papers, the reported success rate (99% and 90% respectively) is higher than is usual with axillary blocks, suggesting that using a catheter may be a good way of performing the block.

Because of the relatively slow metabolism of amide local analgesic agents, studies have been carried out to measure the plasma concentrations resulting from continuous brachial blocks. Tuominen et al and colleagues[26] found that toxic levels were not reached with either supplementary dosage or with continuous infusion at the rate of 25 mg/hour of bupivacaine through an axillary catheter. In a more recent paper[27] similar findings were reported with continuous infusion of bupivacaine through an interscalene catheter. Although 3 patients out of 40 were described as experiencing mild toxic symptoms, 2 experienced common side-effects of interscalene block (hoarseness and Horner's syndrome) and 1 patient suffered from dizziness (which resolved when the infusion was stopped).

The supraclavicular approach

The supraclavicular approach to the brachial plexus is more consistently successful than either the axillary or the interscalene approaches because the brachial plexus is more tightly grouped on the first rib and the landmarks are better. A smaller volume of local analgesic is required; this may be an advantage with elderly patients. The resulting block gives analgesia for a tourniquet on the upper arm and also of the shoulder joint (although not the skin covering). The block may be used to provide analgesia for reduction of a dislocated shoulder when the classically dropped shoulder provides easier access to the brachial plexus. For surgery of the shoulder it is necessary to inject local analgesic subcutaneously proximal to the shoulder to block branches of the supraclavicular nerves. In obese patients, the supraclavicular fossa often remains free from fat pads and the necessary landmarks are still palpable so that a brachial plexus block may be used in preference to a difficult general anaesthetic.

When performing the block, the modification of approach suggested by Winne et al[17] should be used to avoid any backwards (dorsal) angulation of the needle, which might carry it into the bow of the first rib and cause a pneumothorax. The needle should be short — no more than 4 cm — and of fine gauge since the feel of the tissues is less important with this approach and usually paraesthesiae are elicited before the first rib is contacted. It is best to warn patients that they may feel an 'electric shock' in the arm and ask them to report when it occurs but not to move: if a heavy premedication has been given, patients may simply not notice paraesthesiae and this will not be a dependable end-point. Occasionally the sensation is so brief that patients are uncertain where it was felt: any sensations around the shoulder should be disregarded since they are probably caused by stimulation of branches of the brachial plexus after they have left the plexus, principally the suprascapular nerve, and are a poor guide to the plexus itself. When paraesthesiae have been obtained, injection of local analgesic should begin — slowly at first with a few millilitres of solution. The patient should be warned that the paraesthesiae may become worse briefly and then will disappear. This second sensation seems duller and more long-lasting than the initial paraesthesiae and Winnie[19] suggests that it is provoked by an increase in pressure resulting from injection. If pain occurs that might indicate intraneural injection, the needle should be withdrawn a little and injection recommenced. The development of shoulder tip pain or a fit of coughing suggest pleural irritation and again the needle should be withdrawn and the landmarks checked.

The most significant complication of the supraclavicular approach is a pneumothorax, which has a reported incidence of 0.6–6%. However, De Jong,[28] using the classical 'downwards, inwards and backwards' technique, found an incidence on chest X-ray of 25%. The symptoms and signs of a pneumothorax may not be present for many hours postoperatively as the air leaks only slowly from the lung and therefore patients should be observed overnight in hospital afterwards. If a pneumothorax does develop, it may be treated by simple aspiration through a needle in the first instance, and resort made to a chest drain only if the pneumothorax reforms. Clearly, it is unwise to use this approach in a patient with chronic respiratory disease or as part of an anaesthetic technique that involves automatic ventilation and that might lead to a tension pneumothorax.

The interscalene approach
Finally, the brachial plexus may be blocked by a yet more proximal injection still in the interscalene groove at the level of the cricoid ring (C6). This will provide a block adequate for surgery of the upper arm and shoulder as the injected volume of solution spreads to include elements of the cervical plexus. The ulnar nerve (C8, T1) often escapes blockade because the solution fails to track down the necessary three segments. The likelihood of this is reduced if the injection is made with the patient sitting up supported by a nurse, and if the injection site is massaged downwards on completion. Serious complications have also arisen with this approach caused primarily by inadvertent cervical epidural or spinal block. Phrenic nerve block with hemidiaphragmatic paralysis and recurrent laryngeal nerve block producing a cord palsy are common; thus this approach is best avoided in patients who have respiratory disease — particularly a restrictive ventilatory defect or a contralateral cord palsy.

Peripheral blocks in the arm
More peripheral blocks in the arm may be used alone or to add to an incomplete plexus block. After axillary block, it is often necessary to block the musculocutaneous nerve in the intermuscular groove lateral to the tendon of biceps at the elbow. This is performed by injecting 5 ml of local analgesic solution subcutaneously at the level of the epicondyles, and will provide analgesia of the skin over the dorsolateral aspect of the wrist. It is often required for reduction of a Colles' fracture.

Blocks of ulnar, median and radial nerves at the wrist are occasionally used for suture of skin lacerations of the hand in the casualty department, thus avoiding the need for a plexus block. More commonly, however, such surgery will involve formal exploration of the wound under a tourniquet and more proximal analgesia will be required. Median nerve block at the wrist should not be performed in patients who have symptoms of carpal tunnel compression.

Intravenous regional analgesia
Intravenous regional analgesia (IVRA) is an important area of local analgesia if only because of the very large number of such blocks administered each year: the clutch of broken arms produced by the first icy pavements of winter would probably be unmanageable without such a simple technique. It follows that IVRA is often performed by junior staff, many of them non-anaesthetists. The procedure is quick and reliable, requiring only the ability to insert a needle into a vein. Nevertheless, meticulous care of equipment and close attention to detail are necessary if IVRA is to be used safely and the best results achieved. In this respect, anaesthetists must set standards and educate orthopaedic and accident and emergency colleagues as to the correct procedures. For all its simplicity, IVRA is not without risk; Grice et al[29] record that by 1986 the technique had been associated with at least 7 deaths, 2 cardiopulmonary arrests, 10 generalized seizures and many milder toxic symptoms. These mishaps have occurred through the escape of local analgesic into the systemic circulation,

either because of failure or early release of the tourniquet or through leakage of the solution beneath the tourniquet. A Health Notice (Hazard) issued by the Department of Health in 1982 drew attention to tourniquet failure and made plain the requirement to maintain the equipment, paying particular attention to hoses, connections and the accuracy of the pressure gauge. This notice also required the presence of someone (not necessarily an anaesthetist) whose sole duty was to supervise the tourniquet: the casualty officer should not perform both the block and carry out the procedure without adequate assistance.

Leakage past the tourniquet has been reported by many workers and radiocontrast studies show that this leakage commonly occurs through the venous system although further routes of possible leakage are the interosseous circulation, which will bypass the tourniquet[30] and the failure of a tourniquet to occulude clacified arteries.[31] After a near clinical disaster, experimental work was carried out by El Hassan, et al[32] to determine the factors that were associated with leakage of solution beneath the tourniquet. They found that in order to minimize the risk of leakage, the injection site should be distal, that is, in the hand rather than in the antecubital fossa; the injection should be performed slowly over 90 seconds to allow run-off of the solution; the volume of blood in the arm should be reduced as much as possible by exsanguination with an Esmark bandage to create room for the volume of injectate and an adequate pressure should be maintained in the tourniquet. These suggestions were confirmed in a later paper by Grice et al.[29]

It was also found that tourniquet width was important — the narrower the tourniquet, the higher the pressure required to prevent venous leakage beneath it since vessels beneath the tourniquet acted as collapsible 'spillover' resistors. Davis et al[33] found that narrow tourniquets (5–6 cm wide), as included in proprietary double cuffs for Bier's block, required a pressure 58 mm Hg higher than wide (12–14 cm) tourniquets to occlude vessels. Grice et al[29] considered that a pressure of at least 300 mm Hg was necessary for safe use of IVRA. However, when reporting a case of nerve damage produced by a tourniquet, Larsen and Hommelgaard[34] recommended lower pressures and related the necessary pressure to the arterial occlusion pressure. They suggested that the tourniquet pressure should be equal to the arterial occlusion pressure + 100 mm Hg and that the tourniquet time should not be greater than 2 hours. They also recommended that the double cuff tourniquet should not be used for obese patients. The suitability of tourniquet techniques in patients with burns has also been questioned by Pfeifer[35] when reporting the case of a 14-year-old burned boy who developed renal failure after rhabdomyolysis occurred in the ischaemic limb. However, the tourniquet pressure used for this case was 520 mmHg, which may itself have been cause enough.

IVRA is suitable only for procedures of the forearm and hand that can be completed within the tourniquet time limit: for more proximal surgery the bulky tourniquet begins to intrude upon the surgical field. For fine work on the hand many surgeons are unhappy with the degree of exsanguination that is possible with an awake patient and full sensation in the arm. Mottling of the arm after induction of the block is caused by poor exsanguination and better results are obtained if exsanguination is carried up and over the lower tourniquet when a double cuff is being used. In the leg, a thigh tourniquet is required for adequate vascular occlusion but the dose of local analgesic required for that bulk of tissue is hopelessly toxic: if the tourniquet is applied to the lower leg, then vascular occlusion is not obtained because the vessels lie protected between the tibia and fibula. Despite this, heroic efforts continue to be made to adapt IVRA for use in the leg.[36,37] Davis & Walford[38] were able to measure plasma concentrations of bupivacaine leaking out from beneath a leg tourniquet even before surgery had begun, and discovered that the loss of local analgesic tended to produce a patchy block.

Although prilocaine is the most suitable agent for IVRA because of its low systemic toxicity it is clear that other more toxic agents continue to be used. It is alas all too easy to imagine the disaster cascade in action when a harrassed junior doctor performs a Bier's block in casualty for a forearm fracture, where no exsanguination is carried out because the limb is painful, the only vein immediately available is in the antecubital fossa, the injection is made hurriedly because there are many other things to do and no help is available because everyone else is busy.

INTERCOSTAL NERVE BLOCKS

Intercostal nerve blocks are an alternative to thoracic extradural block for the provision of analgesia after rib fractures or upper abdominal surgery and long-lasting analgesia is possible, either with repeated injections or by the insertion of catheters. In a well-controlled prospective study Engberg and Wiklund[39] found that the incidence of postoperative complications was halved after subcostal incisions when intercostal blocks were used for analgesia compared with centrally acting analgesics. Interestingly, no difference in complication rate was found for midline upper abdominal incisions, although the patients had less pain and were more comfortable. Shelley and Park[40] used a modified technique in children and found that the need for opioid analgesia after liver transplantation was markedly reduced; indeed, 56% of children required no additional analgesia to the block. After one patient developed a pneumothorax, their technique was modified so that instead of approaching the rib directly as in the conventional approach, they approached the rib tangentially (Fig. 4.4) so that the needle was much less likely to enter the pleura. This seems to be a worthwhile change in technique for all intercostal blocks and will improve safety.

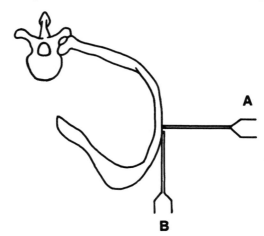

Fig. 4.4 A safer approach for intercostal blockade. The traditional approach ('A') can easily lead to a pneumothorax. A tangential approach ('B') is less likely to do so. Reproduced from Shelley and Park[38] 1987,[40] with permission.

Reservations about intercostal block have arisen from the unpredictable spread of injected local analgesic — particularly if the block is inserted under direct vision at thoracotomy dorsally near the neck of the rib. At this point, the intercostal space is continuous with the paravertebral space and the extradural space so that the possibility exists for injected solution to travel up or down the paravertebral space and to cross the midline through the epidural space. Sury & Bingham[41] reported total spinal block following such an injection, while extensive sympathetic blockade occurred in the case reported by Skretting.[42] The possibility of unexpected spread should therefore be remembered — especially when the block is performed during thoractomy and a minimum volume of local analgesic employed.

REGIONAL ANALGESIA IN THE LEG

Innervation of the leg is by three major trunks (femoral, sciatic and obturator) and many other cutaneous branches entering the thigh. Analgesia for proximal operations on the thigh, therefore, is often best provided by central neural blockade, while peripheral blocks in the leg are more useful for operations of the lower leg and foot.

Femoral nerve block

Extensive analgesia of the anterolateral thigh and knee results from the femoral paravascular block described by Winnie et al.[8] For this block, 20 ml of solution are injected proximally, lateral to the femoral artery (usually a clear landmark) and spread down the leg is prevented by pressure distally. The solution spreads proximally in the plane of the femoral nerve and reaches further branches of the lumbosacral plexus — the obturator nerve and the lateral cutaneous nerve of the thigh. Although the lateral cutaneous nerve of the thigh is easily blocked elsewhere as it enters the thigh medial to the anterior superior iliac spine, the obturator nerve is relatively inaccessible and other approaches have a poor success rate. The inguinal paravascular block is useful for muscle biopsy of the thigh as described earlier, for surgery of the knee to provide postoperative analgesia and also for postoperative analgesia after stripping of varicose veins when virtually the whole territory involved is supplied by the saphenous branch of the femoral nerve. Although the inguinal paravascular block is very effective in providing analgesia after arthroscopy, the block tends to last too long for day surgery, even when lignocaine is used, and patients do not recover quadriceps power quickly enough to go home the same day. For day-case arthroscopies, therefore, the choice of regional analgesia lies between local infiltration of the arthroscope track combined with distension of the knee with bupivacaine and spinal analgesia. Local infiltration will be acceptable only if the surgeon is content to operate without a tourniquet, which some find difficult because relatively minor bleeding quickly obscures the field of view.

Sciatic nerve block

There are many approaches to the sciatic nerve and none is reliable. In the buttock and upper thigh, the nerve is deep-seated and poorly related to landmarks and computerized tomography (CT) studies reveal considerable variation in location. It is necessary to use a long (8–10 cm) needle and best results are obtained by using a nerve stimulator. It is desirable to use insulated needles with the nerve stimulator but inexpensive intravenous cannulae will serve.[43,44] However, the sciatic nerve is easily damaged as it is a large structure and is often transfixed by the needle. It is preferable, therefore, to use a needle with a straight-cut tip and to avoid using needles with a cutting bevel designed to pierce skin. In the series quoted by Edmonds-Seal et al[3] 2 patients had long-lasting neurological sequelae probably caused by trauma to the nerve. Selander et al[45] published photomicrographs showing damage to nerve trunks with disruption of nerve fibres, which resulted from impaling the trunks with a cutting needle.

When using a nerve stimulator, the needle should be advanced towards the nerve until a motor response is obtained with minimum stimulus. Accurate positioning of the needle may be confirmed by injecting 2 ml of 2% lignocaine and looking for the abolition of the motor response as described by Raj[46] before injecting the therapeutic dose. Because of the physical size of the sciatic nerve, high concentrations of local analgesic are required to produce effective blockade and the latency of onset of the block is long (20–40 min.). The depth of the injection and the likelihood that multiple attempts will be required make this a block best performed in the anaesthetized or heavily sedated patient.

Ankle block
Ankle block is a consistently successful and useful peripheral nerve block. It may be used to avoid general anaesthesia in diabetic patients who need debridement of ulcers of the foot or the amputation of toes, or in patients with peripheral vascular disease who are undergoing similar procedures. Ankle block is also useful to to provide postoperative analgesia following surgery to excise bunions or straighten toes — procedures that give rise to much pain. When injecting deeply to block the deep branch of the anterior tibial nerve and the posterior tibial nerve, it is important both to aspirate before injecting, as each nerve accompanies an artery, and also to withdraw the needle before injection if the bone is contacted. If a subperiosteal injection is made, it is relatively ineffective and gives rise to much pain postoperatively.

REGIONAL ANALGESIA IN CHILDREN
There has been growing interest in better provision of analgesia for children, fuelled recently by articles in the medical and lay press about the neonate's response to pain. These articles question existing techniques of anaesthesia that are more concerned with the systemic toxicity of powerful analgesics in small babies than with the need for analgesia. Often the analgesic problem can be bypassed by using regional analgesia.

Arthur and McNicol[47] reviewed the pharmacokinetics of local analgesic drugs in children. Their greater cardiac output leads to a more rapid mobilization of an injected agent and earlier peak blood concentrations. There is also a greater rate of metabolism since the liver is relatively larger in children as a percentage of body weight[48] and also contains more metabolic sites for the breakdown of drugs. These arguments, however, do not apply to infants of less than 1 year, especially neonates in whom plasma protein concentrations are lower thus reducing potential binding sites for local analgesic drugs and increasing the concentration of free agent. Plasma pseudocholinesterase concentrations are also reduced, limiting metabolism of procaine whilst metabolism of other local analgesic is greatly reduced.

As ever, the greatest difficulty in paediatric anaesthetic practice is the calculation of

Table 4.1 Scheme of maximum safe dosage of anaesthetic for children (From Arthur and McNicol (1986),[47] with permission.)

Agent	Proprietary name	Maximum safe dose
Lignocaine	Lidothesin	7 mg/kg
	Xylocaine	
Priolocaine	Citanest	8 mg/kg
Bupivacaine	Marcain	2 mg/kg
Cinchocaine	Nupercaine	0.4 mg/kg
Etidocaine	Duranest	4 mg/kg

dosage required. Arthur & McNiol[47] suggest a scheme of maximum safe dosage for children of more than 1 year (Table 4.1). For children younger than this greatly enhanced toxicity of local analgesics should be expected and dosage per kilogram body weight reduced.

With careful preparation and gentle handling, children will accept regional analgesic techniques. Serlo and Haapanemi[49] reported a high success rate and excellent acceptance of regional techniques in 199 paediatric patients. Of these, 157 receive a brachial plexus block. The children were heavily premedicated and the techniques chosen did not require the co-operation of the patient (techniques are often easier because landmarks are more easily identified and the tissues are more distinctive). The contrast between the difficulty of a caudal block in a child and the same block in an adult is striking.

In association with light general anesthesia, regional blocks serve to diminish the physiological assault of surgery, reduce dosage of general anaesthetic agents and provide a calm pain-free postoperative interval. It is wise to warn children about any postoperative loss of sensation or power and tell them how soon these will return.

Replantation procedures, especially of the hand and digits, are especially successful and worthwhile in children: the loss of thumb or forefinger may be made good by the transplantation of a great toe to create a useable hand later. Good regional analgesia from a plexus block is an important contribution to the success of surgery and the postoperative management.

Various techniques of regional analgesia have been suggested for the common paediatric operations of circumcision, orchidopexy and inguinal hernia repair; penile block, ilioinguinal and iliohypogastric block, caudal block. However, in a well-reasoned letter Fell et al[50] made a plea for simplicity and in a subsequent paper[51] it was found that simple infiltration of wound edges was as effective in providing pain relief as caudal block. Tree-Trakarn et al[52] found that simple topical application of lignocaine after circumcision was effective in reducing pain and tenderness. These workers used a charming self-explanatory linear analogue scale (Fig. 4.5), which could prove useful in other studies of pain in children.

Preparation for any needling procedure in children (or nervous adults) is helped by the use of EMLA (Eutetic Mixture of Local Analgesic) cream. The cream should be applied to the site and covered by an occlusive dressing: better results are obtained if the cream is applied 2 hours or more before the procedure rather than 1 hour before, as is recommended. The surface analgesia then permits deeper injection of local

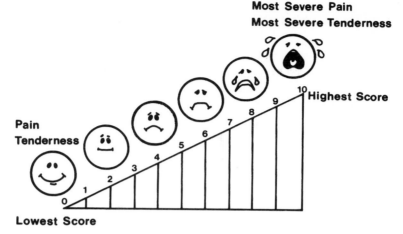

Fig. 4.5   A simple linear analogue pain diagram for use with children. From Tree-Traken et al[51] (1987)[52] with permission.

analgesic prior to the insertion of an intravenous cannula or a regional block needle. EMLA cream squirted into the external auditory meatus and retained for 2 hours also produces adequate analgesia of the tympanic membrane for tympanotomy.[53]

CONCLUSION

The techniques of regional analgesia have no mystique, they represent only applied anatomy. For the anaesthetist, the blocks are interesting to perform and are a very useful part of the repertoire. For the patient there are many advantages: recovery from sedation or light general anaesthesia is swift; postoperative vomiting and nausea are diminished and the analgesia resulting from the block can transform the postoperative period.

APPENDIX

The European Society of Regional Anaesthesia exists to promote the wider use of local and regional anaesthetic techniques. Information about membership and meetings can be obtained from Dr J.H. McClure, Department of Anaesthetics, The Royal Infirmary, Edinburgh EH3 9YW, Scotland.

REFERENCES

1.   Scott D B 1984 The use of local anaesthesia in the A and E department. Royal College of Surgeons' anniversary forum: the anaesthetist in the accident and emergency department
2.   Fanard L, Van Steenberge A, Demeire X, Van der Puyl F 1988 Comparison between propofol and midazolam as sedative agents for surgery under regional anaesthesia. Anaesthesia 43 (suppl.): 87–89
3.   Edmonds-Seal J, Paterson G M C, Loach A B 1980 Local nerve blocks for postoperative analgesia. Journal of the Royal Society of Medicine 73: 111–115
4.   McQuay H, Carroll D, Moore R A, 1988 Postoperative orthopaedic pain: the effect of opiates and local anaesthetic blocks. Pain 33: 291–295

5. Wall P D 1988 The prevention of postoperative pain. Pain 33: 289–290
6. Newman R J, Radda S K 1983 The myotoxicity of bupivacaine, a 31P NMR investigation. British Journal of Pharmacology 79: 395–399
7. Gielen M J M, Viering W 1986 Three-in-one lumbar plexus block for muscle biopsy in malignant hyperthermia patients: amide local anaesthetic agents may be used safely. Acta Anaesthesiologica Scandinavica 30: 581–583
8. Winnie A P, Ramamurthy S, Durrani Z 1973 The inguinal paravascular technic of lumbar plexus anesthesia: the 3-in-1 block. Anesthesia and Analgesia 52: 989–996
9. Cooke E D, Lloyd M J, Bowcock S A, Pilcher M F 1977 Intravenous lignocaine in prevention of deep venous thrombosis after elective hip surgery. Lancet 2: 797–799
10. Luostarinen V, Evers H, Lyytikainen M-T, Scheinin A, Wahlen A 1981 Antihthrombotic effects of lidocaine and related compounds on laser-induced microvascular injury. Acta Anaesthesiologica Scandinavica 25: 9–11
11. Borg T, Modig J 1985 Potential antithrombotic effects of local anaesthetics due to their inhibition of platelet aggregation. Acta Anaesthesiologica Scandinavica 29: 739–742
12. Winnie A P, Tay C H, Patel K P, Ramamurthy S, Durrani Z 1977 Pharmacokinetics of local analgesics during plexus blocks. Anesthesia and Analgesia 56: 852–861
13. Selander D 1987 Axillary plexus block: paresthetic or perivascular? Anesthesiology 66: 726–728
14. Bryce-Smith R 1976 Practical regional anaesthesia Lee J A, Bryce-Smith R (eds) Excerpta Medica and Elsevier, New York
15. Vester-Andersen T, Husum B, Lindeborg T, Borits L, Gothgen I 1984 Perivascular axillary block IV: blockade following 40, 50, 60 ml of mepivacaine 1% with adrenaline. Acta Anaesthesiologica Scandinavica 28: 99–105
16. Ang E T, Lassale B, Goldfarb G 1984 Continuous axillary brachial plexus block — a clinical and anatomical study. Anaesthesia and Analgesia 63: 680–684
17. Winnie A P 1975 Regional anesthesia. Surgical Clinics of North America 55: 861–892
18. Erikson E 1969 Illustrated handbook of local anaesthesia Munksgaard, Copenhagen
19. Winnie A P 1983 Plexus anesthesia, vol. 1: Perivascular technics of brachial plexus block. Churchill Livingstone, Edinburgh
20. Vester-Andersen T, Broby-Johansen U, Bro-Rasmussen F 1986 Perivascular axillary block VI: the distribution of gelatine solution injected into the axillary neurovascular sheath of cadavers. Acta Anaesthesiologica Scandinavica 30: 18–22
21. Thompson G E, Rorie D K 1983 Functional anatomy of the brachial plexus sheaths. Anesthesiology 59: 117–122
22. Partridge B L, Katz J, benirschke K 1987 Functional anatomy of the brachial plexus sheath: implications for anaesthesia. Anesthesiology 66: 743–747
23. Selander D 1977 Catheter technique in axillary plexus block Acta Anaesthesiologica Scandinavica 21: 324–329
24. Plancarte A, Amascua C, Marron M, San Miguel P, Aldrete J A 1987 Continuous brachial plexus block introducing catheters through a Tuohy needle in the axilla. Anesthesiology 67: 3A A287
25. Gaumann D. Lennon r L. Wedel D J 1987 Axillary plexus block: proximal catheter technique for postoperative pain management. Anaesthesiology 67: 3A A242
26. Tuominen M K. Rosenberg P H. Kalso E 1983 Blood levels of bupivacaine after single dose and during continuous infusion in axillary plexus block. Acta Anaesthesiologica Scandinavica 27: 303–306
27. Tuominen M K. Pitkanen Mt. Rosenberg P H 1986 Continuous interscalene brachial plexus block with bupivacaine for postoperative pain relief. Anesthesiology 65: 3A A197
28. de Jong R H 1977 Local anaesthetics. Thomas, Springfield
29. Grice S C, Morell R C, Balestrieri F J, Stump D A, Howard G 1986 Intravenous regional anaesthesia: evaluation and prevention of leakage under the tourniquet. Anesthesiology 65: 316–320
30. Cotev S, Robin G C 1966 Experimental studies on intravenous regional analgesia using radioactive lignocaine. British Journal of Anaesthesia 38: 936–939
31. Jeyaseelan S, Stevenson T M, Pfitzner J 1981 Tourniquet failure and arterial calcification: case report and theoretical dangers. Anaesthesia 36: 48–51
32. El Hassan K M, Hutton P, Black A M S 1984 Venous pressure and arm volume schanges during simulated Bier's block. Anaesthesia 39: 229–236
33. Davis A H, Hall I D, Wilkey A D, Smith J E, Walford A J, Kale V R 1984 Intravenous regional anaesthesia. The danger of the congested arm and the value of occlusion pressure. Anaesthesia 39: 416–422
34. Larsen U T, Hommelgaard P 1987 Pneumatic tourniquet paralysis following intravenous regional analgesia. Anaesthesia 42: 526–529

35. Pfeiffer P M 1986 Acute rhabdomyolysis following surgery for burns — possible role of tourniquet ischaemia. Anaesthesia 41: 614–619
36. Fagg P S 1987 Intravenous anaesthesia for lower limb orthopaedic surgery. Annals of the Royal College of Surgeons of England 69: 274–276
37. Valli H, Rosenberg P H 1986 Intravenous regional anesthesia below the knee: a cross-over study with prilocaine in volunteers. Anaesthesia 41: 1196–1202
38. Davis J A H, Walford A J 1986 Intravenous regional anaesthesia for foot surgery. Acta Anaesthesiologica Scandinavica 30: 145–147
39. Engberg G, Wiklund L 1988 Pulmonary complications after upper abdominal surgery: their prevention with intercostal blocks. Acta Anaesthesiologica Scandinavica 32: 1–9
40. Shelly M P, Park G R 1987 Intercostal nerve blockade for children. Anaesthesia 42: 541–545
41. Sury M R J, Bingham R M 1986 Accidental spinal anaesthesia following intercostal nerve blockade: a case report. Anaesthesia 41: 401–404
42. Skretting P 1981 Hypotension after intercostal nerve block during thoracotomy under general anaesthesia. British Journal of Anaesthesia 53: 527–531
43. Smith B E, Fischer H B J, Scott P V 1984 Continuous sciatic nerve block. Anaesthesia 39: 155–158
44. Hansen M, Bendixen D, Hartman F 1988 Modified intravenous cannula used for nerve stimulation. British Journal of Anaesthesia 60: 347
45. Selander D, Dhuner K G, Lundborg G 1977 Peripheral nerve injury due to injection needles used for regional anaesthesia Acta Anaesthesiologica Scandinavica 21: 182–188
46. Raj P P 1983 Mechanical aids. In: Henderson J J, Nimmo W S (eds) Practical regional anaesthesia. Blackwell, Oxford
47. Arthur D S, McNicol L R 1986 Local anaesthetic techniques in paediatric surgery. British Journal of Anaesthesia 58: 760–778
48. Rylance G 1981 Clinical pharmacology: drugs in children. British Medical Journal 282: 50–51
49. Serlo W, Haapanemi L 1985 Regional anaesthesia in paediatric surgery. Acta Anaesthesiologica Scandinavica 29: 283–286
50. Fell D, Derringtson M C, Wandless J G 1987 Caudal and ilioinguinal, iliohypogastric nerve blocks in children. Anesthesiology 67: 1020
51. Fell D, Derrington M C, Taylor E, Wandless J G 1988 Paediatric postoperative analgesia. Anaesthesia 43: 107–111
52. Tree-Trakarn T, Pirayavaraporn S, Lertakyamanee J 1987 Topical analgesia for relief of post-circumcision pain. Anesthesiology 67: 395–399

5. Sedation techniques

S.M. Willatts and K.L. Kong

Many unpleasant procedures disturb patients but cannot truly be said to warrant general anesthesia. Indeed, general anaesthesia may add considerably to the risk of the procedure as well as be demanding of skilled staff and facilities. Sedation techniques are valuable and widely used. This subject is enormous and we therefore propose to consider only a few circumstances. Firstly, some consideration will be given to the suitability of agents most commonly used for sedation, then certain techniques for their use will be discussed.

SEDATIVE AGENTS

Sedation is chiefly produced by use of analgesic drugs or intravenous or inhalational anaesthetic agents in concentrations lower than those required to induce anaesthesia. The ideal sedative drug should have a short half-life, inactive metabolites, be excreted independently of normal hepatic or renal function, should have no adverse effect on the cardiovascular or central nervous system, nor any interaction with other drugs and have no toxic effects on other organs. It might also be inexpensive, readily stored and easy to use.

Opioids

Narcotic analgesic or opioid drugs are those that bind to any of a variety of receptors to produce some agonist effect. Most opioids produce sedation, often with euphoria, as well as analgesia and have been used for this effect for hundred of years.

Side-effects of opioids may be useful, as in the respiratory depression caused by morphine and to a greater extent by phenoperidine, when patients require controlled ventilation or unwanted, such as the hypotension that can occur with a single dose of morphine. Significant hypotension and cardiac dysrhythmia can occur after administration of virtually all narcotic analgesics.

Morphine. This reduces both venous and arterial tone in humans, induces bradycardia by vagal stimulation and releases histamine although it causes little myocardial depression in healthy patients. Other disadvantages of this group of drugs include meiosis, making assessment of pupillary signs more difficult, reduction of gastric emptying and impaired intestinal absorption, stimulation of the chemoreceptor trigger zone and development of tolerance with long-term use. Morphine is widely used at present. Both morphine and fentanyl are mu-receptor agonists with high efficacy. Morphine administered intravenously is extensively taken up by the tissues, is not very lipid soluble and therefore crosses the blood-brain barrier relatively slowly. Its elimination half-life is 1.5–4 h (Table 5.1); furthermore 90% is excreted conjugated with glucuronide.

83

Table 5.1   Approximate distribution and elimination half-lives of opioid agents in normal patients.

Agent	Distribution half-life (min)	Elimination half-life (h)
Morphine	25	1.5–4
— glucuronides		3–6
Fentanyl	3	2–5
Alfentanil	3	1.5–3.5
Phenoperidine	3	1.5–4
Pethidine	7	3–6.5
Nalbuphine	2	3.5–4

In patients with hypotension, the profound fall in liver blood flow markedly reduces morphine clearance.[1] However, other factors such as sepsis, age and inotropic therapy also affect morphine elimination.[2] Hypercapnoea reduces the volume of distribution of morphine thereby potentiating its effect.[3]

Pethidine. This drug has a potential advantage in that it produces less spasm of the Sphincter of Oddi than morphine. Prolonged use at high dosage results in accumulation of the metabolite norpethidine, which has convulsant properties.

Phenoperidine. This drug is relatively long acting and produces profound respiratory depression. Cardiovascular collapse has been reported.[4] Some reduction of cortisol occurs after prologed use but of greatest concern is the increase in intracranial pressure (ICP), which has been reported and seems to be related to its vasodilating effect.[5]

Fentanyl. Used in high doses, this synthetic narcotic has the added potential advantage of reducing the stress response to trauma. Fentanyl is highly fat-soluble and is sequestered in muscle and stomach to be released at a later time with recurrence of respiratory depression. Despite a short distribution half-life, after repeated or prolonged administration, clearance depends solely on metabolism.

Alfentanil. This drug is shorter acting than fentanyl, with a half-life of 100 min but the duration of action is prolonged in some patients.[6]

Intravenous Anaesthetics
These drugs may be administered by continuous intravenous infusion to produce sedation; the usual aim being to permit rapid awakening at the end of the procedure. In the past, both Althesin and etomidate were popular for this purpose but the former provoked anaphylactoid reactions and was withdrawn and the latter depresses steroidogenesis[7] and cannot therefore be recommended for this purpose.

Barbiturates

These drugs are cheap, readily available and easy to use but their prolonged cumulative effect prevents rapid recovery. Barbiturates lower ICP but direct myocardial depression as well as vasodilatation reduce cerebral perfusion pressure. While they may offer some protection against cerebral ischaemia in animals, even if given 1 hour after the insult, the use of high doses in the head-injured human patient increases mortality from sepsis and ARDS.[8-10] Nevertheless, they have a valuable anticonvulsant action with the exception of methohexitone.

Methohexitone. Despite the drawback mentioned above, methohexitone has been widely used for sedation during painful procedures of short duration such as nerve blocks, but it causes pain on injection, excitation and cardiovascular depression. Addition of an opiate reduces the excitatory phenomena but increases respiratory depression.

Propofol. Chemically 2,6-di-iso-propyl phenol, it is the most recent addition to this group of drugs. Its main advantage is rapid recovery after even prolonged infusion without depression of steriodogenesis. Disadvantages include pain on injection and cardiovascular depression from the vasodilator action.

Ketamine. This is a derivative of phencyclidine that produces dissociative analgesia and sedation. It has been used alone or with other agents for postoperative analgesia and sedation. Widespread acceptance is precluded by many disadvantages.

Benzodiazepines

Diazepam. This drug is formulated in propylene glycol and may produce marked pain on injection and thrombophlebitis. Its more recent formulation in fat emulsion, as Diazemuls® is painless on injection. While diazepam is a useful sedative, amnesic and anticonvulsant drug, its metabolite desmethyl diazepam is also sedative and prolonged recovery may be expected.

Midazolam. This is a non-irritant water-soluble benzodiazepine that can be administered into peripheral veins. Like diazepam there is wide variation in the dose required to produce sedation. Midazolam gives rise to more anterograde amnesia than diazepam. Haemodynamic disturbances are not severe. However, in some patients (slow metabolizers), recovery from midazolam sedation by infusion is prolonged (Table 5.2). In addition, patients receiving prolonged infusions of midazolam develop cumulation of the active hydroxy-metabolite.

Lorazepam. This drug has no active metabolites but is relatively long-acting.

There is a suggestion that benzodiazepine opiate antagonism occurs.[11] This is supported by clinical observation and animal studies. However, in a study by Korttila et al,[12] intramuscular administration of pethidine potentiated the amnesic effects of diazepam for painful stimuli, prolonged the amnesic action for visual stimuli and improved patient acceptance of the intravenous regional technique.

Some of the problems of the prolonged action of benzodiazepines may be overcome

Table 5.2   Approximate elimination half-lives of benzodiazepines in normal patients

Agent	Elimination half-life (h)
Diazepam	30–56
Desmethyl diazepam	46–78
Lorazepam	10–20
Temazepam	10–16
Midazolam	
— normal patients	1–4
— slow metabolizers	8–22

by use of the specific benzodiazepine antagonist, flumazenil. Flumazenil has been compared with placebo in 60 women who had undergone laparoscopy using midazolam as the premedicant (7.5 mg orally) and the induction agent. An initial dose of midazolam 0.2 mg/kg was supplemented by 0.1 mg/kg when needed. The effects of flumazenil were statistically better than placebo for up to 30 min after administration. Patients were alert, co-operative and had good recall after awakening, with a stable arterial blood pressure and heart rate and no significant side-effects.[13] Sage et al[14] confirmed these findings in patients after prostatic surgery under subarachnoid anaesthesia with midazolam sedation. No anxiety states were found but the effects of flumazenil wore off before those of midazolam and after initial complete awakening, re-sedation occurred in the treated group. Similar results are found in patients undergoing oral surgery.[15] Patients with benzodiazepine overdose recover more quickly with flumazenil.

In 32 patients undergoing genito-urinary surgery with deep sedation provided by diazepam, aminophylline 60–120 mg was shown to reverse sedation rapidly when compared with saline. The effect persisted through the 2 hours of the study and it therefore appears that aminophylline also antagonizes diazepam sedation. In the circumstances of this study there were no cardiovascular side-effects nor anxiety after administration of the aminophylline.[16] This effect of aminophylline is probably mediated by adenosine receptor blockade.

Chlormethiazole
Chlormethiazole is a sedative drug used most commonly in delerium tremens and pre-eclampsia. Recovery is rapid after short infusions. After prolonged infusions, however, recovery is delayed owing to accumulation. After short infusions, rapid wakening is attributed to redistribution of the drug but after 48 h infusion, recovery is much slower with a drug elimination half-life of 3.5–12.1 h.[17] Clearance in the critically ill is likely to be further reduced. Chlormethiazole is available commercially in a 0.8% solution. Greater concentrations produce thrombophlebitis. Large fluid volumes are therefore required in some circumstances to achieve adequate sedation with the possibility of water overload. The drug has no analgesic properties and may also increase upper airway secretions, with nasal irritation, and produce pronounced tachycardia.

Anaesthetic Gases And Vapours

Nitrous oxide. This was used extensively for postoperative analgesia and sedation until it was appreciated that bone marrow depression occurred with prolonged use[18,19] (see also Chapter 2). In critically ill patients this occurs after relatively short exposures.

Isoflurane. This newer volatile agent has many of the features of an ideal sedative. It is minimally metabolized (0.2%), excreted rapidly via the lungs, has little or no recognized organ toxicity, nor interaction with other drugs. At low concentration there is minimal reduction of blood pressure. Preliminary results are encouraging.

SEDATION FOR LOCAL AND REGIONAL ANALGESIA

Some anaesthetists use drugs that are appropriate for premedication in fairly heavy dosage, while others prefer benzodiazepines or propofol. There is little to choose between individual benzodiazepines. Because of this, Herregods et al[20] compared midazolam 0.15 mg/kg with diazepam 0.2 mg/kg, both given by intravenous bolus injection. They found no difference between the two drugs with regard to heart rate, blood pressure, respiratory rate and incidence or duration of apnoea, or recovery, although midazolam gave less pain on injection and better sedation at 60 min than diazepam.

Tubal ligation has been performed under local infiltration block with diazepam and pentazocine supplementation. Lorazepam and diazepam were both found to be unsatisfactory sedative agents as adjuncts to epidural analgesia for Caesarean section. Inadequate sedation was common and 10% of the diazepam patients and 36% of those receiving lorazepam had symptoms of delirium. The dosage was 0.05 mg/kg lorazepam and 0.1 mg/kg diazepam.[21]

Triazolam, one of the newer benzodiazepine drugs, has been used for pre- and intra-operative sedation in patients undergoing plastic surgery as an out-patient procedure under local analgesia. Triazolam has a very short duration of action and gave satisfactory sedation in 96% of 251 patients, all of whom also received intravenous diazepam for its amnesic action.[22] However, it is difficult to see how the authors could separate the effects of the two benzodiazepines. Lorazepam supplementation for transurethral prostatectomy performed under spinal analgesia produced a co-operative drowsy patient with significant amnesia for the operation. Benzodiazepines used in appropriate dosage have no significant effect on the airway or cardiovascular system. Addition of morphine to the regimen further reduces the pain and discomfort associated with the procedure.

A similar approach has been used to produce conscious sedation in patients requiring otolaryngological procedures under local analgesia. Diazepam is given intravenously and the dose titrated against eye signs. This is followed by fentanyl in a dose that maintains verbal contact between the patient and the surgeon.[23]

It appears that subanaesthetic combinations of ketamine with nitrous oxide and diazepam give no higher incidence of hallucinations than when fentanyl is substituted for ketamine.[24] Low-dose ketamine with diazepam may produce a slight increase in pulse rate and blood pressure but does not produce unpleasant recollections.

In the USA, plastic surgical and other procedures normally confined to the hospital environment are being performed in the 'office'. It is claimed that sedation with ketamine and diazepam can, in some cases, eliminate the need for local techniques.[25] Dissociative analgesia occurs but there is the danger of airway obstruction, which may be difficult to deal with in a single-handed practice. The lack of untoward effects after ketamine-diazepam combinations is confirmed by Korttila et al[26] in patients undergoing lower abdominal or extremity surgery under epidural, spinal or brachial plexus block.

Chlormethiazole as a supplement to nerve block gives controlled sedation — particularly if given as a two-stage infusion. A loading dose of 1520 mg is given over 30 min followed by a maintenance rate of 10 mg/min. There is no adverse effect on mental function in the elderly.[27] A comparison of chlormethiazole with diazepam[28] showed that the desired level of sedation was easier to maintain by altering the rate of the chlormethiazole infusion than by giving repeated doses of diazepam. Sinclair et al[29] studied the cardiovascular effects of chlormethiazole infusion at 30–49 ml/min in 6 patients undergoing extradural analgesia. During the infusion, there were small reductions in mean arterial blood pressure and left ventricular ejection time, which were statistically significant, but cardiac output did not fall. Patient acceptance was high and the authors concluded that there were no adverse cardiovascular effects.

Propofol was compared with methohexitone in the provision of light general anaesthesia for patients undergoing surgery with spinal block.[30] Intermittent bolus injection was a feasible way of maintaining anaesthesia. A mean infusion rate of 0.13 mg/kg. min^{-1} propofol and 0.089 mg/kg. min^{-1} methohexitone was required. Propofol produced smoother anaesthesia with significantly fewer excitatory side-effects and less pain on injection than methohexitone, but cardiovascular and respiratory depression commonly occurred. Recovery was rapid with both agents but minor postoperative sequelae were commoner after methohexitone. Clearly many sedative drugs can be suitable, benzodiazepines are widely used but there is little to choose between them.

SEDATION FOR RADIOLOGICAL PROCEDURES

Many radiological procedures require analgesia that can be given intramuscularly as a premedication or intravenously during the procedure. Anxiolytic drugs may be given in a similar fasion to allay fear caused by complex and often noisy machinery. Use of benzodiazepines alone for painful procedures is unsatisfactory and results in a restless confused patient. Local analgesia is provided by infiltration.

Computerized axial tomography and nuclear magnetic imaging

The major requirement for such investigations is that the patient keeps still. Most of these investigations can be performed without any anaesthesia or sedation although about 5% will require general anaesthesia. In neurosurgical patients, especially babies, who may be unco-operative, there is little alternative to general anaesthesia. A great variety of intravenous sedative techniques have been described for adults but can lead to difficulty with the airway. Any airway obstruction in patients with raised intracranial pressure (ICP) is dangerous and may precipitate tentorial herniation. Therefore general anaesthesia is often safer, although an infusion of propofol is readily reversible owing to the rapid recovery time. Information on the effect of this drug on ICP is, however, limited — especially in patients where ICP is raised and the reduction in arterial blood pressure that occurs will reduce cerebral perfusion.

Neonates requiring cerebral computerized axial tomography (CAT) should be immobilized. Oral, intramuscular and rectal medication is unsuitable. Repeated sedation for such procedures has resulted in respiratory arrest.[31] Therefore general anaesthesia with hyperventilation is most appropriate. However, in a large series reported by Strain et al,[32] 5134 paediatric patients were reviewed retrospectively. Operators preferred intravenous pentobarbitone (Nembutal®); recovery time was not prolonged and there were only 2 sedation failures and no sedation-related complications.

A further prospective study of 582 paediatric cranial computed tomography (CAT) scans compared sedation with either oral chloral hydrate 80 mg/kg or an intramuscular 'APPS' preparation of atropine, pethidine, promethazine and quinalbarbitone (Seconal®) with intravenous supplements as required. The CAT examination failed in 15% in the chloral hydrate group and 12% in the APPS group. Complications, mostly minor, occurred in 3.5%. Rectal thiopentone has been used for this purpose and certainly produces rapid-onset, short-duration sedation but respiratory depression is a disadvantage.[33] Chlormethiazole is an effective sedative in children.[34]

An advantage of sedation rather than general anaesthesia with controlled ventilation is that spontaneously breathing patients tend to maintain their body temperature much better than paralysed ones. This is important as the CAT scanner tends to be housed in an air-conditioned room with the attendant danger of hypothermia.[35] Nevertheless, controlled hyperventilation is the treatment of choice where there is any increase in intracranial pressure.

Cerebral angiography

This is almost always performed under local analgesia with premedication, unless general anaesthesia is indicated because of failure to co-operate or the presence of raised ICP. Benzodiazepine sedation or a neurolept technique is appropriate if ICP is not raised. However, in a study of the effects of sedation with pentazocine (30 mg) and midazolam (5–22.5 mg) in 21 patients undergoing cerebral angiography, arterial carbon dioxide was shown to rise signficantly. Where ICP is already raised, this could lead to a dangerous further increase.[36] Moreover, marked cerebral vasodilatation results in poor quality angiograms.

SEDATION FOR NEUROSURGICAL PROCEDURES

Stereotactic surgery

Application of cold (using a cryprobe), or heat (using a radiofrequency current) is used by neurosurgeons to make a discrete lesion within the brain, often in the absence of direct vision. The lesion must be accurately positioned and therefore its location must be tested in a co-operative patient. Nevertheless, insertion of the needle may be both painful and tedious such that some form of analgesia and sedation are required.

The sitting position may be used for stereotactic surgery with its attendant problems of hypotension and air embolus. Vomiting or fitting may follow the injection of water-soluble contrast media to locate the site of the needle. There is little pain during the procedure although discomfort occurs during fixation of the head frame, making the burr holes and stripping the dura. If the electroencephalogram (e.e.g.) is to be recorded, drugs such as diazepam and barbiturates should be avoided. Ketamine should be avoided as it causes alternate high-delta and fast activity, and may provoke fits in epileptic patients. Where the surgery is being performed for Parkinson's disease, phenothiazines should be omitted as they may attenuate the tremor, which is being used to monitor the effects of surgery. If these patients are on L-dopa, which is decarboxylated to dopamine, there may be problems with anaesthesia but not usually with sedative techniques.

Local analgesia with sedation is the most suitable technique in co-operative patients, although these operations often take several hours. This is not appropriate for children or the psychiatrically disturbed. A neuroleptic technique has been used successfully since neither droperidol nor the narcotics phenoperidine or fentanyl have a prolonged effect on tremor or the e.e.g. This method supplies good operating conditions, sedation and analgesia. Doses should be titrated against patient response to a maximum of $250\,\mu$g fentanyl and 15 mg droperidol. There may be loss of patient co-operation. A scalp block is required in addition to sedation.

Epilepsy Surgery

When anticonvulsant medication fails and neurophysiological investigation reveals an epileptiform focus, surgery may be indicated to remove the focus. In this situation, e.e.g. recording is used to identify the focus initially and methohexitone may be useful at this time to stimulate a convulsion. The requirements for this procedure are the same as those for stereotactic surgery.

Trigeminal neuralgia and radiofrequency lesion

Trigeminal neuralgia produces severe pain in one of the divisions of the fifth nerve, which can be extremely disabling and medical treatment often proves inadequate.

A radiofrequency lesion is produced by insertion of a needle through the foramen ovale under X-ray control. The fifth nerve is stimulated to locate the relevant division for thermocoagulation and one or more lesions are subsequently made. There is considerable pain as the needle is inserted through the foramen and some form of analgesia or sedation is required but the patient should awaken rapidly and co-operate during the period of stimulation of the relevant division for accurate localization. Heavy sedation with neuroleptanalgesia alone may suffice, although it is difficult to obtain subsequent patient co-operation. The combination of local analgesia with heavy premedication produces similar problems, especially in the elderly in whom most of these cases arise and can induce confusion, which is counterproductive. Narcotic analgesics in high dosage induce vomiting, which is highly undesirable when the needle is in place. Owing to these difficulties with sedative techniques, a brief period of general anaesthesia with a short-acting intravenous induction agent such as propofol is the technique of choice. Diazemuls® may be supplemented by a narcotic analgesic but again patients often remain drowsy and unco-operative after insertion of the needle.

The same sedation techniques can be used for treatment of hemifacial spasm, which results from lesions of the facial nerve, and for percutaneous cordotomy, which is usually performed for uncontrolled pain from malignant disease.

Carotid Endarterectomy

Most of these procedures are performed under general anaesthesia. However, a neurolept technique with droperidol and fentanyl in combination with cervical plexus block can be useful. Motor function can be tested during carotid clamping and the operation can proceed without a shunt in most patients.[37]

SEDATION IN ECLAMPSIA

The most serious need for sedation in obstetric patients occurs in eclampsia and pre-eclamptic toxaemia (p.e.t.), which are a major cause of maternal mortality and morbidity. Sedation may be needed to supplement control of the hypertension and convulsions. In untreated eclampsia, death occurs from coma, respiratory or cardiac failure. However, deaths related to eclampsia also result from excessive sedation in a condition where cerebral and laryngeal oedema are common and there is a special danger during recovery from anaesthesia.[38] Continuous neurological assessment is very important because of the risk of cerebrovascular accident.

Management includes bedrest in a quiet environment, often supplemented by mild sedation with benzodiazepines and antihypertensive treatment with hydrallazine. If p.e.t. is severe the aim is prevention of convulsions, control of blood pressure and expeditious delivery with minimum trauma to mother or fetus.

In the UK, anticonvulsant prophylaxis is often supplied by an infusion of diazepam or chlormethiazole. Diazepam produces loss of beat-to-beat variation in the fetal heart during intravenous infusion. In high dosage there is delayed onset of the baby's respiration, apnoea, hypotonia and hypothermia.[39,40] Intravenous chlormethiazole requires a large volume for infusion with potential for worsening cerebral oedema, especially in the presence of impaired renal function. It crosses the placenta, producing some short-term respiratory depression in the fetus and sedation.[41] A recent study[42] does not suggest that a major problem occurs with the effects of chlormethiazole on placental vascular resistance with clinical doses.

Magnesium sulphate is a poor sedative agent but is used as the main anticonvulsant in the USA, although it is associated with cardiorespiratory arrest if an overdose is given. Magnesium sulphate reduces the release of acetylcholine at the neuromuscular junction and therefore increases sensitivity to neuromuscular blocking drugs. It also crosses the placenta and gives rise to fetal hypotonia. High concentrations in the newborn produce respiratory depression and apnoea.

A recent study by Slater et al[43] used high-dose intravenous phenytoin (10.8–18 mg/kg) for anticonvulsant prophylaxis in 2 eclamptic patients and 24 with moderate to severe p.e.t. There were no major maternal or fetal side-effects. Plasma phenytoin was within the therapeutic range (7–20 mg/l) at 30 min and 6 hours after the infusion in all patients and remained there in 21 patients for 24 h. Phenytoin may cause acute hypotension but this is rare if administered slowly (25 mg/min). Newborn infants exposed to phenytoin have bleeding tendencies during the first day of life caused by reduced levels of vitamin K-dependent clotting factors.

Pain relief is an adjunct to sedation. Epidural analgesia can be used during labour provided there is no coagulopathy. It should never be used as a method of lowering blood pressure but with fluid preloading will have a beneficial effect on placental blood flow.

SEDATION FOR OPHTHALMIC SURGERY

Conscious sedation with local anaesthesia and retrobulbar block is a valuable combination for eye surgery. Insertion of the retrobulbar block is painful and the patient benefits from short-acting analgesia and a benzodiazepine. The aim is an awake, co-operative and relaxed patient who is completely pain free.[44]

Cataract surgery is commonly performed on an elderly population with coexisting disease. Thus local techniques supplemented by sedation are useful. The increasing use of day surgery centres has lead to more studies in this field. Intravenous sedation with benzodiazepines and fentanyl is popular but there is a wide variation in dose requirement. Gilbert et al[45] used a fixed dose of methohexitone and nalbuphine or fentanyl and diazepam. There was no difference between the two regimens with regard to side-effects, intraocular pressure or postoperative nausea and vomiting. Nalbuphine and methohexitone resulted in some prolongation of recovery but better sedation at the time of insertion of the nerve block, lack of recall of its insertion and better operating conditions and patient acceptability. The incidence of intra-operative vomiting was high but reduced by intravenous droperidol. Other workers have used a small dose of thiopentone just prior to insertion of the block.[46]

SEDATION FOR DENTISTY

In a survey of the use of general anaesthesia and sedation in the general dental service in East Anglia, Kemp and Broadway[47] reported that the highest percentage (42%) of general anaesthetics were administered by consultant anaesthetists, but a significant number (35%) were given by dentally qualified practitioners.

Simple sedation (as defined by the Wylie Report[48]), coupled with local block, is a safe alternative for dental surgery. The advantages of such a regimen are minimal effects on vital signs, maintenance of protective reflexes and patient co-operation, minimal requirement for monitoring and rapid recovery to street fitness. Inhalation sedation falls within this category of simple sedation. The Seward Report[49] recommended an upper limit of 30% nitrous oxide be set when used by a suitably trained practitioner with trained assistance in the absence of a second qualified doctor or dentist. Intravenous sedation is an important part of current dental practice. The use of intermittent intravenous methohexitone or other intravenous induction agents by personnel untrained in the administration of general anaesthesia is not compatible with current concepts of safety and has been largely abandoned. The Jørgensen technique, which employed the use of pentobarbitone, pethidine and hyoscine to achieve drowsiness and sedation, suffered from the disadvantages of a variable recovery time with severe hangover effects. This combination of three powerful central depressant drugs can no longer be recommended when simpler alternatives are available.

Intravenous and oral agents

Since the introduction of injectable diazepam into dentistry in the late 1960s, diazepam has been the intravenous sedative agent used most widely. The drug is given at a rate of 2.5 mg every 30 s until drowsiness, slurred speech and drooping eyelids occur; the usual dose being between 10–20 mg. At this point local analgesia is administered. The advantages of diazepam are its wide margin of safety and the useful degree of anterograde amnesia lasting up to 30 min. Its new formulation in Intralipid® (Diazemuls®) is free from the problems of pain on injection and venous thrombosis. Although most patients appear normal after an hour, some postural unsteadiness and hypotension may be demonstrable, and complete recovery may take several hours. Patients should always be accompanied home and the same postoperative restrictions as for full general anaesthesia apply.

Intravenous midazolam (0.1–0.17 mg/kg) has been claimed to be better than intravenous diazepam with a faster onset of sedation, a quicker recovery, more profound amnesia and fewer side-effects.[50] Dixon et al,[51] however, found an increased incidence of drowsiness, unsteadiness and forgetfulness in patients given intravenous midazolam (0.14 mg/kg) compared to those given intravenous diazepam (0.29 mg/kg) for sedation in conservative dentistry. The authors also observed an increased incidence of partial airway obstruction in those patients given intravenous midazolam and concluded that there was insufficient evidence to choose midazolam in preference to Diazemuls® unless the profound amnesic effect of midazolam is desired.

Sedatives administered by mouth can be as effective as those given intravenously and have the advantages of greater patient acceptability, ease of administration, safety and few sequelae. O'Boyle et al[52] compared oral midazolam with intravenous diazepam in outpatient oral surgery and found oral midazolam to be a safe alternative to intravenous diazepam for conscious sedation in outpatients undergoing minor surgical procedures. Temazepam, a benzodiazepine with a short duration of action and no active metabolites has been reformulated as an elixir, which is thought to be more rapidly absorbed than the original gelatin capsules. Significantly greater plasma concentrations of temazepam have been found after the oral administration of the elixir when compared with the capsules. Hosie and Brooke[53] compared temazepam elixir 30 mg given orally one hour pre-operatively with intravenous diazemuls (maximum of 20 mg) for minor oral surgical procedures. They found temazepam elixir to be a safe and effective alternative method of sedation in dental out-patients. Patients who received oral temazepam showed less amnesia but a quicker recovery compared with those who received intravenous diazemuls.

The disadvantages of oral medication is that the effect of a single dose of the drug cannot be accurately predicted, and incremental addition by the oral route is difficult, making precise control of sedation impossible. Thus oral sedation seems best suited for mild anxiety states.

Diazepam in children has been disappointing. Oral diazepam is no more effective than an inert placebo in helping nervous children cope with dentistry.[54] Sedation techniques are often unsatisfactory in this age group and full general anaesthesia is often the only option.

The problem of slow recovery to 'street fitness' and the variability of drug response associated with the use of benzodiazepines in out-patients have prompted some practitioners to use narcotic analgesics to supplement diazepam sedation. Corall et al[55] reported that the addition of 30 mg of pentazocine significantly reduced the mean dose of diazepam required to produce sedation, and significantly reduced the occurrence of apparent lack of sedation at a maximum dose of 20 mg diazepam. Although pentazocine supplementation of diazepam sedation did not alter the recovery times, the authors reported the rare occurrence of severe respiratory depression necessitating resuscitation. This emphasizes the dangers of using techniques employing a combination of drugs in dental sedation, which may lead the practitioner into difficulties unless skilled in the techniques of cardiopulmonary resuscitation.

Inhalational agents

The use of nitrous oxide as a sedative in dentistry was repopularized by the work of Langa[56] in the technique known as relative analgesia. In this method, nitrous oxide is supplied in variable concentrations by the operator according to his assessment of the patient's needs. However, the attention of the operator is divided between performing the dental treatment and monitoring the patient's condition and adjusting the concentration of nitrous oxide supplied.

Inhalation sedation refers to the technique whereby the inhalational agent is supplied in a preselected fixed concentration so that there is no possibility of the patient losing consciousness. The mixture is supplied at a relatively high flow rate through a nasal mask and the patient can regulate the depth of sedation by either breathing through the nose or the mouth, or both. The advantages of the technique are numerous. It is a safe and effective method, producing a relaxed, comfortable and co-operative patient. The level of sedation produced is easily controlled with a rapid recovery. The technique can be performed by any dental practitioner with adequate training. Verbal response ensures that the level of sedation is not excessive.

Edmunds and Rosen[57] reported the results of a field trial of the use of a fixed concentration of 25% nitrous oxide to produce sedation in 394 anxious dental patients treated on 1005 occasions. Of these patients, 99% were treated successfully without any incidence of loss of consciousness. These included 47 children treated on 88 occasions.

The major disadvantage of the technique is the toxic effects of nitrous oxide on prolonged exposure. Occupational exposure to nitrous oxide has been shown to cause depression of vitamin B_{12} activity, resulting in measurable changes in the bone marrow secondary to impaired synthesis of dexoyribonucleic acid.[58] The alternative agents, trichloroethylene and methoxyflurane, in subanaesthetic concentrations, have proved less satisfactory because of slow uptake and excretion. Recently, Parbrook et al[59] investigated the sedative effects of subanaesthetic concentrations of isoflurane and found it to be an effective alternative to nitrous oxide for inhalation sedation in dentistry.

It should be remembered that the success of any sedation technique in dental surgery depends largely on the skill of the dental surgeon in patient management, operative manipulation and his ability to achieve painless but totally effective local analgesia. Most patients with a phobia of dental treatment can be helped by the simple and safe sedative techniques described. The small numbers of failures may then be referred to centres where more complex techniques including general anaesthesia are available.

SEDATION FOR CARDIAC CATHETERIZATION

Cardiac catherization is usually accomplished with heavy sedation in adults but small children present greater problems. Small infants and children may require emergency catheterization. A recent review[60] of this topic suggests that paediatric catherization may be performed under general anaesthesia, with sedation or with no medication at all. Sedation has the advantage that it allows the child to tolerate the often prolonged procedure without distress and restlessness. It enables the child to breathe room air making shunt calculations more accurate and, provided small doses of sedatives are used, hypercapnoea and hypoxia are avoided. Further supplements may be required if sedation wears off during a prolonged procedure. A wide variety of sedatives have been used, but most depress cardiovascular function and increase pulmonary artery pressure. The Toronto mixture (pethidine, chlorpromazine and promethazine) has been popular since its introduction in 1958, but barbiturates, opioids, phenothiazines, benzodiazepines and neuroleptic agents have all been used successfully. Supplementary doses are commonly required during the procedure.

SEDATION FOR ENDOSCOPY

Although upper gastro-intestinal endoscopy can be performed without sedation, the use of sedative drugs increases patient acceptability and facilitates the examination.[61] Long-acting amnesia is undesirable, although amnesia during the unpleasant endoscopic procedure itself is an advantage since many such procedures have to be repeated frequently. Intravenous diazepam (0.15 mg/kg) is widely used for this purpose and its new formulation in emulsion (Diazemuls®) has minimal irritant effects on the veins.

Intravenous midazolam is an effective alternative to diazepam in allowing quick yet safe endoscopy. Whitwam et al[62] compared intravenous midazolam 0.07 mg/kg with diazepam 0.15 mg/kg for sedation during upper gastrointestinal endoscopy. Although patients who received midazolam had a faster onset of effect and a greater degree of amnesia, there was no difference in the degree of sedation, ease of endoscopy and speed of recovery in the two groups of patients. Douglas et al[63] found oral temazepam, in a fixed dosage (20 mg), as effective as titrated doses of intravenous diazepam in achieving sedation and patient co-operation for upper gastrointestinal endoscopy. Although oral administration is safe and simple, it requires good planning to ensure optimal sedation at the time of endoscopy.

Boldy et al[64] assessed the combination of intravenous Diazemuls® (10 mg) with pethidine (50–75 mg) plus reversal with intravenous naloxone (0.4 mg) for sedation in endoscopic procedures. They found the technique to produce significantly better patient cooperation than Diazemuls® alone without any significant delay in recovery. However, the use of an opioid such as pethidine in out-patient endoscopic procedures and the routine 'prophylactic' use of naloxone (which is itself not without side-effects) cannot be recommended.

Bronchoscopy under local anaesthesia is often a disagreeable and frightening examination and diazepam has been recommended for sedation.[65] However, all the commonly available benzodiazepines are useful. They produce good patient co-operation, cardiovascular stability and a comparable speed of recovery.

The management of patients who require painful procedures may be improved by the addition of an analgesic to benzodiazepine sedation techniques. Sury and Cole[66] compared nalbuphine 0.2 mg/kg and midazolam 0.05 mg/kg with midazolam 0.05 mg/kg alone for day-case fibreoptic bronchoscopy. They found that nalbuphine increased patient comfort during bronchoscopy but this was achieved at the expense of nausea, dizziness and prolonged recovery. In the nalbuphine group, 2 patients developed obstructive apnoea; the sedative properties of nalbuphine may have contributed to this. The authors concluded that sedation with a nalbuphine-midazolam combination should be reserved for prolonged painful procedures when benzodiazepines alone are inadequate, and emphasized the need for full resuscitation and recovery facilities.

SEDATION FOR VENTILATED PATIENTS REQUIRING INTENSIVE THERAPY

Increased awareness of the potential dangers of sedative drugs and of the importance of optimizing their use has heightened interest in sedative regimens for the critically ill.

Attention to details such as the use of nasotracheal rather than orotracheal intubation, having adequate windows in the intensive care unit, and frequent communication and reassurance can do much to allay anxiety in the critically ill patient. Although there is no substitute for caring and sympathetic nurses and doctors to ensure patient comfort on the intensive care unit (ICU), pharmacological intervention is often required for humanitarian and medical reasons.

Many patients will experience pain and will therefore need adequate analgesia. This can effectively be provided by intravenous opioids or by regional analgesia. Most patients requiring mechanical ventilation will need sedation to allay anxiety, encourage sleep and to facilitate controlled mechanical ventilation. Sedative drugs are also useful in minimizing distress during uncomfortable procedures, in obtunding the physiological responses to stress (such as tachycardia and hypertension), and to lower intracranial pressure and therefore potentially improve cerebral perfusion in neuro-surgical patients. In a recent postal survey,[67] opioids and benzodiazepines were found to be used in combination by 60% of ICUs in the UK. Papaveretum and phenoperidine were the most commonly used opioids, and diazepam (Diazemuls®) and midazolam were the most commonly used benzodiazepines.

The major concern in critically ill patients is to avoid excessive sedation and its complications. The regular monitoring of the depth of sedation is therefore an important clinical consideration.

Assessment of sedation

Methods of assessing sedation must take into account both the depth as well as the quality of sedation. Deep sedation is no longer thought to be desirable and the ideal level of sedation to aim for is that at which the patient is comfortable and co-operative and would rouse spontaneously from sleep or be so roused if required.

Physiological variables such as heart rate and blood pressure are inaccurate indices of the depth of sedation in the ICU patient, since changes in these physiological variables are induced by numerous other factors such as hypotension and septicaemia. Linear analogue scales are subjective and do not give reproducible results between different observers. They are of unproven accuracy in controlling sedative regimens. The Glasgow coma scale employs a weighting system to describe pathological neurological responses. However, it is not applicable to the intact, sedated brain.

Simple descriptive terms such as 'good' or 'poor' sedation are imprecise and are open to varied interpretation by different observers. Categorization allows greater specificity in defining depth of sedation. Scoring systems that use different graded identifiable clinical end-points, such as that described by Ramsay et al,[68] are of practical value in assessing sedation in the ventilated patient. Analysis of the e.e.g., such as power spectral analysis and cerebral function monitoring, provide an objective assessment of sedation. Changes in the amplitude and the distribution of frequencies of the power spectrum may be related to changes in the depth of sedation. However, electrical monitoring of sedation is expensive and further developments in this field are necessary if these techniques are to be useful. Evans et al[69] demonstrated a correlation between lower oesophageal contractility (LOC), clinical signs of anaesthesia and dose of anaesthetic. Measurement of LOC has also been advocated as an objective measure of depth of sedation in ICU patients. However, the number of drugs and disease processes that affect the oesophagus in the critically ill is enormous. The application of the technique is also limited by the large interindividual variability in the response of the oesophagus to the anaesthetic agents.

The measurement of severity of illness is an important aspect of the assessment of sedation in the critically ill. Physiological disturbances such as reduced organ perfusion and tissue oxygenation affect the brain. These components of cerebral depression must therefore be taken into consideration.

Several groups of drugs are available for sedation on the intensive care unit. Unfortunately, all have disadvantages when given continuously to critically ill patients. While there are clear advantages for continuous infusions of drugs to maintain a constant level of sedation in most patients receiving intensive therapy, there are also disadvantages to this practice. The rate of infusion must be reduced in patients with impaired renal and hepatic function and reduced organ perfusion. Single small intravenous doses of sedative or analgesic drugs may then be given as a supplement for stimulating or painful procedures.

Opioids

The narcotic analgesics might seem ideal drugs for use in intensive care. The resultant euphoria, drowsiness and analgesia are all useful in patients who require sedation and are in pain. However, opioids also cause nausea and vomiting, decreased gastrointestinal motility, truncal rigidity and prolonged ventilatory depression.

Morphine provides effective analgesia and sedation in a large proportion of patients receiving intensive care. Large doses of morphine may however reduce immunocompetence and may be associated with an increased risk of infection.[70] Although its elimination half-life is 1.5–4 h in normal subjects, this is markedly increased in patients with impaired liver function or reduced liver blood flow.[1] Recently, Osborne and colleagues[71] drew attention to the severe and prolonged ventilatory depression and delayed recovery in patients with impaired renal function as a result of the accumulation of active morphine 6 glucuronide.

Papaveretum has similar advantages and disadvantages to those of morphine. It is, however, more sedative than morphine alone and is the most commonly used opioid[67] in 33% of ICUs in 1987. Synthetic narcotic analgesics (e.g. fentanyl and phenoperidine) are popular because of the resultant profound ventilatory depression that facilitates controlled mechanical ventilation. Recent reports of the effects of phenoperidine on intracranial pressure are disconcerting.[5] Bingham and Hinds[72] in a study of the effects of intermittent intravenous 1–2 mg doses of phenoperidine in patients with traumatic coma found a reduction in mean arterial pressure and consequently in the cerebral perfusion pressure. In some instances, the reduction in cerebral perfusion pressure was considerable. They concluded that intermittent doses of phenoperidine should be avoided in traumatic coma and other opioids used with caution.

The newer opioid alfentanil has been shown to provide useful sedation in the ventilated patient in intensive care.[73] The advantages of alfentanil are its short elimination half-life (about 100 min), rapid onset of action, potent analgesic effects and lack of depressant effects on the cardiovascular system. However, additional sedation with benzodiazepines may be required. Clearance of the drug is reduced in children, the elderly, and in cirrhotics, with the potential danger of prolonged ventilatory depression. Its detailed pharmacokinetics have not been studied in the critically ill patient.

Intravenous anaesthetic agents

Barbiturates are generally unsuitable for the sedation of intensive care patients because of cumulative effects and the increased incidence of sepsis. Barbiturates lower the intracranial pressure but direct myocardial depression and peripheral vasodilatation reduce the systemic arterial pressure and therefore the cerebral perfusion pressure. Although they may offer some protection against cerebral ischaemia, their prolonged effects make repeated neurological assessments, including the diagnosis of brain stem death, very difficult. They are, however, very cheap, readily available and have a useful anticonvulsant action.

Ketamine has potent analgesic as well as sedative properties. The successful use of ketamine infusions at 5–25 μg/kg. min^{-1} to achieve both sedation and bronchodilatation in asthmatic patients in intensive care has recently been highlighted.[74] The major disadvantages of ketamine sedation are hallucinatory side-effects and accumulation of the metabolites. The concurrent use of benzodiazepines will attenuate the unwanted central nervous system side-effects but with the attendant disadvantages of the benzodiazepines themselves. Used cautiously, ketamine may be a valuable sedative agent for ventilated asthmatics.

Propofol (2,6-di-isopropylphenol), a substituted phenol, has been widely investigated both for induction and maintenance of anaesthesia. Patients have demonstrated impressively rapid and clear headed recovery with a minimum of early postoperative morbidity such as headache, confusion, restlessness, nausea and vomiting. Its use has recently been extended into the intensive care unit for the sedation of critically ill patients. Newman and colleagues[75] found propofol to be an effective agent when used as a continuous infusion in 10 general intensive care patients who displayed a range of illness severity, as determined by the APACHE II score. Sedation was readily achieved and maintained by an initial loading dose of 1 mg/kg (if required) followed by an infusion of 1–3 mg/kg. h^{-1}. The most significant advantage of the technique is that propofol provides a controllable level of sedation with a rapid recovery in most cases. In another study, Grounds et al[76] compared an infusion of propofol (mean 54.83 mg/h, s.e.m. 4.57) with intermittent incremental 2.5 mg doses of midazolam to achieve adequate sedation in 60 patients. Although the results of the study showed early promise, the study itself was disappointingly flawed. It is hardly surprising that patients receiving intermittent doses of a drug should be less satisfactorily sedated than those receiving a continuous infusion. It is also not surprising that those patients who received intermittent doses of midazolam should require more papaveretum, which, in turn, could account for the delayed recovery in this group of patients. The authors also drew the unsupported conclusion that propofol infusion is suitable for the sedation of patients receiving intensive therapy when their study was conducted entirely in post cardiac surgical patients.

Propofol is known to depress the respiratory and cardiovascular systems, especially when given by the higher infusion rates used in general anaesthesia. The major difficulty with its use in intensive care is that critically ill patients are particularly sensitive to the cardiovascular depressant effects of the drug, even at low doses. In the study by Newman and colleagues,[75] of the 3 patients who received a loading dose of propofol, 2 of them showed marked decreases in mean arterial pressure of 40% and 53%. In a further 3 patients, the infusion rate had to be reduced because of a continuing downward trend in arterial pressure. A recent, large multicentre study comparing midazolam with propofol[77], confirms the ease of control of sedation with propofol and the rapid recovery on discontinuation of the infusion.

Benzodiazepines

In some patients, the desired level of sedation is impossible to achieve with benzodiazepines. Attempts to control the agitated patient by increasing the dose results in oversedation. Benzodiazepine sedation also reduces the time in rapid eye movement (REM) sleep. Until the introduction of midazolam, diazepam was the most widely used benzodiazepine for sedation in the intensive care unit although lorazepam also produced satisfactory sedation.

Midazolam, a water soluble benzodiazepine, has been shown to provide satisfactory sedation in postoperative cardiac patients with maintenance of cardiovascular stability with intravenous infusions at 2 mg/h. The vasodilatation produced in these patients may also be an advantage.[78] Midazolam showed promise in early pharmacokinetic studies. In critically ill patients, however, the half-life of midazolam is markedly increased and becomes highly unpredictable. Critically ill patients may show prolonged recovery from midazolam for a variety of reasons. Hepatic clearance of midazolam is decreased in critically ill patients with impaired liver function or impaired perfusion. Elderly patients and patients on enzyme-inhibiting drugs, such as cimetidine, will demonstrate a reduced hepatic clearance of midazolam. Patients in chronic renal failure, those having had major operative procedures and the elderly have an increased volume of distribution of the drug. In 1986, Dundee and colleagues[79] reported a prolonged elimination half-life of between 8 and 22 h in 6% of a group of 217 patients given 0.3 mg/kg of midazolam. The metabolism of midazolam in man involves hydroxylation by hepatic microsomal enzymes and subsequent conjugation with glucuronic acid before renal excretion. The hydroxy metabolites of midazolam have sedative properties although their contribution to the overall clinical effects of midazolam is not established nor is their relative potency or precise duration of effect.

Flumazenil (Anexate or RO15–1788)

This is a synthetic imidazodiazepine that is a specific benzodiazepine receptor antagonist. It antagonizes the behavioural and the CNS electrophysiological effects of benzodiazepines with recovery to full orientation. The potential dangers of its use include the precipitation of convulsions in epileptics and withdrawal symptoms in patients dependent on benzodiazepines. There is also the risk of re-sedation following antagonism of midazolam sedation owing to its short elimination half-life (0.9 ± 0.2 h). There has been limited experience with the use of flumazenil in reversing midazolam sedation in the critically ill. From the sparse clinical data available, a prolonged infusion of flumazenil for several hours may be required before spontaneous wakefulness may be maintained.[80] The rapid reversal of midazolam sedation by flumazenil in patients with severe head injuries increases the intracranial pressure and may lead to dangerous decreases in cerebral perfusion pressure.[81]

Inhalational Agents

Nitrous oxide

The useful sedative properties of nitrous oxide were recognized as long ago as the early 1950s, when this gas was used to sedate paralysed patients with severe tetanus who required long-term mechanical ventilation. Although nitrous oxide is, in many ways, an ideal agent for the sedation of mechanically ventilated patients, it interferes with the metabolism of vitamin B_{12} causing bone-marrow depression and other toxic effects (see Chapter 2).

Isoflurane

The physicochemical properties of isoflurane suggest that it would approximate very closely to the ideal sedative agent. Its low blood solubility facilitates control of anaesthetic depth (and possibly depth of sedation), and ensures rapid recovery from anaesthesia. Isoflurane is minimally metabolized (0.2%) and therefore nephrotoxicity and hepatotoxicity are extremely unlikely. The elimination of isoflurane is independent of normal renal or hepatic function — a highly desirable property of a sedative drug for use in the critically ill patient. Kong and Willatts[82] have shown that isoflurane is a useful agent for sedating ventilated patients in the intensive care unit. When compared with midazolam, isoflurane produces satisfactory sedation for a greater proportion of time with a more rapid recovery. Results to date demonstrate that isoflurane sedation for up to 24 h has no adverse effects on hepatic, renal and adrenocortical function.

CONCLUSION

Uncontrolled sedation can be dangerous, particularly where there is only one practitioner present. Patients should always have a full history taken, asking particularly about evidence of previous adverse reactions to drugs and about allergies. A clinical examination will alert the operator to other potential complications but nevertheless there is wide variation in patient response to sedatives. As more surgery is performed on a day-case basis with techniques that include sedation, assessment of recovery is of great importance. Wherever sedation is practised, someone skilled in management of the unconscious patient and all aspects of resuscitation must be immediately available.

REFERENCES

1. Macnab M S P, Macrae D J, Guy E, Grant I S, Feely J 1986 Profound reduction in morphine clearance and liver blood flow in shock. Intensive Care Medicine 12: 366–369
2. Samuel I O, Morrison J D, Dundee J W 1980 Central haemodynamic and forearm vascular effects of morphine in patients after open heart surgery. British Journal of Anaesthesia 52: 1237
3. Finck A D, Berkowitz B A, Hempstead J, Ngai S H 1977 Pharmacokinetics of morphine: effects of hypercarbia on serum and brain morphine concentrations in the dog. Anesthesiology 47: 407–410
4. Green D W 1981 Severe cardiovascular collapse following phenoperidine. Anaesthesia 36: 617
5. Grummitt R M, Goat V A 1984 Intracranial pressure after phenoperidine. Anaesthesia 39: 565
6. Yate P M, Thomas D, Short S M, et al. 1986 Comparison of infusions of alfentanil or pethidine for sedation of ventilated patients on the ITU. British Journal of Anaesthesia 58: 1091–1099
7. Fellows I W, Bastow M D, Byrne A J, Allison S P 1983 Adrenocortical suppression in multiply injured patients: a complication of etomidate treatment. British Medical Journal 287: 1835
8. Belopavlovic M, Buchtal A 1980 Barbiturate therapy in the management of cerebral ischaemia. Anaesthesia 35: 271
9. Michenfelder J D 1982 Barbiturates for brain resuscitation: yes and no. Anesthesiology 57: 74–5
10. Ward J D, Becker D P, Miller J D, 1985 Failure of prophylactic barbiturate coma in the treatment of severe head injury. Journal of Neurosurgery 62: 383–388
11. McDonald C F, Thomson S A, Scott N C, Scott W, 1986 Benzodiazepine-opiate antagonism — a problem of intensive-care therapy. Intensive Care Medicine 12: 39–42
12. Korttila K, Tarkkanen L, Aittimaki J, Hyoyt P 1981 The influence of intramuscularly administered pethidine on the amnesic effects of intravenous diazepam during intravenous regional anaesthesia. Acta Anaesthesiologica Scandinavica 25: 323–327
13. Alon E, Baitella L, Hossli G 1987 Double blind study of the reversal of midazolam-supplemented general anaesthesia with Ro15-1788. British Journal of Anaesthesia 59: 455–458
14. Sage D J, Close A, Boas R A 1987 Reversal of midazolam sedation with anexate. British Journal of Anaesthesia 59: 459–464
15. Rodrigo M R C, Rosenquist J B 1987 The effect of RO 15-1788 (Anexate) on conscious sedation produced with midazolam. Anaesthesia and Intensive Care 15: 185–192
16. Arvidsson S, Niemand D, Martinall S, Ekstrom-Jodal B 1984 Aminophylline reversal of diazepam sedation. Anaesthesia 39: 806–809
17. Scott D B, Beamish D, Hudson I N, Jostell K-G 1980 Prolonged infusion of chlormethiazole in intensive care. British Journal of Anaesthesia 52: 541–545
18. Nunn J F, Sharer N M, Gorchein A, Jones J A 1982 Megaloblastic haemopoiesis after multiple short-term exposure to nitrous oxide. Lancet 1: 1379
19. Sharer N M, Nunn J F, Royston J P, Chanarin I 1983 Effects of chronic exposure to nitrous oxide on methionine synthase activity. British Journal of Anaesthesia 55: 693
20. Herregods L, Mortier E, Donadoni R, Rolly G 1987 A comparison of midazolam and diazepam for sedation during locoregional anaesthesia. Acta Anaesthesiologica Belgica 38: 97–102
21. Ong B Y, Pickering B G, Palahniuk R J, Cumming M 1982 Lorazepam and diazepam as adjuncts to epidural anaesthesia for caesarian section. Canadian Anaesthetist Society Journal 29: 31–34
22. Riefkohl R, Kosanin R 1984 Experience with triazolam as a pre-operative sedative for out-patient surgery under local anaesthesia. Anaesthesia and Plastic Surgery 8: 155–157
23. Scamman F L, Klein S L, Choi W W 1985 Conscious sedation for procedures under local or topical anaesthesia. Annals of Otology, Rhinology and Laryngology 94: 21–24
24. Tucker M R, Hann J R, Phillips C L 1984 Subanaesthetic doses of ketamine, diazepam and nitrous oxide for adult outpatient sedation. Journal of Oral and Maxillofacial Surgery 42: 668–672
25. Vinnik C A 1981 An intravenous dissociation technique for outpatient plastic surgery: tranquility in the office surgical facility. Plastic and Reconstructive Surgery 67: 799–805
26. Korttila K, Levanen J 1978 Untoward effects of ketamine combined with diazepam for supplementing conduction anaesthesia in young and middle-aged adults. Acta Anaesthesiologica Scandinavica 22: 640–648

27. Marley J E, Ward S 1980 Chlormethiazole as sleep cover for the elderly. Intravenous infusion during local anaesthesia. Anaesthesia 35: 386–390
28. Seow L T, Mather L E, Cousins M J 1985 Comparison of the efficacy of chlormethiazole and diazepam as iv sedatives for supplementation of extradural anaesthesia. British Journal of Anaesthesia 57: 747–752
29. Sinclair C J, Fagan D, Scott D B 1985 Cardiovascular effects of chlormethiazole infusion in combination with extradural anaesthesia. British Journal of Anaesthesia 57: 587–590
30. Mackenzie N, Grant I S 1985 Comparison of propofol with methohexitone in the provision of anaesthesia for surgery under regional blockade. British Journal of Anaesthesia 57: 1167–1172
31. Abel M 1987 Respiratory failure in a newborn infant following repeated sedation for computerized tomography. Klinische Padiatrie 199: 52–54
32. Strain J D, Harvey L A, Foley L C, Campbell J B 1986 Intravenously administered pentobarbital sodium for sedation in paediatric CT. Radiology 161: 105–108
33. White T J, Siegel R L, Burckhart G J, Ramey D R 1979 Rectal thiopentone for sedation of children for computed tomography. Journal of Computer-Assisted Tomography 3: 286–288
34. Stanley T V 1985 Chlormethiazole: an effective oral sedative for cranial CT scans in children. Australian Paediatric Journal 21: 191–192
35. Walters F J M 1987 Anaesthesia for neuroradiology. British Journal of Hospital Medicine 38: 351–356
36. Spargo P M, Howard W V, Saunders D A 1985 Sedation and cerebral angiography. The effects of pentazocine and midazolam on arterial carbon dioxide tension. Anaesthesia 40: 901–903
37. Erwin D, Pick M J, Taylor G W 1980 Anaesthesia for carotid artery surgery. Anaesthesia 35: 246–249
38. Bleyer W A, Skinner A L 1976 Fatal neonatal haemorrhage after maternal anticonvulsant therapy. Journal of the American Medical Association 235: 626–627
39. Rowlatt R J 1978 Effect of maternal diazepam on the newborn. British Medical Journal 1: 985
40. Cree J E, Meyer J, Hailey B M 1973 Diazepam in labour: its metabolism and effect on the clinical condition and thermogenesis of the newborn. British Medical Journal 4: 251–255
41. Johnson R A 1976 Adverse neonatal reaction to maternal administration of chlormethiazole and diazoxide. British Medical Journal 1: 943
42. Allen J, Maigaard S, Christensen F, Andreasen F 1987 Effects of thiopentone or chlormethiazole on human placental stem villous arteries. British Journal of Anaesthesia 59: 1273–1277
43. Slater R M, Wilcox F L, Smith W D, Donnai P 1987 Phenytoin infusion in severe pre-eclampsia. Lancet 1: 1417–1421
44. Shane S M 1982 Conscious sedation and behavioural modification with local standby anaesthesia for ophthalmological surgery. Ophthalmic Surgery 13: 50–52
45. Gilbert J, Holt J E, Johnston J, Sabo B A, Weaver J S 1987 Intravenous sedation for cataract surgery. Anaesthesia 42: 1063–69
46. Vindhya P K, Sheets J H, Tolia N H, Tomlinson L J 1987 Retrobulbar block using pentothal as a sedative for ambulatory cataract surgery. Journal of Cataract and Refractive Surgery 13: 321–322
47. Kemp F M, Broadway E S 1986 Use of general anaesthesia and sedation in the general dental service in East Anglia. British Dental Journal 161: 364–366
48. Wylie W D (Chairman) 1978 Report of the Working Party on Training in Dental Anaesthesia. London: Royal College of Surgeons of England
49. Seward G R (Chairman) 1981 Inter-Faculty Working Party Considering the Implementation of the Wylie Report. London: Royal College of Surgeons of England
50. Aun C, Flynn P J, Richards J, Major E 1984 A comparison of midazolam and diazepam for intravenous sedation in dentistry. Anaesthesia 139: 589–593
51. Dixon R A, Kenyon C, Marsh D R G, Thornton J A 1986 Midazolam in conservative dentistry. A cross over trial. Anaesthesia 41: 276–281
52. O'Boyle C A, Harris D, Barry H 1987 Comparison of midazolam by mouth and diazepam iv in outpatient oral surgery. British Journal of Anaesthesia 59: 746–754
53. Hosie H E, Brook I M 1987 Oral sedation with temazepam: a practical alternative for use in dentistry? British Dental Journal 162: 190–193
54. Lindsay S J E, Yates J A 1985 The effectiveness of oral diazepam in anxious child dental patients. British Dental Journal 159: 149–153
55. Corall I M, Strunin L, Ward M E, 1979 Sedation for outpatient conservative dentistry: a trial of pentazocine supplementation to diazepam and local anaesthetic techniques. Anaesthesia 34: 855–858
56. Langa H 1968 Relative Analgesia in Dental Practice: Inhalation Analgesia with Nitrous Oxide, Ch. 3. W B Saunders, Philadelphia, pp. 34–56
57. Edmunds D H, Rosen M 1984 Inhalation sedation with 25% nitrous oxide: report of a field trial. Anaesthesia 39: 138–142

58. Sweeney B, Bingham R M, Amos R 1985 Toxicity of bone marrow in dentists exposed to nitrous oxide. British Medical Journal 291: 567–569
59. Parbrook G D, James J, Braid D P 1987 Inhalational sedation with isoflurane: an alternative to nitrous oxide sedation in dentistry. British Dental Journal 163: 88–92
60. O'Higgins J 1988 The anaesthetist and paediatric cardiac catheterization. British Journal of Hospital Medicine 40: 58–63
61. Hoare A M, Hawkins C F 1976 Upper gastrointestinal endoscopy with and without sedation: patients' opinions. British Medical Journal 2: 20
62. Whitwam J G, Al-Khudhairi D, McCloy R F 1983 Comparison of midazolam and diazepam in doses of comparable potency during gastroscopy. British Journal of Anaesthesia 55: 773–777
63. Douglas J G, Nimmo W S, Wanless R, 1980 Sedation for upper gastrointestinal endoscopy. A comparison of oral temazepam and i.v. diazepam. British Journal of Anaesthesia 52: 811–815
64. Boldy D A R, English J S C, Lang G S, Hoare A M 1984 Sedation for endoscopy: a comparison between diazepam and diazepam plus pethidine with naloxone reversal. British Journal of Anaesthesia 56: 1109–1112
65. Editorial 1976 Sedation for minor procedures. Drugs and Therapeutics Bulletin 14: 19
66. Sury M R J, Cole P V 1988 Nalbuphine combined with midazolam for outpatient sedation. An assessment in fibreoptic bronchoscopy patients. Anaesthesia 43: 285–288
67. Bion J F, Ledingham IMcA 1987 Sedation in intensive care — a postal survey. Intensive Care Medicine 13: 215–216
68. Ramsay M A E, Savege T M, Simpson B R I, Goodwin R 1974 Controlled sedation with alphaxolone-alphadolone. British Medical Journal 2: 656–658
69. Evans J M, Bithell J F and Vlachonikolis I G 1987 Relationship between lower oesophageal contractility, clinical signs and halothane concentration during general anaesthesia and surgery in man. British Journal of Anaesthesia 59: 1346–1355
70. Tubaro E, Borelli G, Croce C, Cavallo G, Santiangeli C. 1983 Effect of morphine on resistance to infection. Journal of Infectious Diseases 148: 656–666
71. Osborne R J, Joel S P, Slevin M L 1986 Morphine intoxication in renal failure: the role of morphine-6-glucuronide. British Medical Journal 292: 1548–1549
72. Bingham R M, Hinds C J 1987 Influence of bolus doses of phenoperidine on intracranial pressure and systemic arterial pressure in traumatic coma. British Journal of Anaesthesia 59: 592–595
73. Cohen A T, Kelly D R 1987 Assessment of alfentanil by intravenous infusion as long-term sedation in intensive care. Anaesthesia 42: 545–548
74. Park G R, Manara A R, Mendel L, Bareman P E 1987 Ketamine infusion. Its use as a sedative, inotrope and bronchodilator in a critically ill patient. Anaesthesia 42: 980–983
75. Newman L H, McDonald J C, Wallace P G M, Ledingham I McA 1987 Propofol infusion for sedation in intensive care. Anaesthesia 42: 929–937
76. Grounds R M, Lalor J M, Lumley J, Royston D, Morgan M 1987 Propofol infusion for sedation in the intensive care unit: preliminary report. British Medical Journal 294: 397–400
77. Aitkenhead A R, Pepperman M P, Willatts S M, Coates D P et al 1989 A randomized prospective comparison between propofol and midazolam for 24 hours sedation in the intensive care unit, in preparation
78. Westphal L M, Cheng E Y, White P F 1987 Use of midazolam infusion for sedation following cardiac surgery. Anesthesiology 67: 257–262
79. Dundee J W, Collier P S, Carlisle R J T, Harper K W 1986 Prolonged midazolam elimination half-life. British Journal of Clinical Pharmacology 21: 425–429
80. Geller E, Halpern P, Leykin Y 1986 Midazolam infusion and benzodiazepine antagonist for sedation in ICU — a preliminary report. Anesthesiology 65: A65
81. Chiolero R L, Ravussin P, Anderes J P de Tribolet N, Freeman J 1986 Midazolam reversal with RO15-1788 in patients with severe head injury. Anesthesiology 65: A358
82. Kong K L, Willatts S M 1988 Isoflurane for sedation of ventilated patients in intensive care. Clinical Pharmacology and Therapeutics 43: 142

6. Fluid therapy

K. Hillman

Recent advances in the field of fluid therapy have probably not been as spectacular as in other areas of anaesthesia. Advances in this area have had a much lower profile than, for example, new anaesthetic drugs and patient monitoring. There are possible explanations for this neglect. Firstly, there do not appear to be many problems associated with our current way of giving fluids in the peri-operative period — a bottle or two of crystalloid solution running in the background during an operation is usually sufficient. A bolus of a few hundred millilitres may be necessary in the face of a falling arterial pressure, and 2–3 litres of a salt-containing solution is usually adequate in the postoperative period until the patient can tolerate oral fluids. While the impression remains that there are few problems with this approach there appears to be little impetus for change. Moreover, fluids are not confined to any particular organ in an era of increasing specialization where motivation for research is largely generated from within these organ-based specialities. Finally, and perhaps cynically, there are very few new and expensive fluids being used on a widespread basis, making private funding for research in these days of financial stringency, difficult.

Nevertheless, there have been advances in our approach to fluid therapy, particularly the monitoring of fluid administration. Assessment and monitoring of the body fluid status can now be performed more accurately. There is an increased range of blood products and colloids available and much more about the dangers of overexpansion of the interstitial space (ISS) is known. With an increased awareness of basic physiology and knowledge of the dangers of poor fluid therapy, a more rational approach is being employed. New drugs and procedures, such as haemofiltration, make manipulation of body fluid spaces possible. Complex fluid problems, such as those accompanying septicaemia and extensive gastrointestinal losses, require a more logical approach based on sound physiological principles and recent advances in drugs and technology.

ASSESSMENT OF BODY WATER

Rationale fluid therapy is based on the accurate estimation of the body fluid status. Body water compromises approximately 40 l in a 70 kg adult.[1] The fluid is distributed into three spaces: the intravascular space (IVS); the ISS; and the intracellular space (ICS) (Fig. 6.1). The IVS and ICS are commonly classified as extracellular fluid (ECF). While the ECF contains a similar concentration of water and electrolytes as the fluid in the IVS, there is a vast difference in the composition and function between the IVS and ISS. Circulating fluid in the IVS contains protein molecules that, because they are largely contained within that space by the capillary endothelial cells, exert a colloid oncotic pressure (COP) relative to the ISS. This tends to cause water to move

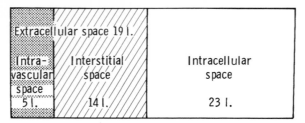

Fig. 6.1   Body fluid compartments representing the approximate volume of the bodies three fluid compartments in an average 70 kg male. (From Twigley and Hillman,[30] with permission from Academic Press Inc. (London) Ltd.)

from the ISS to IVS and, according to Starling's hypothesis, is counteracted by the hydrostatic pressure exerted within small vessels, causing fluid to move from the IVS to ISS. The predominant cation in the ECF is sodium and the predominant cation in the ICS is potassium. The nature of cell membranes and the sodium/potassium pump ensure that this distribution is maintained.

The circulating volume is readily amenable to clinical estimation (Table 6.1). Measurements such as pulse rate, blood pressure, peripheral perfusion, urine output, central venous pressure (CVP), pulmonary artery wedge pressure (PAWP) and cardiac output (CO) all indirectly indicate the volume of the IVS. In the clinical setting a fluid challenge of 200–300 ml is given before and after measuring as many of these variables as possible in order to estimate the adequacy of the circulating volume.[2] Although the volume of the IVS is only about 5 l, it is the space that is most amenable to volume estimation. The remaining 35 litres of fluid in the ISS and ICS is far more difficult to estimate. Guidelines such as tissue turgor, dryness of mucosa, serum sodium, clinical history, fluid balance charts and chest X-ray are used to estimate the ISS and ICS. Some of the shortcomings and strengths of body fluid measurements will now be discussed.

Intravascular space

Pulse rate
The pulse rate, under the influence of the autonomic nervous system and circulating catecholamines, rises with hypovolaemia. A pulse rate of over 100 beats/min correlates well with significant intra-operative bleeding.[3] This is most evident in fit, young, bleeding patients. Drugs such as anaesthetic agents, beta-adrenoceptor blocking drugs and inotropes, as well as light anaesthesia and underlying cardiac disease, can all cause bradyarrhythmias and tachyarrhythmias, which can also influence heart rate. Nevertheless, pulse rate is normally a simple and reliable guide to blood loss.

Blood pressure
As well as producing hydraulic changes within the cardiovascular system, hypovolaemia stimulates pressure receptors; through a neuro-endocrine response this causes an increase in stroke volume, heart rate and systemic vascular resistance, all of which help to maintain blood pressure.[4] The reflex is strongest in young patients who notoriously maintain blood pressure in the face of extreme hypovolaemia. However, under the effects of anaesthesia and in older patients, hypotension occurs with smaller fluid losses. Hypotension tends to track hypovolaemia in these circumstances.

Table 6.1   Assessment of intravascular volume (From Hillman,[38] with permission.)

Direct measurement
   Isotopic dilution technique

Indirect measurement

Vascular pressure	Central venous pressure	(CVP)
	Pulmonary artery wedge pressure	(PAWP)
	Arterial blood pressure	(BP)
	Dynamic mean systemic filling pressure	
Blood flow	Cardiac output	
Organ blood flow		
Brain	Decreased level of consciousness	
Kidney	Oliguria	
Skin	Decreased peripheral temperature	
	Doppler flow measurement	
	Transcutaneous partial pressure of oxygen ($PtcO_2$)	
Heart rate		
Haematocrit		

Peripheral perfusion

Peripheral perfusion decreases with hypovolaemia owing to decreased flow as a result of neuro-endocrine responses and reduced circulating blood volume. There is a crude but reliable relationship between the degree of hypovolaemia and the degree of peripheral shutdown.[3] The simultaneous measurement of core and peripheral skin temperature is a guide to the degree of peripheral shutdown. This can be quantified in a slightly more accurate fashion by measuring skin blood flow using the Doppler technique.[5,6] Alternatively, transcutaneous measurement of tissue oxygen tension ($PtcO_2$) tracks peripheral cardiovascular impairment when oxygenation is normal.[7]

Central venous pressure

Central venous pressure (CVP) is a time-honoured method for estimating the circulating volume. Normal CVP values are quoted as being anywhere between 4 and 17 cmH$_2$O. It is sobering to note that this may also be the normal range of pressures in a circulation that has come to a standstill. So- called 'normal values' can be associated with normal, increased or reduced blood volumes.[3,8,9] In life, the CVP is a reflection of the ability of the right heart to cope with venous return at the moment of measurement. Many factors apart from blood volume will affect it. These include the tone of the venous walls, raised pulmonary artery pressure secondary to pulmonary pathology, right ventricular compliance, atrial compliance, tricuspid valve function, as well as factors affecting intrathoracic pressure such as intermittent positive pressure ventilation (IPPV) and positive end-expiratory pressure (PEEP). For example, under conditions of high sympathetic tone as may exist in hypovolaemia, the CVP could rise.[10] The infusion of fluid in these circumstances may paradoxically decrease the CVP.[11] At best, CVP measurements are a guide to blood volume when used in association with a fluid challenge and in conjunction with other indicators of the IVS. Even in these circumstances the CVP measurements should be cautiously interpreted during resuscitation from severe haemorrhage.

Dynamic mean filling pressure

The concept of a 'normal' blood volume is only relevant when considered in the light of the size of the vascular tree in which it is contained. In order to take into account the influence of blood volume upon cardiovascular dynamics the compliance of the vessel walls must also be considered. The concept of mean circulatory filling pressure, developed by Guyton, Polizo and Armstrong,[12] describes the relationship between blood volume and circulatory compliance. Its clinical usefulness is limited by the fact that circulation must be allowed to come to static equilibrium by stopping the heart. Using mathematical modelling,[13,14] readily available cardiovascular measurements (CO, mean blood pressure and right atrial pressure) as well as height, weight and age, a similar estimate of intravascular volume requirements has been developed — the dynamic mean systemic filling pressure.[14] As well as a useful physiological concept, this measurement may help to overcome the shortcomings of other pressure readings within the circulation.

Urine output

The hourly urine output is a reflection of blood volume. During hypovolaemia there is a decrease and an internal redistribution of renal blood flow. Like other estimates of the IVS it is subject to other factors such as underlying renal disease and drugs such as diuretics, anaesthetic agents and inotropes. Increased intrathoracic pressure can result in a marked decrease in renal blood flow probably because of decreased renal venous pressure and decreased arterial supply as a result of decreased CO.[15] Ideally PEEP levels and the peak inspiratory pressure therefore should be reduced during controlled mechanical ventilation and, where possible, a ventilatory mode using spontaneous breathing such as intermittent mandatory ventilation (IMV) or continuous positive airways pressure (CPAP) should be employed.

Increased intra-abdominal pressure can also reduce urine output.[16] All postoperative patients with suspected raised intra-abdominal pressure as a result of ileus, ascites or bleeding should probably have their intravesical pressure monitored as a reflection of intra-abdominal pressure. This is easily performed by: connecting a CVP manometer recording set into the urinary catheter via a needle or cannula; running in 50 ml of sterile isotonic saline; clamping the urinary catheter distal to the measuring line; and recording the pressure from the level of the pubic symphysis. The intravesicle pressure measured with this technique correlates well with intra-abdominal pressure.[16] With pressures of 25–30 cm H_2O, oliguria supervenes, and above 30 cm H_2O renal failure and anuria becomes inevitable. Where possible, surgery may be indicated to reduce the intra-abdominal pressure.[16]

Haematocrit

Like other estimates of IVS, the haematocrit is influenced by many factors other than blood volume. The haematocrit will, of course, be normal after severe acute blood loss. Following blood loss the haematocrit will decrease depending on the extent of sequestration of fluid from the ISS and on how much clear fluid has been used to resuscitate the patient. The blood volume may, in fact, be normal while the haematrocrit is extremely low. Thus, the haematocrit is a crude and indirect estimate of blood volume but a very useful measurement of red blood cell loss. Similar shortcomings exist in techniques that rely on mass density measurements as a way of monitoring blood volume.[17] The mass density relies on plasma/red blood cell fractions and is therefore subject to the same limitations as haematocrit measurements.

Direct measurement of blood loss

Intra-operative estimation of blood volume is helped by the fact that blood loss is very amenable to direct measurement. Swab weighing and suction bottle measurements are the most common techniques employed. Indicator dilution methods are less frequently used. The latter technique uses swabs and drapes washed in a known volume of solvent and an amount of indicator whose concentration in the patient's undiluted blood is known. The indicator is measured in the resulting solution and estimates of blood loss made. The same principle is used for determining the volume of irrigating fluid.

The pulmonary artery catheter

The introduction of the pulmonary artery catheter by Swan et al[18] quickly led to its widespread use in anaesthesia and intensive care. At one time, to 'Ganz' somebody or to put a 'Swan' in became almost synonymous with an anaesthetist's 'standing' among his colleagues and associated with macho inferences of clinical 'oneupmanship'. There was an implication that the number of catheterizations per annum correlated with the clinical standing of a department. After nearly 20 years of clinical usage and despite billions of dollars being spent on the device, there is almost no evidence that it has made any difference to mortality. In fact, the only two studies that have looked scientifically at this issue have shown no benefit associated with the use of the catheter.[19,20] This has prompted caution about the use of the pulmonary artery catheter in several recent editorials.[21-23]

Not only has it not been shown to decrease mortality, but it may have contributed to a significantly increased mortality.[23] Therefore one must carefully weigh the risks of its usage against potential benefits during anaesthesia. The benefits are clouded by challenges to basic beliefs such as the validity of Starling's Law of the heart[24] and the meaning of derived values such as systemic vascular resistance[25] and pulmonary vascular resistance.[26] Even direct measurements such as pulmonary artery wedge pressure (PAWP) and cardiac output (CO) are very difficult to interpret.[27]

Pulmonary artery wedge pressure

The PAWP is meant to be a reflection of left ventricular end diastolic volume (LVEDV) and thus an indicator of the preload of the heart, which, in turn, estimates blood volume. Apart from the disadvantages of the pulmonary artery catheter already discussed, there are many assumptions and physiological traps in the relationship between PAWP and blood volume. The many steps in assuming that PAWP reflects left atrial pressure (LAP), left ventricular end diastolic pressure (LVEDP) and LVEDV have recently been challenged.[28] In the clinical situation, there is often a poor correlation between changes in blood volume and PAWP.[8,9] The exact role of PAWP in anaesthesia has not been established. There is little place for its use in acute fluid resuscitation and caution must be exercised, even in fine tuning the circulation, to prevent pulmonary oedema.[29] It could be that, like the CVP, it is best used together with other indicators of blood volume during a fluid challenge.

Cardiac output

The CO can be measured by the thermodilution technique using a pulmonary artery catheter. Its relevance in anaesthesia is probably limited. There are less invasive and equally useful indicators of pre-operative cardiac function. There is almost no role for CO determinations as an estimate of intra-operative blood volume as it is not accurately correlated with it.[9] Because of the poor correlation of blood volume with CO its use in resuscitation is also limited. It may have a place for fine tuning the blood volume in conjunction with other measurements and as part of a fluid challenge.

Interstitial and intracellular space

Although the ISS has traditionally been associated with the IVS and considered part of the ECF, it is more appropriate, in terms of clinical assessment, to consider the ISS and ICS together. While there are many shortcomings in estimating the relatively small IVS volume, clinical assessment of the ISS and ICS remain even more difficult.[30] It is important to remember the relative shortcomings of body fluid assessment when prescribing fluids to replenish any fluid compartments.

History

Any pre-operative assessment includes a history of fluid losses. These would include excessive gastrointestinal tract losses, an ileus, lack of oral intake, presence of a fever, and so on. A knowledge of the composition of body fluids is essential to understand from which compartment the fluid may have come. For example, bile and pancreatic fluid has a sodium concentration similar to the ECF; the loss therefore would be mainly from the ISS and only partly from the IVS. Fluid from excessive sweating and other forms of insensible loss contains little sodium, thus the fluid loss would be mainly from the cells with losses from the ISS and IVS proportional to the sodium concentration. Thirst is a non-specific finding indicating water depletion, an increased osmolar load or acute intravascular volume depletion.[31]

Fluid balance charts

Nursing staff spend an enormous amount of time and effort on keeping accurate fluid balance records. The charts have historically been an integral part of peri-operative management. Unfortunately they are sometimes interpreted on the basis of single 'in' and 'out' figures. What comes out does not necessarily have anything to do with what goes in, and vice versa. Even in the normal basal resting state, there are more unrecordable 'outs' and 'ins' than recordable ones.[32] The unrecordable fluid gains and losses include water of oxidation, insensible losses, as well as intestinal and wound sequestration. At best, fluid balance charts are a rough estimate of major losses and gains and certainly not accurate enough to deserve attempts to computerize their information.

Skin turgor

Skin turgor supposedly correlates with total body water (TBW). Whether it is fluid in the ISS or the ICS that is pinched between the forefinger and thumb, is, of course, impossible to say. The range of normal skin turgor is extensive — especially with age. The skin of a newborn is very elastic compared with that of the elderly mainly because of the higher percentage of water in the newborn.[33] Extremes of turgor, such as with dehydration and peripheral oedema, are clinically relevant signs but tissue turgor is an otherwise crude and probably meaningless estimate of ISS or ICS, or both. Similarly, the presence of dry mucous membranes is a non-specific finding that may indicate TBW deficit.[34]

Chest X-ray
Extravascular lung water (EVLW) probably representing the ISS of the lung correlates reasonably well with the degree of opacification of the chest X-ray.[35] However, the origin of the EVLW cannot always be determined on the chest X-ray. Thus, the EVLW may be related to cardiogenic or non-cardiogenic pulmonary oedema. Moreover, it is often difficult to distinguish EVLW from other respiratory pathology on chest X-ray appearance alone. The chest X-ray is also extremely useful for determining intravascular volume. The width of the large systemic vessels that form most of the upper mediastinal density on chest X-ray correlates strongly with the volume of the IVS.[36]

Serium sodium
Assuming blood glucose is normal, the determinants of serum sodium (Nas) are the exchangeable stores of sodium (Nae), the exchangeable stores of potassium (Ke) and the TWB.[37]

$$\text{Na}s \propto \frac{\text{Na}e + \text{K}e}{\text{TBW}}$$

The most clinically significant of these is the TBW. The serum sodium is inversely proportional to body water. Most sodium disturbances in the clinical situation are related to excessive or diminished water rather than sodium deficiency or excess. Serum sodium is the most important clinical determinant of TBW status.[38]

Measurement of interstitial space pressure
When giving a fluid such as isotonic saline or Ringer's lactate, which is distributed mainly to the ISS, it is more logical to measure the pressure in that space rather than IVS pressures. This can be achieved by using an implantable capsule that has been allowed to equilibrate with the ISS[39] or by a wick directly implanted in the ISS.[40] These techniques are mainly experimental with, as yet, little widespread application in clinical practice. The closest estimate in widespread clinical use is tissue turgor with all of its shortcomings.

PRINCIPLES OF FLUID REPLACEMENT

We have to acknowledge and live with the shortcomings in measurements of body fluid compartments. This is because when we choose a particular fluid and administer a certain amount, that decision is based on our clinical assessment of the three body spaces.

Non-ionic solutions
Water, which has a solute able to be metabolized and usually added to achieve iso-osmolality, is distributed proportionately over the three body spaces. Examples include

Table 6.2   Composition of commonly used IV solutions (From Hillman,[38] with permission.)

	Na (mmol/l)	K (mmol/l)	Ca (mmol/l)	Mg (mmol/l)	Cl (mmol/l)	Lactate (mmol/l)	Dextrose (g/100 ml)	pH	Osmolality (mmol)
0.9% Saline	154	—	—	—	154	—	—	5.0	308
0.4% Saline	77	—	—	—	77	—	—	5.2	154
Hartmann's solution (Ringer's lactate)	131	5	1	1	112	29	—	6.5	280
4.3% Dextrose in 0.18% NaCl	31	—	—	—	31	—	43	4.0	300
5.0% Dextrose	—	—	—	—	—	—	50	4.0	278
2.5% Dextrose in 0.45% NaCl	75	—	—	—	75	—	25	4.0	280
3.75% Dextrose in 0.225% NaCl	37.5	—	—	—	37.5	—	37.5	4.0	280

the dextrose-containing solutions and amino-acid solutions. A very small percentage of these solutions will be distributed to the IVS, while most will be distributed to the ICS and a smaller volume to the ISS. These solutions are rarely used in the intra-operative period because intracellular dehydration is rarely a problem. However, TBW depletion may be considered in patients with long-term fluid problems such as gastrointestinal losses. When necessary, 5% dextrose solution is used to replenish the ICS and is titrated against the serum sodium in the absence of hyperglycaemia or facti-tious hyponatraemia.[14,37] Intracellular dehydration is rarely a life-threatening prob-lem. In fact, unless hypernatraemia is acute, it should be slowly corrected, enabling osmolar gradients between different fluid spaces adequate time to equilibrate.[41] Water loss is often accompanied by intracellular ion losses, such as potassium, magnesium and phosphate. These would have to be regularly measured and replaced during resuscitation.

Sodium-containing solutions
Sodium-containing solutions have been the mainstay of peri-operative fluid therapy (Table 6.2). They are often used for pre-operative resuscitation, intra-operative fluid maintenance and postoperative replacement. The sodium ion is confined mainly to the ECF by the nature of the cell membrane and the sodium/potassium pump. Therefore, depending on the sodium concentration, these fluids will be confined to the ECF. Solutions containing approximately isotonic amounts of sodium such as isotonic saline, Ringer's lactate or Hartmann's solution will be almost entirely confined to the ECF. Because the ISS is approximately three times the size of the IVS, three quarters of administered fluid will be distributed to the ISS and one quarter to the IVS. Thus isotonic saline is more efficient in resuscitating the IVS than 5% dex-trose, where only approximately one-eighth is distributed to the IVS. However, just as 5% dextrose is largely distributed to the ICS, isotonic saline solutions are mainly distributed to the ISS[30] and therefore not as efficient as a colloid in rehydrating the IVS.

As the concentration of sodium in salt-containing solutions is decreased, there is an increasing amount of water available for distribution to the cells. Depending on the sodium concentration, dextrose/saline solutions will be distributed proportionately between the ECF and intracellular fluid. Thus, this type of solution is more suitable for peri-operative fluid replacement than for intravascular resuscitation.

Table 6.3 Physiochemical properties of various colloids (From Sadder & Horsey,[48] with permission.)

Colloid	Mw*	Mn†	Mw/Mn	Colloid (%)	Na⁺ (mmol/l)	Cl⁻ (mmol/l)	K⁺ (mmol/l)	Ca²⁺ (mmol/l)	Citrate (mmol/l)
Succinylated gelatin	35 000	22 600	1.5	4.0	154	125	0.4	0.4	—
Urea-linked gelatin	35 000	24 500	1.4	3.5	145	145	5.1	6.26	—
Dextran 70 in 0.9% NaCl	70 000	39 000	1.9	6.0	154	154	—	—	—
Human albumin solution	69 000	69 000	1.0	4.5	varies	varies	<2	—	4–10
Hydroxyethyl starch 450/0.7	450 000	70 000	6.4	6.0	154	154	—	—	—

*Mw Molecular weight (weight average)
†Mn Molecular weight (number average)

Blood products and colloids

Colloids or plasma substitutes are fluids; and because they contain oncotic particles they are largely confined to the IVS. Blood and blood products such as albumin solutions exert their oncotic pressure through large protein molecules. Artificial colloid solutions contain other large molecules such as gelatins, dextrans or hydroxyethyl starch. All colloid solutions and blood products expand the plasma volume. However, the term 'plasma expander' is usually confined to a solution that has a higher oncotic pressure than blood. Extracellular fluid is thus mobilized from the ISS to the IVS and the plasma volume expands by an amount greater than the infused fluid.

Just as isotonic amounts of sodium confine a fluid to the ECF, iso-oncotic solutions confine fluids to IVS. This makes colloid solutions ideal for replacing intravascular fluid. Measurements such as blood pressure, pulse rate, CVP, urine output, core versus peripheral temperature and PAWP, are all estimates of intravascular volume and should be used to titrate fluids such as colloid or blood, which are largely confined to that space.[42]

Colloids

The first colloids were manufactured from substances such as acacia, gelatin and pectin in the early part of this century[43-45] They gradually fell out of fashion after reports of anaphyloid reactions and other complications. Interest was rekindled during the World War II with increased demand for the fluid resuscitation of battle casualties.

This lead to the development, by the German Army, of a polyvinylpyrrolidone compound, which had such a long half-life that it is probably still circulating in survivors.[46] After the war dextran solutions were developed in Sweden,[47] many new modified gelatin solutions were manufactured[48] and hydroxyethylated derivatives of starch became available.[49]

Modified gelatins. The earlier gelatin solutions would become viscous and gel at low temperatures. To overcome this problem, the gelatin molecules were modified to retain large molecules while avoiding the gel effect at low temperature. During the manufacturing process, the gelatin is exposed to either heat denaturation or chemical hydrolysis and then modified to form larger molecules by linking the molecules using a succinylated method[50] as for 'Gelofusine®' or by using urea-linking[51] as for 'Haemaccel®'. Not only do these solutions have various types of large molecules, but they are also suspended in different solutions (Table 6.3). Over 60% of modified gelatin molecules are excreted in urine but they do not appear to accumulate in the presence of renal failure.[52] Approximately 10% remains in the circulation at 24 h but small amounts may still be detected after a week. Small amounts are metabolized or excreted in faeces. Large amounts can be used for resuscitation[53] since it does not appear to affect haemostasis, cross-matching techniques or renal function.[54] While rapid infusion of Haemaccel® is associated with histamine release,[55] the incidence of allergic reactions[56] is less than 0.146% and reports of life-threatening reactions significantly less than with dextran solutions. Because of the relatively high calcium concentration, the urea-linked gelatin solutions should be avoided in the presence of hypercalcaemia. The relatively short half-life of modified gelatins compared with other solutions can be a disadvantage in that they do not remain in the IVS for so long. However, this property may be used to advantage in the initial resuscitation of acute haemorrhage while blood is being cross-matched.

Dextrans. Dextran is a polysaccharide that is produced by the action of the bacterium, *Leuconostoc messenteroides,* on sucrose.[47] They are classified according to molecular weight. The high molecular weight solutions, dextran 150 and 110 are no longer produced. Dextran 70 (Macrodex®) and dextran 40 (Rheomacrodex®) have an average molecular weight of 70 000 and 40 000 respectively.

Because of the larger molecules and longer intravascular half-life, dextran 70 is more suitable than dextran 40 for fluid resuscitation and is made up in either 0.9% saline or 5% dextrose solution. Approximately 40% of dextran 70 is excreted in the kidneys. The half-life is about 12 h, and after 24 h approximately 30% remains in the plasma and another 30% is found in extravascular fluid.[57]

Since dextran-40 molecules block renal tubules and cause renal failure[58] its use is limited in hypovolaemia. However, rouleaux formation and interference with blood cross-matching techniques are not a problem with currently available dextrans.[54] Nevertheless, the effects of dextrans on haemostasis limit its use to less than 1.5 g/kg every 24 h or approximately 1500 ml. This limits the use of any dextran solution for resuscitation and hypovolaemia, where the upper limits of potential fluid loss are unpredictable. Moreover, dextrans have the highest incidence of serious anaphylactoid reactions,[56] and even when used for prophylaxis against thrombo-embolism, the risk of the treatment can exceed the risk of thrombo-embolism.[59]

Hydroxyetheyl starch. Hydroxyethyl starch (HES) is a molecular polymer manufactured by hydrolysing corn. Currently, there are three commercially available solutions: high molecular weight HES (HES 450/0.7); medium molecular weight HES (HES 200/0.5) and low molecular weight HES (HES 40/0.5). The figures respectively refer to the molecular weight and the degree of molecular substitution (see Table 6.3). The high molecular weight compound (HES 450/0.7) is most commonly used for resuscitation. Because its average particle size (70 000) is similar to albumin it has a longer half-life in plasma than other colloids.[49] Approximately 40% remains in plasma after 24 h and 40% is excreted in urine.[57] While it is mainly the smaller molecules that are lost in the urine, larger ones are slowly hydrolysed by plasma α-amylase and cleared, once their size falls below renal threshhold.[57] About 30% of the dose leaves the IVS and is deposited in the reticulo-endothelial system; mostly the liver and spleen.[57]

Like all colloids, HES is associated with a small frequency of serious anaphylactoid reactions.[56] Hydroxyethyl starch does not appear to influence renal function[60] and, while haemostasis is affected,[57] this does not appear to be clinically significant in the small number of series so far.[61,62]

Blood products
Blood is obviously an ideal replacement fluid for the IVS and is essential in all cases of severe haemorrhage. When the transfusion of red blood cells is not essential, derivatives of blood, based on human albumin and other plasma proteins, can be used. The most commonly used fluid is a solution of fractionated and pasteurized human plasma. It has a protein and electrolyte concentration similar to plasma. The half-life of the protein is reduced by the manufacturing process, but at about 5–10 days is still longer than other colloid solutions.[54] While rare, there have been reports of allergic reactions — probably related to kinin activity, which activates the kallikrein-kinin system.[63,64] Plasma protein solution is free from transmittable disease, has a long shelf-life and is a very efficient fluid for resuscitation of the circulating volume.[65] However, it is more than ten times the cost of other colloids and availability is limited by the number of blood donors.

Artificial blood. Despite more than 20 years of research on this interesting group of compounds, there is still no satisfactory solution for widespread clinical use. Perfluorochemicals, which are capable of carrying oxygen, have been used success-fully in animals[66] — and in clinical practice.[67,68] The perfluorochemicals act both as a colloid and oxygen-carrying solution. Their shortcomings are related to the linear oxygen dissociation curve and poor oxygen carriage unless used in the presence of high oxygen tensions. At a PaO_2 of 73 kPa (550 mmHg), 5.5 ml of oxygen is carried per 100 ml of solution[69] and therefore, in the more physiological range of PaO_2, only minimal amounts of oxygen are carried. Complications such as hypoxia,[70] anaphylac-toid reactions,[71] and possible immune suppression[72] have already been reported. More extensive clinical trials are needed to determine the usefulness and complications of the perfluorochemicals.

COMPLICATIONS OF EXPANSION OF THE INTERSTITIAL SPACE

Since Shires, Williams and Brown's studies,[73] cystalloid solutions have become the mainstay of fluid used in the perioperative period. They demonstrated that the extracellular volume decreased during surgery and suggested it may be as a result of an internal redistribution possibly resulting from wound oedema or an ileus. However, there are many technical difficulties in measuring the volume of the ECF and, while some studies have supported their findings, others have criticized their technique and conclusions.[30] Nevertheless, it is probably true to say that our peri-operative fluid therapy is still based on Shires' original conclusions. It is still common in the intra-operative period to titrate a crystalloid solution, which is essentially distributed to the ISS, against measurements made of the IVS (Fig. 6.2). The expansion of the ISS may be exacerbated by further crystalloid solution being prescribed in the post-operative period in the face of a neuro-endocrine stress response,[74] which results in salt and water retention. Therefore, our peri-operative fluid therapy, while aimed at prevent-ing hypovolaemia and maintaining overall fluid volume usually results in expansion of the ISS.

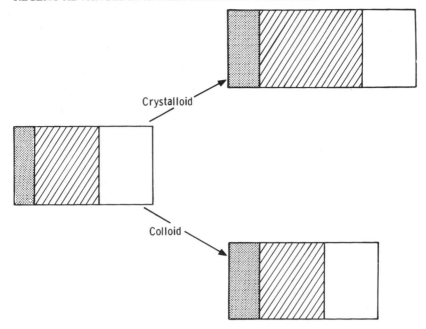

Fig. 6.2   Resuscitation of the correct body space. The dotted area represents the IVS, the striped area the ISS and the plain area, the ICS. The diagram on the left represents a patient with hypovolaemia. When resuscitated with crystalloid (top right), the volume of the IVS can be eventually corrected but with inevitable over-expansion of the ISS. Whereas if a colloid is used for resuscitation it is largely confined to the IVS. (From Twigley and Hillman,[30] with permission from Academic Press Inc (London) Ltd.)

Expansion of the ISS can disrupt lymphatic drainage, which, in turn, can cause excessive accumulation of fluid in the ISS. The removal and concentration of protein in lymphatics reduces the COP in the ISS and facilitates fluid movement into the IVS, helping to create a negative pressure in the ISS.[75] The lymphatic pump itself can contribute to this negative pressure of approximately -6 mmHg. The negative pressure in the ISS is critical for the integrity of cellular architecture, which becomes disrupted in oedematous states. The negative state of the ISS and lymphatic drainage guarantees no excess fluid accumulation, which would otherwise interfere with cellular diffusion and may even result in capillary occlusion. The lymphatics can increase their flow rate by up to 10–50 times the normal. However, once ISS pressure becomes slightly positive, further flow is impeded by distortion of flap valves and collapse of delicate lymph channels by the surrounding fluid.

During simple, uncomplicated anaesthesia, transient increases in the ISS volume and pressure are probably not clinically significant. However, even a relatively small expansion of the ISS may cause complications.

As little as 1 litre of isotonic saline can reduce lung compliance.[76] When crystalloid solutions are used to resuscitate the IVS in major surgery or in the critically ill, significant expansion of the ISS occurs; this can result in overt hypoxia and pulmonary oedema.[77-80]

Increasingly, we are finding that expansion of the ISS in peripheral tissues is no longer simply a theoretical problem. Peripheral oedema can markedly decrease oxygen consumption.[78,81,82] This may be related to the increased distance between cells and capillaries impeding oxygen transport or it may perhaps be the result of occlusion of the thin-walled capillaries by increased ISS pressure. The peripheral oedema is not confined to the skin but is found in many other tissues such as the muscle and the gastrointestinal tract.[83]

Peripheral oedema can also contribute to delayed wound healing. Doubling the volume of the ISS decreases oxygen delivery to such an extent that capillary blood flow needs to be increased by 20-fold to maintain the same oxygen tension.[84] The lowered tissue oxygen levels and oedema are associated with considerable delays in wound healing.[85]

COLLOID VERSUS CRYSTALLOID CONTROVERSY

Much of the controversy surrounding the so-called colloid versus crystalloid controversy is based on the erroneous premise that they are different fluids designed for the same purposes. This is entirely misleading. Crystalloids are distributed over the entire ECF and because the ISS is by far the largest component of the ECF, the fluid is mainly distributed to that space. Whereas colloids, because they contain colloid osmotic molecules, are mainly confined to the IVS. It would, therefore, seem logical that if the IVS is depleted to any great extent, a colloid should be used. Similarly, where the ISS is depleted to any great extent, then a crystalloid should be used. If a crystalloid is titrated against intravascular measurements such as blood pressure and PAWP, then most will be distributed to another compartment that is probably not being monitored. Thus compared with crystalloid solutions, colloids will be more efficient in replacing the IVS.[81] Furthermore, in order to achieve adequate resuscitation when a crystalloid is titrated against measurements of the IVS, there must be an overexpansion of the ISS. This causes increased hypoxia and decreased oxygen consumption when crystalloids are compared with colloids.[78,81,86,87] Whether this matters or not when only small amounts of crystalloid are used to replenish the IVS is debatable. Meticulous use of the most appropriate fluid titrated against relevant end-points becomes increasingly important as greater amounts of fluid are used.[42] The body's own homeostatic mechanisms, including thirst, an intact gastrointestinal tract, normal renal function and adequate clearance by the lymphatics of excessive interstitial fluid, probably prevent significant pulmonary and peripheral oedema from developing in relatively healthy patients requiring small volumes of fluid. However, when any of these mechanisms are compromised and the body can no longer compensate, meticulous attention must then be paid to the right fluid in the right amount.

MANIPULATION OF BODY FLUID SPACES[2]

Our technique is to administer fluid mainly by the intravenous route in the peri-operative period. The fluid is distributed to the three fluid spaces according to the concentration of sodium and oncotic particles. Removing fluid is usually more difficult. Fluid in the IVS is relatively easy to remove by venesection or, more commonly nowadays, by creating a larger intravascular volume with vasodilators, thereby creating a

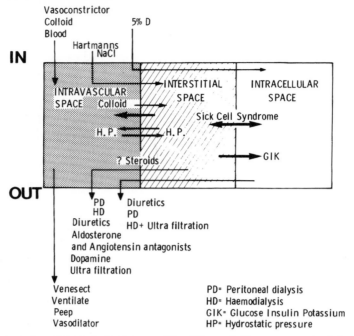

Fig. 6.3 Manipulation of the body fluid spaces. The different fluid compartments of the body and how they can be manipulated. Infused fluids are represented at the top of the diagram and at the bottom are the various techniques used to reduce relative fluid volumes. The various forces that can operate across fluid spaces are represented within the diagram. PD = pertineal dialysis; HD = haemodialysis; HP = hydrostatic pressure; GIK = glucose, insulin and potassium. (From Twigley and Hillman,[30] with permission from Academic Press Inc. (London) Ltd.)

relative hypovolaemia. A similar effect occurs with sympathetic nerve blockade as a result of drugs or spinal and epidural anaesthesia. Similarly, the circulatory tree can be vasoconstricted by drugs such as sympathetic α-adrenergic agonists.

Overexpansion of the ISS and ICS is usually as a result of iatrogenic over-transfusion or renal failure. This can be potentiated by the neuro-endocrine activity associated with the stress response in the peri-operative period or, for example, in disease states such as congestive heart failure and liver failure. Removal of fluid from the ISS and ICS is far more difficult than removal from the IVS.

Initially we restrict salt-containing fluid intake. If the renal excretory mechanism is intact we can use diuretics or aldosterone and angiotensin-antagonizing drugs. This usually encourages salt and water excretion in variable amounts. An osmotic diuretic such as mannitol would cause diuresis of a fluid with the same osmolality as serum and a urinary sodium concentration of approximately 50 mmol/l, whereas a loop diuretic such as frusemide would cause diuresis of a fluid with a very variable electrolyte concentration. Thus, if one wanted to cause excretion of water from a patient with acute hyponatraemia as a result of glycine bladder washouts during a transurethral prostatectomy, an osmotic diuretic to encourage water excretion together with a hypernatraemic solution to replace sodium, would be suitable.

If the renal excretion mechanism is not intact, more invasive techniques for fluid and electrolyte excretion must be employed. These include renal replacement techniques such as haemodialysis and haemofiltration. Haemofiltration is being increasingly used in seriously ill patients, for continuous removal of waste products and for fine tuning fluid therapy. Up to 2–3 l/h of fluid can be removed using a simple extracorporal arteriovenous device with a filter in series.[88] Flow can be facilitated by the same sort of pump used to operate haemodialysis. Newer filters now enable continuous haemodialysis and haemofiltration to be instituted by intensive care staff without any complicated machines or specialized renal nursing staff.[88]

The fluid removed during haemofiltration has almost the same electrolyte composition as ECF. This has added a great deal of flexibility when dealing with complicated fluid and electrolyte problems in the peri-operative patient. For example, seriously ill patients often have hypovolaemia as a result of sepsis or multi-trauma, as well as pulmonary and peripheral oedema either as a result of excessive crystalloid therapy or 'leaky' capillaries. This hypothetical patient clearly requires intravascular volume. The most efficient fluid for this purpose is either colloid or blood, depending on the haemoglobin concentration. This would increase the COP and not only prevent further expansion of the ISS but may help to mobilize some of the interstitial fluid into the IVS. Simultaneously the ISS could be reduced either with diuretic or continuous haemofiltration.

THE CHOICE OF FLUID IN CLINICAL PRACTICE

The principles of fluid replacement should be the same whether the patient is shocked, in the peri-operative period or suffering large fluid losses as a result of an osmotic diuresis or gastrointestinal pathology. The first priority is to rapidly and efficiently correct hypovolaemia.[2,89] Less urgently, water losses from the ICS and ISS should be replaced. The major problem in shock is hypovolaemia not salt and water depletion.[82] As colloids and crystalloid solutions contain fixed amounts of sodium, additional amounts are rarely necessary. Simultaneously, electrolyte losses such as potassium, phosphate, calcium and magnesium should be replaced according to regular measurement.

The rate of replacement of water loss depends on the rate at which it occurred. If it occurred over minutes or hours (e.g. as a result of vomiting and diarrhoea) then it can be rapidly replaced. If the losses occur over days or weeks, it should be corrected slowly.[41,89]

There are many occasions in the peri-operative period where no fluid at all is required. Intravenous access can be achieved with a capped cannula for drug access and for emergency use. Apart from the expense of intravenous fluids and the disadvantages of inappropriate fluid prescribing already outlined, intravenous fluid therapy is associated with a high incidence of morbidity ranging from pain and discomfort to septicaemia.[30] There is also the danger of coagulation being accelerated by saline infusions,[90,91] and the risk of salt-containing solutions increasing the risk of deep venous thrombosis.[92]

With a sound knowledge of the physiology that governs fluid distribution as well as the drugs and techniques that facilitate fluid removal and redistribution, even the most complicated fluid problem can be approached with confidence. On the same basis, greater flexibility in peri-operative fluid regimens can be employed. We need no longer necessarily persist with the rigid approach of 1 litre of crystalloid solution running intra-operatively and 2–3 litres of salt-containing solution postoperatively, until the patient can tolerate oral fluids. However, if we do employ such regimens we must fully understand the reason why we are doing it and what the possible shortcomings and disadvantages are.

ACKNOWLEDGEMENT

The author would like to acknowledge the invaluable assistance of Mrs Sue Williams in preparing this manuscript.

REFERENCES

1. Edelman I S, Leibman J 1959 Anatomy of body water and electrolytes. American Journal of Medicine 27: 256
2. Hillman K 1987 Fluid replacement in the critically ill. Medicine International 2: 1567
3. Irvin T T, Modgill V K, Hayter C J, Goligher J C 1972 Clinical assessment of postoperative blood volume. The Lancet i: 446
4. Cowley A W Jnr., Barber W J, Lombard J H, Osborn J L, Liard J F 1986 Relationship between body fluid volumes and arterial pressure. Federation Proceedings 45: 2864
5. Nilsson G E, Tenland T, Oberg P A 1980 Evaluation of a laser doppler flowmeter for measurement of tissue blood flow. IEEE Transactions on Biomedical Engineering 27: 597
6. Waxman K, Formosa P, Soliman H, Tominaga G, Police A, Hyatt J 1987 Laser doppler velocimetry in critically ill patients. Critical Care Medicine 15: 780
7. Tremper K K, Shoemaker W C 1981 Transcutaneous oxygen monitoring of critically ill adults, with and without low flow stock. Critical Care Medicine 9: 706
8. Baek S M, Makabali G G, Bryan-Brown C W, Kusek J M, Shoemaker W C 1975 Plasma expansion in surgical patients with high central venous pressure (CVP); the relationship of blood volume to haematocrit, CVP, pulmonary wedge pressure and cardiorespiratory changes. Surgery 78: 304
9. Shippy C R, Appel P L, Shoemaker W C 1984 Reliability of clinical monitoring to assess blood volume in critically ill patients. Critical Care Medicine 12: 107
10. Landis E M, Hortenstine J C 1950 The functional significance of venous blood pressure. Physiological Reviews 30: 1
11. Weil M H, Shubin H, Rosoff L 1965 Fluid repletion in circulatory shock. Central venous pressure and other practical guides. Journal of the American Medical Association 192: 668
12. Guyton A C, Polizo D, Armstrong G G 1954 Mean circulatory filling pressure measured immediately after cessation of heart pumping. American Journal of Physiology 179: 261
13. Leaning M S, Pullen H E, Carson E R, Finkelstein L 1983 Modelling a complex biological system: the human cardiovascular system. 1. Methodology and model description. Transactions of the Institute of Measurement Control 5: 71
14. Parkin G 1986 Circulatory disorder: intervention and control. In: Cramp D G, Carson E R (eds) The measurement in medicine series, vol 1. Croom Helm, London, p. 313
15. Steinhoff H H, Kohlhoff R J, Falke K J 1984 Facilitation of renal function by intermittent mandatory ventilation. Intensive Care Medicine 10: 59
16. Richards W O, Scovill W, Shin B, Reed W 1983 Acute renal failure associated with increased intra-abdominal pressure. Annals of Surgery 197: 183
17. Hinghofer-Szalkay H, Greenleaf J E 1987 Continuous monitoring of blood volume changes in humans. Journal of Applied Physiology 317: 1003
18. Swan H J C, Ganz W, Forrester J, Marcus H, Diamond G, Chonette D 1970 Catheterization of the heart in man with use of a flow-directed balloon tipped catheter. New England Journal of Medicine 283: 447
19. Gore J M, Goldberg R J, Spodick D H, Alpert J S, Dalen J E 1987 A community-wide assessment of the use of pulmonary artery catheters in patients with acute myocardial infarction. Chest 92: 721
20. Knaus W A, Draper E A, Wagner D P, Zimmerman J E 1986 An evaluation of outcome from intensive care in major medical centres. Annals of Internal Medicine 104: 410
21. Shaver J A 1983 Haemodynamic monitoring in the critically ill patient. New England Journal of Medicine 308: 277

22. Brandsetter R D, Gitler B 1986 Thoughts on the Swan-Ganz Catheter. Chest 89: 5
23. Robin E D 1987 Death by pulmonary artery flow directed catheter (editorial) Time for a moratorium? Chest 92: 727
24. Altschule M D 1986 Reflections on Starling's Laws of the heart. Chest 89: 444
25. Lang R M, Borow K M, Neumann A, Janzen D 1986 Systemic vascular resistance: an unreliable index of left ventricular afterload. Circulation 74: 1114
26. Versprille A 1984 Pulmonary vascular resistance (editorial). Intensive Care Medicine 10: 51
27. Nadeau S, Nobel W H 1986 Misinterpretation of pressure measurements from the pulmonary artery catheter. Canadian Anaesthetist's Society Journal 33: 352
28. Raper R, Sibbald W J 1986 Misled by the wedge. Chest 89: 427
29. Laine G A, Bryan-Brown C W 1986 Pulmonary capillary pressure? (editorial). Critical Care Medicine 14: 76
30. Twigley A J, Hillman K M 1985 The end of the crystalloid era? Anaesthesia 40: 861
31. Phillips P J 1977 Water metabolism. Anaesthesia and Intensive Care 5: 295
32. Gruber U F, Allgower M 1970 Water and electrolyte balance. In: Diem K, Lentner C (eds) Scientific Tables, Ciba-Geigy, Basle
33. Pain R W 1977 Body fluid compartments. Anaesthesia and Intensive Care 5: 284
34. Dorrington K L 1981 Skin turgor: do we understand the clinical sign? The Lancet i: 264
35. Halperin B D, Feeley T W, Mihm F G, Chiles C, Guthaner D F, Blank N E 1985 Evaluation of the portable chest roentgenogram for quantitating extravascular lung water in critically ill adults. Chest 88: 649
36. Pistolesi M, Milne E N C, Miniati M, Giuntini C 1984 The vascular pedicle of the heart and the vena azygos, II: Acquired heart disease. Radiology 152: 9
37. Edelman I S, Leibman J, O'Mara M P 1958 Interrelations between serum sodium concentration, serum osmolality and total exchangeable sodium, total exchangeable potassium and total body water. Journal of Clinical Investigation 69: 389
38. Hillman K M 1989 Fluid therapy. In: Scurr C, Feldman S, Soni N (eds) Scientific Foundations of Anaesthesia, 4th edn. Heinemann, London, in press
39. Guyton A C 1963 A concept of negative interstitial pressure based on pressures in implanted perforated capsules. Circulation Research 12: 399
40. Fadnes H O, Reed R K, Aukland K 1977 Interstitial fluid pressure in rats measured with a modified wick technique. Microvascular Research 14: 27
41. Rose B D 1986 New approach to disturbances in the plasma sodium concentration. American Journal of Medicine 81: 1033
42. Hillman K M 1986 Crystalloid or colloid (editorial). British Journal of Hospital Medicine 35: 217
43. Hogan J J 1915 The use of colloidal (gelatin) solutions in shock. Journal of American Medical Association 64: 721
44. Erglanger J, Gasser H S 1919 Hypertonic gum acacia and glucose in the treatment of secondary traumatic shock. Annals of Surgery 69: 389
45. Bayliss W M 1916 Methods of raising a low arterial pressure. Proceedings of the Royal Society of Britain 80: 380
46. Hecht G, Weese H 1943 Periston, ein neuer Blutflussig- keitsersatz. Munchener medizinische Wochenscrift 90: 11
47. Gronwell A, Inglemann B 1945 Untersuchungen uber Dextran und sein Verhalten bei paranteraler Zufuhr. Acta Physiologica Scandinavica 9: 1
48. Saddler J M, Horsey P J 1987 The new generation gelatins. Anaesthesia 42: 998
49. Thomson W L, Fukushima T, Rutherford R B, Walton R P 1970 Intravascular persistence tissue storage, and excretion of hydroxyethyl starch. Surgery, Gynaecology and Obstetrics 131: 965
50. Tourtelotte D, Williams H E 1958 Acylated gelatins and their preparations. US Patent 2: 827
51. Schmidt-Thome J, Mager A, Schone H H 1962 Zur Chemie eines neuen plasma expanders. Arzneimittel-forschung 12: 378
52. Kohler H, Kirch W, Fuchs P, Stalder K, Distler A 1978 Elimination of hexamethylene diisocyanate cross-linked polypeptides in patients with normal or impaired renal function. European Journal of Clinical Pharmacology 14: 405
53. Lungsgaard-Hansen P, Tschirren B 1978 Modified fluid gelatin as a plasma substitute. In: Jamieson G A, Greenwalt T (eds) Blood substitutes and plasma expanders. Proceedings of the Ninth American Red Cross Annual Scientific Symposium, Liss, Washington, p. 227
54. Isbister J P, Fisher M McD 1980 Adverse effects of plasma volume expanders. Anaesthesia and Intensive Care 8: 145
55. Lorenz W, Doenicke A, Messmer K, Reimann H-J, Thermann M, Lahn W, Berr J, Schmal A, Dormann P, Egenfuss P, Hamelmann H 1976 Histamine release in human subjects by modified gelatin (Haemaccel) and dextran: an explanation for anaphylactoid reactions observed under clinical condition? British Journal of Anaesthesia 48: 151

56. Ring J, Messmer K 1977 Incidence and severity of anaphylactoid reactions to colloid volume substitutes. The Lancet i: 466
57. Mishler J M 1984 Synthetic plasma volume expanders — their pharmacology, safety and clinical efficacy. Clinics in Haematology 13: 75
58. Mailloux L, Swartz C D, Capizzi R, Kim K E, Onesti G, Ramirez O, Brest A N 1967 Acute renal failure after administration of low-molecular-weight dextran. New England Journal of Medicine 277: 1113
59. Paull J 1987 A prospective study of Dextran-induced anaphylactoid reactions in 5745 patients. Anaesthesia and Intensive Care 15: 163.
60. Lee W H Jnr., Cooper N, Weidner M G, Murner E S 1968 Clinical evaluation of a new plasma expander, hydroxyethyl starch. Journal of Trauma 8: 381
61. Mackintyre E, Mackie I J, Ho D, Tinker J, Bullen C, Machin S J 1985 The haemostatic effects of hydroxyethyl starch (HES) used as a volume expander. Intensive Care Medicine 11: 300
62. Shatney C H, Deepika K, Militello P R, Majerus T C, Dawson R B 1983 Efficacy of hetastarch in the resuscitation of patients with multi-system trauma and shock. Archives of Surgery 118: 804
63. Alving B M, Hojima Y, Pisano J J, Mason B L, Buckingham R E, Mozen M M, Finlayson J S 1978 Hypotension associated with prekallikrein activator (Hageman-factor fragments) in plasmaprotein fraction. New England Journal of Medicine 299: 66
64. Coleman R W 1978 Paradoxical hypotension after volume expansion with plasma protein fraction. New England Journal of Medicine 299: 97
65. Thompson W L 1975 Rational use of alumbin and plasma substitutes. The John Hopkins Medical Journal 136: 220
66. Geyer R P 1975 'Bloodless' rats through the use of artificial blood substitutes. Federation Proceedings 34: 1499
67. Mitsuno T, Ohyanagi H, Naito R 1982 Clinical studies of a perfluorochemical whole blood substitute (Fluosol-DA). Annals of Surgery 195: 66
68. Tremper K K, Friedman A E, Levin E M, Lapin R, Camarillo D 1982 The pre-operative treatment of severely anemic patients with a perfluorochemical oxygen-transport fluid, Fluosol-DA. New England Journal of Medicine 307: 277
69. Yokoyama K, Suyama T, Naito R 1980 Development of fluosol-DA and its perspective as a blood substitute. Oxygen and life. Proceedings of the Second Priestley Conference, Royal Society of Chemistry, London, 142 (special publication 39)
70. Police A M, Waxman K, Tominaga G 1985 Pulmonary complications after Fluosol administration to patients with life-threatening blood loss. Critical Care Medicine 13: 96
71. Tremper K K, Vercellotti G M, Hammerschmidt D E 1984 Hemodynamic profile of adverse clinical reactions to fluosol-DA 20%. Critical Care Medicine 12: 428
72. Waxman K, Cheung C K, Mason G R 1984 Hypotensive reaction after infusion of a perfluorochemical emulsion. Critical Care Medicine 12: 609
73. Shires T, Williams J, Brown F 1961 Acute changes in extracellular fluids associated with major surgical procedures. Annals of Surgery 154: 803
74. Moore F E, Ball M R 1952 The metabolic response to surgery, lst edn. Saunders, Philadelphia
75. Guyton A C, Taylor A E, Granger H J, Coleman T G 1971 Interstitial fluid pressure. Physiological Reviews 51: 527
76. Collins J V, Cockrane G M, Davis J, Benatar S R, Clarke J H 1973 Some aspects of pulmonary function after rapid saline infusion in health subjects. Clinical Science and Molecular Medicine 45: 407
77. Boutros A R, Ruess R, Olsen L, Hoyt J L, Baker W H 1979 Comparison of hemodynamic, pulmonary and renal effects of use of three types of fluids after major surgical procedures on the abdominal aorta. Critical Care Medicine 7: 9
78. Rackow E C, Falk J L, Fein I A, Siegel J S, Packman M I, Haupt M T, Kaufman B S, Putnam D 1983 Fluid resuscitation in circulatory shock: a comparison of the cardiorespiratory effects of albumin, hetastarch and saline solutions in patients with hypovolemic and septic shock. Critical Care Medicine 11: 839
79. Shoemaker W C 1976 Comparison of the relative effectiveness of whole blood tranfusions and various types of fluid therapy in resuscitation. Critical Care Medicine 4: 71
80. Skillman J J, Restall D S, Salzman E W 1975 Randomized trial of albumin vs electrolyte solutions during abdominal aortic operations. Surgery 78: 291
81. Hauser C J, Shoemaker W C, Turpin I, Goldberg S J 1980 Oxygen transport responses to colloids and crystalloids in critically ill surgical patients. Surgery, Gynecology and Obstetrics 150: 811
82. Kaufman B S, Rackow E C, Falk J L 1984 The relationship between oxygen delivery and consumption during fluid resuscitation of hypovolemic and septic shock. Chest 85: 336
83. Schott U, Lindbom L-O, Sjostrand U 1988 Hemodynamic effects of colloid concentration in experimental hemorrhage. A comparison of Ringer's lactate, 3% dextran-60 and 6% dextran-70. Critical Care Medicine 16: 346

84. Knisely M H, Reneau D D, Binely D F 1969 The development and use of equations for predicting limits on the rates of oxygen supply to the cells of tissues and organs. Angiology 20: 61

85. Mangalore P P, Hunt T K 1972 Effect of varying oxygen tensions on healing of open wounds. Surgery, Gynecology and Obstetrics 135: 756

86. Brinkmeyer S, Safar P, Motoyama E, Stezoski W 1981 Superiority of colloid over electrolyte solution for fluid resuscitation (severe normovolaemic hemodilution). Critical Care Medicine 9: 369

87. Shoemaker W C, Schluchter M, Hopkins J A, Appel P L, Schwartz L, Chang P 1981 Comparison of the relative effectiveness of colloids and crystalloids in emergency resuscitation. American Journal of Surgery 142: 73

88. Dickson D M, Hillman K M 1989 Continuous renal replacement therapy. Anaesthesia and Intensive Care, in press

89. Hillman K 1987b Fluid resuscitation in diabetic emergencies — a reappraisal. Intensive Care Medicine 13: 4

90. Tocantins L M, Carrol R T, Holburn H R 1951 The clot accelerative effect of dilution on blood and plasma. Relation to the mechanism of coagulation of normal and hemophilic blood. Blood 6: 720

91. Monkhouse F C 1959 Relationship between antithrombin and thrombin levels in plasma and serum. American Journal of Physiology 197: 984

92. Janvrin S B, Davies G, Greenhalgh R M 1980 Postoperative deep vein thrombosis caused by intravenous fluids during surgery. British Journal of Surgery 67: 690

7. Trauma

J.C. Stoddart

The anaesthetist should be involved in the management of the injured patient from the earliest possible stage. As a member of the major accident teams, he or she may need to go to the site of the accident to provide triage and first aid, and will certainly be a member of the receiving team. The anaesthetist will be called to the casualty department to aid the general resuscitation of the individual trauma victim and should possess special skills, which will be needed for the patient suffering from airway obstruction, thoracic or head injuries. He or she is more directly responsible for the patients' safety and well being while in the operating room or Intensive Therapy Unit (ITU).

In this chapter, some recent advances in the treatment of the trauma victim will be reviewed. Some of this information is only obtainable from specialist journals and, where possible, the references given are to review papers.

TRAUMA AND THE RESPIRATORY TRACT

The anaesthetist should play a major role in the assessment and treatment of patients suffering from trauma to the respiratory tract. Such patients frequently have injuries elsewhere and, although this section will concentrate upon the respiratory tract, the whole patient must always be considered.

The upper airway

Injuries to the upper airway are common and they may occasionally be life-threatening. Blunt trauma to the face, maxilla and mandible are most frequently encountered and occasionally they may cause airway difficulties; this type of injury is more often associated with respiratory obstruction after the patient has received surgical treatment under general anaesthesia and is in the ward or recovery room.

Injuries to the larynx and cervical trachea are uncommon and do not often cause airway obstruction.[1] However, in these and many other situations the anaesthetist may need to be able to provide an alternative airway. Endotracheal intubation, perhaps with the aid of the fibreoptic bronchoscope, or the use of the rigid bronchoscope as an airway, are usually possible: the alternatives include emergency trachostomy, which is dangerous — even in skilled hands. Some other methods are discussed below.

Cricothyroidotomy

The cricothyroid membrane is usually visible and palpable and there are few important or dangerous structures in the midline between it and the skin.

In a dire emergency a large intravenous needle or cannula can be inserted into the trachea via the cricothyroid membrane. Oxygen can be insufflated through it, and controlled ventilation is possible by this route.[2] Surgical cricothyroidotomy is much easier than tracheostomy and causes fewer long-term complications[3] although it probably should not be used for elective controlled ventilation.[4]

There are several devices in kit form that are designed for emergency cricothyroidotomy.[5] With some of these a small cuffed tracheostomy tube[6] can be inserted ('Penlon®' cricothyroidotomy cannula; the 'Nu-trake®' set. However, for the short-term relief of dangerous upper airway obstruction, the 'Minitrach®' system has much to recommend it.[7] This device is widely used to aid the clearance of secretions from the tracheobronchial tree after major surgery or for patients with acute on chronic obstructive airways disease. Many complications of its use have been reported (e.g. haemorrhage, surgical emphysema, tracheal injury, tracheo-oesophageal perforation, etc.) and it should not be used casually. Nevertheless it can be of great value. In the author's experience, it has reduced the need for repeated tracheal intubation, bronchoscopy and tracheostomy.

The commercial unit (Portex®) has been modified several times but, essentially, it is a size 4 uncuffed endotracheal tube with an integral collar for its fixing tapes, a 4-mm endotracheal connector, a shrouded scalpel blade and an introducing stilette.

The cricothyroid notch is identified and if possible stabilized between the finger and thumb of the left hand. If it is considered advisable, or necessary, an assistant can gently extend the patients head and at the same time give oxygen by face mask. After infiltration with local anaesthesia, a vertical stab incision is made through the skin and cricothyroid membrane; the stilette is pushed through this in a downward direction and the tube slid over it. After insertion oxygen can be administered by insufflation through the tube, or by controlled ventilation by hand or machine. High-frequency jet ventilation can also be given. The aperture is not large enough to permit spontaneous breathing for long periods but it may be life-saving.

The original endotracheal tube had a tapered tip but in the kit presently available the end of the tube is straight, although rounded, and is not quite so easy to insert. This change was made because it was suggested that the tapered tip caused tracheal mucosal injury during high-frequency jet ventilation.[8]

Chest wall injuries

These are a very common reason for admission to the ITU and it is important to make an early assessment of their severity and significance. Probably the best known classification system is that of Lloyd et al.[9] and this still provides a useful baseline. Patients are placed in one of three categories, depending upon their age, the extent of the thoracic injury and any associated injuries, blood gas disturbance and pre-existing health status. Treatment is also graded, from systemic analgesia and physiotherapy, via tracheostomy and spontaneous ventilation with oxygen enrichment, to heavy sedation and intermittent positive-pressure ventilation.

The respiratory factors that are of primary importance in isolated chest injuries are pain, inability to cough, paradoxical ventilation, pneumothorax and pulmonary contusions. The effects of pre-existing health status and associated injuries are also vitally important but will not be considered here.

It had been thought that patients with fractures to the first and second ribs commonly had aortic arch damage.[10] However, Fermanis and co-workers[11] could find no statistically significant relationship between the two, although they noted that this type of injury was always associated with particularly violent impact.

Pain relief

Pain relief is all that is required by many patients with chest wall injuries even when there is marked paradoxical ventilation but it is often difficult to provide safely. Parenteral opiates are still the mainstay for pain relief but they are often inappropriate in the traumatized patient. This is particularly the case if the patient has a head injury and they often produce undesirable sedation and inability to cough and breathe deeply.

Many alternative methods have been adopted. 'Entonox® inhalation may be useful for patients with mild to moderately severe pain, particularly to facilitate physiotherapy. However, it is of minimal value for persistent severe pain.

In a controlled trial with a paracetamol-codeine combination, transcutaneous electrical nerve stimulation (TENS) has been reported to be very effective.[12] In this study, the electrodes were placed alongside the appropriate rib spaces. It was reported that the patients preferred the TENS to systemic analgesia and there were no side-effects.

A wide variety of regional and local analgesic blockade techniques have been reported. Epidural blockade with bupivacaine has been favoured by the author for many years[10] and its efficacy has been reported in many cases.[13] Epidural opiates have also been used with apparent success. In 1987 Mackenzie et al[14] reported that epidural fentanyl brought about a marked improvement in gas exchange in patients with blunt chest injuries. Good analgesia but with a high incidence of delayed respiratory depression has been reported in several trials of epidural morphine.[15,16]

Intercostal blockade has been practised for many years. A recent development has been that of continuous intercostal block via a catheter inserted at the angle of the rib.[17,18] This technique has many of the advantages of epidural blockade, with few of its disadvantages — particularly those of hypotension and lower limb weakness. It is a very simple technique and it is usually possible to provide good to adequate analgesia[19] covering 5–8 rib spaces with 20 ml 0.5% bupivacaine as a bolus dose, maintained by an infusion of 5–15 ml/h.

The site of action of the local anaesthetic has been investigated by several workers and it has been established that the local anaesthetic tracks outside the parietal pleura.[20] The effective area of spread is not entirely predictable but by trial and error, adequate pain relief can be obtained and maintained for several days.

Intercostal blockade may be followed by a small (or a large) pneumothorax but the analgesia is often still adequate. Reierstad and Stromskag[21] reported upon the use of continuous intrapleural local anaesthesia for postoperative pain and later this technique was shown also to produce chest wall analgesia.[22] The idea of deliberately inserting a catheter through an epidural needle into the hitherto intact pleural space may well be foreign to anaesthetists, but the morbidity rate is said to be very low. It is reported to be a very simple procedure with a high success rate.

If pain relief is effective, most patients with mild to moderately severe injury can be managed without intubation or formal tracheostomy. They are able to cough, expectorate and breathe deeply, and their blood gas exchange improves commensurately. As described above, mini-tracheostomy may be helpful if secretions still tend to accumulate.

Pulmonary contusion

The causes of hypoxia in chest injured patients are multiple; they include under-ventilation, maldistribution (paradoxical ventilation), pneumothorax, coincidental aspiration of gastric contents, lung laceration and accumulation of secretions. However, almost all blunt chest injuries are accompanied by pulmonary contusions, which causes ventilation-perfusion mismatch or shunting. Controlled ventilation with added oxygen plays an important part in treatment but also has disadvantages. Trinkle and colleagues[23] suggested that in many cases this could be avoided by measures that are directed at reducing accumulation of intrapulmonary water (diuretics, fluid restriction) and these sensible recommendations are widely followed.[10] However, when despite this the alveolar to arterial oxygen tension gradient becomes unacceptable ($PaO_2 < 8.0$ kPa; $PAO_2 > 0.5$ kPa) there is little alternative to sedation and controlled ventilation. The indications for intubation were recently reviewed,[24] and were shown to include; a respiratory rate of greater than 25 breaths/min, a pulse rate greater than 100 bpm, relative hypotension (systolic arterial pressure below 100 mmHg) and hypoxia when breathing oxygen-enriched air. The presence of extrathoracic injuries was also shown to be relevant. Most of these factors are similar to those categorized by Lloyd and co-workers.[9]

Secondary infection is a major cause of morbidity and mortality in the injured patient. Contributory factors include: intra-abdominal injury, with splenectomy being particularly important; the endotracheal or tracheostomy tube may be the portal of entry. Chest drainage tubes are often needed and it is still not agreed whether prophylactic antibiotics should be given after such tubes are inserted.[25,26] Provided they are inserted and managed aseptically, it should be possible to avoid infection, and the author does not give antibiotics prophylactically as a routine.

It is commonly recommended that all patients with rib fractures who require coincidental surgery should have a chest drain inserted before the anaesthesia or operation begins, to avoid the risk of tension pneumothorax occurring at a time when it might be difficult to diagnose. Patients who already have a pneumothorax and require IPPV should present no dilemma, but in any case the tube should be removed as soon as possible after the lung has been shown to be fully inflated and bubbling has ceased. The tube is usually clamped for up to 12 hours to allow time for the pneumothorax to re-accumulate, before it is removed.

Myocardial contusion

The importance of myocardial contusion associated with chest trauma was first demonstrated by McDonald and co-workers.[27] This condition is very difficult to diagnose although electrocardiographic and myocardial enzyme abnormalities may be recognised.[28,29] Patients who are at particular risk are those who with central chest trauma, especially injuries to the sternum. It may cause life-threatening arrhythmias or be associated with pericardial tamponade; rarely, delayed ventricular rupture may occur. Damage to a valve cusp, or to chordae tendinae should be apparent when the patient is first seen.

Because of the diagnostic difficulties patients who are at risk of this complication should be given a prophylactic Class 1 anti-arrhythmic drug, such as flecainide. If arrhythmia occurs during treatment, lignocaine infusion is usually effective but cardioversion may be required and this facility should always be available.

HEAD INJURIES

The treatment of the head-injured patient should follow clearly recommended lines including the avoidance of hypoxia, hypotension and anaemia, and also factors that cause raised intracranial pressure (coughing, straining, hypercapnia, fluid overload, etc.). The elimination of convulsive activity is also important.[30] Several additional theraupetic methods are widely used, and over the last few years some of these have undergone intense investigation.

Hyperventilation

One of the responses to hyperventilation hypocapnia is cerebral vasoconstriction. Since the intracranial pressure is partly due to the calibre and content of cerebral blood vessels, if these can be reduced the intracranial pressure should fall.[31] Moderate hyperventilation to a $PaCO_2$ of 4–4.5 kPa is usually recommended. It has been stated that the efficacy of this treatment is limited by secondary lactic acidosis caused by reduced cerebral oxygenation, resulting in vasodilatation.[32] However, a more recent study[33] suggested that the vasoconstrictor effects of moderate hyperventilation persist at least for as long as 48 hours. This effect is more marked in those patients with cerebral hyperaemia and least effective in patients in whom the cerebral blood flow is subnormal.

Hypocapnia is not always accompanied by a fall in intracranial pressure, since the injury may itself cause brain swelling. Diffuse cerebral oedema is much less important than structural brain damage, although a rise in intracranial pressure to above 60 mmHg is always fatal.[34]

Dexamethasone

Dexamethasone has been used for many years in an attempt to reduce the raised intracranial pressure associated with intracerebral space occupying lesions.[35] It appeared logical to extend this to other forms of raised intracranial pressure and it is still widely used for this purpose. Many papers have now appeared reporting well-controlled and well-executed investigations into this form of treatment. The conclusions are unequivocal — dexamethasone is of no value and may be harmful when used for the treatment of raised intracranial pressure after head injury.[36–39]

Barbiturate coma

Barbiturates and other sedative drugs are widely used to depress seizure activity in head-injured patients and others, but some years ago an additional role was proposed. It was believed that heavy sedation would both reduce cerebral metabolic activity and thereby protect cells against hypoxic or ischaemic damage or both, and reduce intracranial pressure.[40] Barbiturates in anaesthetic dosage can reduce intracranial pressure, although this is often accompanied by systemic hypotension, which may endanger cerebral perfusion and always necessitates respiratory support to avoid the hazard of hypoventilation.

However, it is no longer believed that the use of barbiturates or other sedative agents can increase the quality of recovery after diffuse brain injury from either hypoxia or injury.[41,42] Fears have been expressed that vigorous resuscitation may simply increase the number of severely brain damaged survivors although this is still a matter for dispute.[43,44]

It is generally agreed that the first few minutes after the injury determine the outcome, assuming that the treatment thereafter is not itself harmful.[45] The recommendations made by McIver and colleagues[46] with regard to initial resuscitation and particularly to the provision of a guaranteed airway, with or without ventilatory assistance, remain as appropriate today as when they were first written.

Intracranial pressure measurement
Since all forms of insult to the brain may be followed by an increase in intracranial pressure, it is widely recommended, although by no means universally agreed, that this should be routinely measured in those patients with a Glasgow coma score of 8 or less. There are several available methods, including extradural, subdural and intraventricular devices. The intraventricular route is widely agreed to give the most reliable results and although it probably has the highest complication rate it may also be used to drain cerebrospinal fluid. There is also evidence to suggest that there may be regional variations in intracranial pressure, which are not identified by a single monitor.[47] Although when carefully performed it has an acceptable morbidity rate, studies from centres in which head injuries are treated conservatively without the aid of such monitoring aids imply that the results of treatment are as good as, if not better than, from the more invasive units.[43,48]

VOLUME REPLACEMENT

Thirty years ago it was recommended by the Birmingham Accident Hospital that blood lost should be replaced by an equivalent volume of whole blood.[49] Experience has shown that this is neither necessary nor desirable, particularly because of the non-availability, expense and questionable safety of blood product transfusion. The guidelines to transfusion therapy are based upon the realities of circulating blood volume and oxygen delivery, with replacement of coagulation factors and, possible hydrogen ion regulation, as subsidiary questions. The risks of side-effects must be minimized.

The optimum haematocrit
Because blood is a non-Newtonian fluid its rheological properties cannot be simply expressed. Oxygen delivery depends upon mean blood pressure, flow, haemoglobin content and the dimension of the capillaries, with other factors such as intrinsic tissue pressure, oxygen tension gradient and pH being involved. Flow through simple tubes appears to change linearly with haematocrit,[50] with the optimum oxygen transport occurring at haematocrit of 30%. Later work with dogs showed that local and regional compensatory variation in flow and calibre of blood vessels followed changes in haematocrit; these data demonstrated that there was no significant difference in oxygen delivery over the haemocrit range 30–53%[51].

These and other results suggest that, provided the patient has no disease process that restricts cardiac output or makes tachycardia undesirable, a haematocrit of 30% is quite adequate.[52] It is also worth remembering that the oxygen carrying capacity of transfused stored blood may not return to normal for many hours.[53,54]

Crystalloid colloid controversy

For many years, there has been argument as to what is better for resuscitation, electrolyte solutions (saline, Ringer's lactate, etc.), or one of the many so-called colloid solutions (dextran, gelatin, albumin, hydroxyethyl starch, etc). Battlefield experience demonstrated that immediate resuscitation with electrolytes such as Ringer's lactate achieved satisfactory results. However, many investigators showed that electrolyte solution could not be equated with whole blood and that much larger volumes had to be given for the equivalent response. This observation was accompanied by the recognition that much of this volume moved into the tissues and, particularly, the lung.[55,56] Other workers suggested that Ringer's lactate solution was better than other electrolyte solutions if resuscitation was delayed, perhaps partly because it tended to neutralize any metabolic acidaemia present.[57,58] Rackow and co-workers[59] found that albumin or hydroxyethyl starch were more effective than saline in restoring the cardiovascular parameters in bled animals. Tissue oxygen delivery was shown to be better when resuscitation was performed with colloid than with crystalloid.[60]

Although the present consensus is that colloid solutions are better than crystalloid,[56] a balanced resuscitation regimen of crystalloid, colloid and the appropriate amount of red cells to maintain the haematocrit within the range 30–35% is a practical compromise.[57]

Reactions to blood substitutes

Allergic reactions, from skin rashes and rigors, to bronchospasm, cardiocirculatory collapse and death have been recorded with most of the blood substitutes.[61] The incidence of severe reactions was recorded in a prospective trial of more than 200 000 infusions of assorted fluids.[62] This was found to be 0.003% for plasma protein solutions; 0.006% for hydroxyethyl starch; 0.008% for dextran; 0.038% for gelatine solutions. Anxiety has been expressed as to the ultimate fate and biological activity of hydroxyethyl starch, which remains in the body for much longer than the other colloids.

Coagulation factors

When patients receive large volume transfusion, their intrinsic coagulation factor levels are temporarily reduced by dilution, while at the same time the stress that necessitates the transfusion may increase them. The significance of these effects has been widely investigated. Counts and co-workers[63] prospectively recorded the effects of massive transfusion on the coagulation profile of trauma victims. They concluded that the only effect that may require correction was thrombocytopenia below 100 000/ml. Martin and co-workers[64] showed that adding fresh frozen plasma (FFP) as supplements to massive blood transfusion was of no demonstrable value. The use of FFP as coagulant, and as volume replacement has recently been reviewed.[65,66] It was concluded that it is of very little value and has all the hazards of any biological transfusion fluid, and that its use should be severely curtailed — except perhaps in those patients with specific needs, in whom a coagulation factor shortage has been clearly established, or in patients with angioneurotic oedema for whom FFP is the treatment of choice.

Autotransfusion
The practice of collecting the patient's own blood from the pelvic cavity during surgery for ruptured ectopic pregnancy, and re-transfusing it, was followed for many years. Recently, because of the non-availability of blood, the increasing extent of operative surgery, and worries about the transmission of diseases such as AIDS, blood salvage and re-transfusion have become more widely practised.[67,68] Commercial devices are available (e.g. Solcotrans®, Haemonetics®) and blood has been safely and satisfactorily re-used after aortic surgery[69] from the mediastinum and thorax[70] and after liver transplantation.[71] Napoli and colleagues[72] demonstrated experimentally that levels of coagulation factors were adequate after re-transfusion from experimental haemothorax. Protagonists of this technique state that it allows the use of banked blood to be reduced very significantly.

Increasingly, patients who are to undergo elective major surgery are being offered the opportunity to donate 1–2 units of their own blood 2–3 weeks before the proposed operation, for re-use if necessary. This creates few administrative problems and will probably become a standard practice.[73]

THE PULMONARY EFFECTS OF NON-THORACIC TRAUMA

The adult respiratory distress syndrome (ARDS) is the lungs' response to a systemic injury. This could be a major limb, abdominal or pelvic injury, burns or extensive surgical procedure. ARDS has also been reported in association with acute pancreatitis, fat embolism syndrome, haemodialysis and the use of the extracorporeal membrane oxygenator. In some of these conditions, the respiratory disturbance is preceded by signs of systemic sepsis.[74]

The cardinal features of ARDS are hypoxia, reduced pulmonary compliance and functional residual capacity and the appearance of widespread infiltrates on the chest radiograph. The sequence of events is thought to be as follows:

1. Tissue injury and/or endotoxin activate the complement cascade.
2. Complement C5 α encourages the margination of polymorphonuclear leukocytes within the pulmonary capillary so they adhere to the endothelium and release leukocyte membrane phospholipid and proteases. This process is associated with the appearance of oxygen free radicals (O_2^{2-}, peroxide), which are themselves toxic to the capillary endothelium. Arachidonic acid is also released. This is an intermediary in the formation of eicosonoids, such as leukotrienes, which increase capillary permeability, and prostaglandins (particularly $F_2\alpha$) which are vasoactive.
3. Tissue damage may also lead to platelet aggregation, resulting in microembolism and the release of histamine and serotonin.[75,76]

The results of these processes are transient pulmonary hypertension, intravascular thrombosis and increased pulmonary capillary permeability. This is followed by the accumulation of protein-containing fluid in the pulmonary interstitium and ultimately, in the alveolar air spaces. Fibronectin may be incriminated, and the coagulation cascade may also be activated, giving rise to disseminated intravascular coagulation.

The term ARDS should only be used if no other cause of lung pathology is known. For example, patients with pneumonia (including aspiration pneumonia), with direct pulmonary trauma (contusion, haemorrhage) or with cardiogenic pulmonary oedema are, by definition, not suffering from ARDS. Alternatively, patients who develop the clinical and laboratory features of ARDS at a later stage in their illness may have an underlying cause. This is almost always severe infection outside the respiratory tract.

Diagnostic features
These are usually said to be a low pulmonary artery wedge pressure and the identification of protein and proteases in alveolar lavage fluid. This description emphasises the central role of the polymorphonuclear leukocyte; however, a similar condition has been seen in patients with extreme granulocytopenia, where other leukocytes may be incriminated.[77]

Incidence and mortality
It has been stated[78] that there are from 10 000–15 000 cases of ARDS in the UK each year, with a mortality rate of 60–90%. This may be an overestimate since the term is often used loosely. By definition, ARDS does not occur as an isolated process, and death is usually the result of multiple organ failure rather than hypoxia alone.[79]

Treatment
The objectives are, to achieve acceptable (if not ideal) blood gas exchange with the smallest penalty. This usually involves controlled ventilation with oxygen-enriched air to maintain the arterial oxygen tension at or above 8.0 kPa (60 mmHg).

Although positive end-expiratory pressure (PEEP) is usually recommended there is no evidence[80] that its early application delays or prevents the onset of ARDS and the undesirable effects of PEEP are well known.[81,82] Other methods of achieving gas exchange such as reversed I : E ratios[83] and high frequency ventilation[84] are being tried.

Fluid overload must be avoided and diuretics and dopamine are usually given. In oliguric and anuric patients, haemofiltration can readily achieve large fluid losses if this is felt to be useful.[85]

Hypoalbuminaemia is common, and it is usual to give intravenous albumin supplements, although it is widely suspected that much of this soon exudes into the pulmonary intersitium.

Drug therapy
Every effort should be made to prevent secondary bacterial pneumonia, thus systemic antibiotics may be given. There is some evidence that the incidence of such infections is reduced by the prophylactic use of oral, intragastric and intravenous antibiotics for all patients at risk.[86,87] If this is confirmed it will be very helpful since secondary bacterial pneumonia is a hazardous feature in many cases.

Recently, a multicentre trial has confirmed earlier work that corticosteroids are of no value and may be harmful.[88] Prostaglandins,[89] prostacyclin and prostaglandin inhibitors[90] have all been used but, as yet, with little evidence of long-term benefit. Prospective trails of the effects of some of these agents are in progress at present.

Treatment of the underlying cause

This must be identified and treated if possible. Repeated laparotomy and wide re-excision of damaged or infected tissue may be required. Unless the cause can be found, the prognosis is bad, although, as stated earlier, acute respiratory failure alone is only rarely the cause of death.

TRAUMA SCORING SYSTEMS

Attempts to validate therapeutic methods and establish prognostic criteria are increasingly being made for clinical and administrative purposes. Two of the best known of these are the injury severity score[91] and the APACHE system.[92,93]

The injury severity score is based upon the quantification of the three most severely injured parts of the body, on a scale of 1–5. Each number is then squared before being summated as it was recognized that the significance of multiple injuries was greater than the sum of individual injuries. This system has recently been re-evaluated and shown to provide reliable prognostic data.[94]

The APACHE system (Acute Physiology and Chronic Health Evaluation) is also well known. It was based upon an analysis of 5030 patients in the intensive care units of 13 American hospitals. This also is a numerical system that quantifies variation from the normal range of 13 readily measured parameters. It includes the effects of age and intercurrent disease.

Although such systems provide valuable tools for comparing treatment methods and the efficiency of different units, neither can predict the outcome with 100% certainty. In addition, the systems are based upon the results obtained from dated treatment methods, some of which may now have been superseded and perhaps, improved. Nevertheless, it should be possible by the general use of this type of analysis to quantify and validate the commonly used treatment programmes.

REFERENCES

1. Angood P B, Attia E L, Brown R A, Mulder D S 1986 Extrinsic civilian trauma to the larynx and cervical trachea — important predictors of long-term mortality. Journal of Trauma 26(10): 869–873
2. Spoerel W E, Shahvari M B G, Singh N B 1971 Transtracheal ventilation. British Journal of Anaesthesia 43: 932–939
3. Van Hasselt E J, Bruining H A, Hoeve L J 1985 Elective cricothyroidotomy. Intensive Care Medicine 11: 207–209
4. Brantigan C O, Grow J B 1976 Cricothyroidotomy: elective use in respiratory problems requiring tracheostomy. Journal of Thoracic and Cardiovascular Surgery 71: 72
5. Ravlo O, Bach V, Lybecker H, 1987 A comparison between two emergency cricothyroidotomy instruments. Acta Anaesthesiology Scandinavica 31: 317–319
6. Weiss S 1983 A new emergency cricothyroidotomy instrument. Journal of Trauma 23: 155–158
7. Matthews H R, Hopkinson R B 1984 Treatment of sputum retention by mini tracheostomy. British Journal of Surgery 71: 147–148
8. Portex Ltd., Personal communication.
9. Lloyd J W, Crampton Smith A, O'Connor B T 1965 Classification of chest injuries as an aid to treatment. British Medical Journal 1: 1518–1520
10. Stoddart J C 1985 The management of chest injuries In: Stoddart J C Trauma and the anaesthetist. Ch. 4. Bailliere Tindall, London, p. 189
11. Fermanis G G, Deane S A, Fitzgerald P M 1985 The significance of first and second rib fractures. Australian and New Zealand Journal of Surgery 55: 383–386
12. Sloan J P, Muwanga C L, Waters E A, 1986 Multiple rib fractures: transcutaneous nerve stimulation versus conventional analgesia. Journal of Trauma 26(12): 1120–1122

13. Worthley L I G 1985 Thoracic epidural in the management of chest trauma. Intensive Care Medicine 11: 312–315
14. McKenzie R C, Shackford S R, Hoyt D B, Karagianes T G 1987 Continuous epidural fentanyl analgesia; ventilatory function improvement with routine use in treatment of blunt chest injury. Journal of Trauma 27(11): 1207–1210
15. McCaughey W, Graham J L 1982 Respiratory depression of epidural morphine. Anaesthesia 37(10): 990–995
16. Sandler A N, Chavaz P, Whiting W 1986 Respiratory depression following epidural morphine: a clinical study. Canadian Anaesthestic Society Journal 33(5) 542–549
17. O'Kelly E, Garry B 1981 Continuous pain relief for multiple fractured ribs. British Journal of Anaesthesia 53: 989–991
18. Murphy D F 1983 Intercostal nerve blockade for fractured ribs and postoperative analgesia: description of a new technique. Regional Anaesthesia 8: 151–153
19. Johansson A, Reuck H, Aspelin P, Jacobsen H 1985 Multiple intercostal blocks by a single injection: a clinical and radiological investigation. Acta Anaesthesiologica Scandinavica 29: 524–528
20. Crossley A W A, Hosie H E 1987 Radiographic study of intercostal nerve blockade in healthy volunteers. British Journal of Anaesthesia 59: 149–154
21. Reierstad F, Stromskag K E 1986 Intrapleural catheter in the management of post-operative pain. Regional Anaesthesia 11: 89–91
22. Rocco A, Reierstad F, Gudman J, McKay W 1987 Intrapleural administration of local anaesthetics for pain relief in patients with multiple rib fractures. Regional Anaesthesia 12(1): 10–14
23. Trinkle J K, Richardson J D, Franz J L, 1975 Management of flail chest without mechanical ventilation. Annals of Thoracic Surgery 19: 355–359
24. Barone J E, Pizzi W F, Nealson T F, Richman H 1986 Indication for intubation in blunt chest trauma. Journal of Trauma 26 (4): 334–337
25. Stone H H, Symas P N, Hooper A 1981 Cefamandol for prophylaxis against infection in closed-tube thoracostomy. Journal of Trauma 26(11):975–977
26. Lo Curto J J, Tischler C D, Swan K G, 1986 Tube tracheostomy and trauma: antibiotics or not? Journal of Trauma 26 (12): 1067–1072
27. McDonald R C, O'Neill D, Hanning C D, Ledingham I McA 1981 Myocardial contusion in blunt chest trauma: a 10-year review Intensive Care Medicine 7: 261–268
28. Tengler M L 1985 The spectrum of myocardial trauma. Journal of Trauma 25: 620–627
29. Muwanga C L, Cole R P, Sloan J P, 1986 Cardiac contusion in patients wearing seat belts. Injury 17: 37–39
30. Moss E, Gibson J S, McDowall D G, Gibson R M 1983 Intensive management of severe head injuries. Anaesthesia 38(3): 214–225
31. Greenberg J H, Alava A, Reivich M, 1978 Local cerebral blood volume response to carbon dioxide in man. Circulation Research 43: 324–331
32. James J E, Lanfitt T W, Kumar V S, 1977 Treatment of intracranial hypertension: analysis of 105 consecutive continuous recordings of intracranial pressure. Acta Neurochircurgica 36: 189–200
33. Obrist W D, Langfitt T W, Jaggi J L, 1984 Cerebral blood flow and metabolism in comatose patients with acute head injury. Journal of Neurosurgery 61: 241–253
34. Miller J D, 1979 Barbiturates and raised intracranial pressure. Annals of Neurology 6: 189–193
35. Galicich J H, French L A 1961 The use of dexamethasone in the treatment of cerebral oedema resulting from brain tumours and brain surgery. American Practitioner 12: 169–174
36. Braakman R, Schouten H J A, Blaauw van Dischoeck M, 1983 Megadose steroids in severe head injury: results of a prospective double-blind clinical trial. Journal of Neurosurgery 57: 326–330
37. Sollman W P, Hussein S, Stolke D 1985 Results of management of severe craniocerebral trauma with and without dexamethasone. Neurochirurgica (Stuttgart) 28: 46–50
38. Dearden N M, Gibson J S, McDowall D G, 1986 Effect of high-dose dexamethasone on outcome from severe head injury. Journal of Neurosurgery 64: 81–88
39. Fanconi S, Kloti J, Meuli M, 1988 Dexamethasone therapy and endogenous cortisol production in severe paediatric head injury. Intensive Care Medicine 14: 163–166
40. Breivik H, Safar P, Sand P, 1978 Clinical feasibility trials of barbiturate therapy after cardiac arrest. Critical Care Medicine 6: 228–244
41. Ward J D, Becker D B, Miller J D, 1985 Failure of prophylactic barbiturate coma in the treatment of severe head injury. Journal of Neurosurgery 62: 383–388
42. Abramson N S 1987 Barbiturates and brain ischaemia, again. Intensive Care Medicine 13: 221–222
43. Gelpke G J, Braakman R, Habbema D F, Hilden J 1983 Comparison of outcome in two series of patients with severe head injuries. Journal of Neurosurgery 59: 745–750

44. Miller J D, 1985 Aggressive medical care of severe head injury — is it justified ethically and economically? In: Warlow C, Garfield J (eds.) Dilemmas in the management of the neurological patient. Churchill Livingstone, Edinburgh
45. Miller J D, Sweet R C, Naraya R, Becker D P 1978 Early insults to the injured brain. Journal of the American Medical Association 240(5): 439–442
46. McIver I N, Frew I J C, Matheson J C 1958 The role of respiratory insufficiency in the mortality of severe head injuries. Lancet 1: 390–393
47. Takizawa H, Gabra-Sanders T, Miller J D 1986 Analysis of changes in intracranial pressure — volume index at different locations in the craniospinal axis during supratentorial epidural balloon inflation. Neurosurgery 19: 1–8
48. Stuart F F, Merry G S, Smith J A, Yelland J D N 1983 Severe head injury managed without intracranial pressure monitoring. Journal of Neurosurgery 59: 601–605
49. Ruscoe Clarke A 1957 Recent advances in haemorrhage and shock. British Medical Journal 2: 721–726
50. Crowell J W, Smith E E 1967 Determinant of the optimal haematocrit. Journal of Applied Physiology 22(3): 501–504
51. Fan F, Chen R Y Z, Schmessler G B, Chien S 1980 Effects of haematocrit variations on regional hemodynamics and oxygen transport in the dog. American Journal of Physiology 238(7): 545–549
52. Messmer K F W 1987 Acceptable hematocrit levels in surgical patients. World Journal of Surgery 11: 41–45
53. McConn R, Derrick J B 1972 The respiratory function of blood. Anesthesiology 36(2): 119–128
54. Guy J T, Branberg P A, Metz E N, 1974 Oxygen delivery following transfusion of stored blood: 1. Normal rats. Journal of Applied Physiology 37(1): 60–63
55. Virgilio R W, Rice C L, Smith D E, 1979 Crystalloid verse colloid resuscitation: is one better? Surgery 2: 129–139
56. Twigley A J, Hillman K M 1985 The end of the crystalloid era? — a new approach to peri-operative fluid administration. Anaesthesia 40(9): 860–871
57. Horton J, Landreneau R, Tuggle D 1985 Cardiac response to fluid resuscitation from hemorrhagic shock. Surgery, Gynecology, Obstetrics 160: 444–452
58. Traverso L W, Lee W P, Langford M J 1986 Fluid resuscitation after an otherwise fatal hemorrhage: 1. Crystalloid solution. Journal of Trauma 26. 2. 168–175
59. Rackow E C, Falk J L, Fein A, 1983 Fluid resuscitation in circulatory shock: a comparison of the cardiorespiratory effects of albumin hetastarch and saline solution in patients with hypovolemic and septic shock. Critical Care Medicine 11 (11): 839–850
60. Smith J A R, Normal N J 1982 The fluid of choice for resuscitation of severe shock. British Journal of Surgery 69: 702–705
61. Messmer K F W 1987 The use of plasma substitutes with special attention to their side-effects World Journal of Surgery 11: 69–74
62. Ring J, Messmer K 1977 Incidence and severity of anaphyladoid reactions to colloid substitutes. Lancet 1: 466–469
63. Counts R B, Haisch C, Simon T L, 1979 Haemostasis in massively transfused trauma patients. Annals of Surgery 190(1): 91–99
64. Martin D J, Lucas C E, Ledgerwood A M, 1985 Fresh frozen plasma supplements to massive red blood cell transfusion. Annals of Surgery 202: 505–511
65. Consensus Conference 1985 Fresh frozen plasma: indications and risks. Journal of the American Medical Association 253: 551–555
66. Jones J 1987 Abuse of fresh frozen plasma. British Medical Journal 295(2): 287
67. Orr M D 1982 Autotransfusion: intra-operative scavenging. International Anesthesiology Clinics 20: 97–119
68. Davies M J, Cronin K D 1984 Blood conservation in elective surgery. Anaesthesia and Intensive Care 12: 229–235
69. Clifford P C, Kruger A R, Smith A, Chant A D B, Webster J H H 1987 Salvage autotransfusion in aortic surgery: initial studies using a disposable reservoir. British Journal of Surgery 74: 755–757
70. Solem J O, Steen S, Tengborm L, 1987 Mediastinal drainage blood. Scandinavian Journal of Thoracic and Cardiovascular Surgery 21: 149–152
71. Dale R F, Lindop M J, Farman J V, Smith M E 1986 Autotransfusion: an experience of 76 cases. Annals of the Royal College of Surgeons of England 68: 295–297
72. Napoli V M, Symbas P J, Symbas P N, Vroon D U 1987 Autotransfusion from experimental hemothorax: levels of coagulation factors. Journal of Trauma 27(3) 296–300
73. Surgenor D M 1987 The patients blood is the safest blood. New England Journal of Medicine 316(9) 542
74. Bernard F, Brigham K 1985 The adult respiratory distress syndrome. Annual Review of Medicine 36: 195–205

75. Till G O, Johnson K S, Kimkel R, Ward P A 1982 Intravascular activation of complement and acute lung injury. Journal of Clinical Investigation 69: 1126–1135
76. Tate R M, Repine J E 1983 Neutrophils and the adult respiratory distress syndrome. American Review of Respiratory Disease 128: 552–559
77. Laute M D, Simon R H, Flint A, Kneller J B 1986 Adult respiratory distress syndrome in neutropenic patients. American Journal of Medicine 80: 1022–1026
78. Editorial 1986 Adult respiratory distress syndrome. Lancet 1: 301–303
79. Stoddart J C 1988 The management of multi-organ failure in the ITU. In: Carter D C (ed.) Peri-operative care, British Medical Bulletin 44 (2) Churchill Livingstone, London, pp. 473–498
80. Pepe P E, Hudson L D, Carrico C J 1984 Early application of positive end-expiratory pressure in patients at risk for the adult respiratory distress syndrome. New England Journal of Medicine, 311: 281–286
81. Domek S J, Lynch J P, Weg J G, Dantzker D C 1980 The dependence of oxygen uptake on oxygen delivery in the adult respiratory distress syndrome. American Review of Respiratory Disease 122: 387–395
82. Rounds J, Brody J S 1984 Putting PEEP in perspective. New England Journal of Medicine 311: 323–325
83. Cole A G H, Weller S F, Sykes M K 1984 Inverse ratio ventilation compared with PEEP in adult respiratory failure Intensive Care Medicine 10(5): 227–232
84. Wattwil L M, Sjostrand V H, Borg U R 1983 Comparative studies of IPPV and HFPPV with PEEP in critical care medicine: 1. A clinical evaluation. Intensive Care Medicine 11(1): 30–37
85. Gotloib L, Barzilay E, Shustak A, Lev A 1984 Sequential hemofiltration in non-oliguric high capillary permeability pulmonary oedema of severe sepsis: preliminary report. Critical Care Medicine 12: 997–1000
86. Stoutenbeek C P, Van Saene H K F, Miranda D R, Zandstra D F 1984 The effect of selective decontamination of the digestive tract on colonization and infection rate in multiple trauma patients. Intensive Care Medicine 10(4): 185–192
87. Ledingham I McA, Alcock S R, Eastaway A T, 1988 Triple regimen of selective decontamination of the digestive tract, systemic cefotaxime and microbiological surveillance for prevention of acquired infection in intensive care. Lancet 1: 785–790
88. Sprung C L, Caralis P V, Marcial E H 1984 The effects of high-dose corticosteroids in patients with septic shock New England. Journal of Medicine 311: 1137–1143
89. Tokioka H, Kobayashi O, Ohta U, 1985 The acute effects of prostaglandin E_1 on the pulmonary circulation and oxygen delivery in patients with the adult respiratory distress syndrome. Intensive Care Medicine 11: 61–64
90. Kerstein M D, Crivello M 1986 Reversal of histopathological pulmonary changes with indomethacin Surgery, Gynecology, Obstetrics 151: 786–790
91. Baker S P, O'Neill B, Haddon W, Long W B 1974 The injury severity score: a method for describing patients with multiple injuries and evaluating emergency care. Journal of Trauma 14(3): 187–196
92. Knaus W A, Zimmerman J E, Wagner D P, Draper E A, Lawrence D 1981 APACHE: acute physiology and chronic health evaluation: a physiologically based classification system. Critical Care Medicine 9: 591–597
93. Knaus W A, Draper E A, Wagner D P, Zimmerman J E 1985 Prognosis in acute organ failure. Annals of Surgery 202: 685–693
94. Champion H R, Gainer P S, Yackee E 1986 A progress report on the trauma score in predicting a fatal outcome. Journal of Trauma 26(10) 927–931

8. Anaesthesia for craniofacial surgery

V.A. Goat

Craniofacial surgery can be defined as the surgical correction of disorders affecting the base of the skull, the orbits and the upper face. Until recently, this complex anatomical territory fell into 'no mans land' with several major surgical specialities performing part of the surgery but no one speciality able to provide a comprehensive surgical service for the patient. Consequently, results were poor and the incidence of morbidity and mortality unacceptably high. In the 1960s, Dr Paul Tessier pioneered the establishment of multidisciplinary teams; these were composed of plastic, neurosurgical, maxillofacial, ear, nose and throat (ENT) and ophthalmic surgeons who worked together to manage these complex problems. Since this time, several craniofacial teams have been established.

The anesthetist is an important member of this multidisciplinary team, who must be aware of the complexity of the surgery and be able to recognize and manage problems that may arise during the procedure. Although the number of anaesthetists involved in craniofacial reconstruction in the UK is small, the anaesthetic principles involved can be applied to most major head and neck surgery, and some of the more common problems are dealt with outside the craniofacial centres. It is also likely that at sometime during his or her career, the anaesthetist will encounter patients with major craniofacial abnormalities, presenting for unrelated surgery and anesthesia.

Three major groups of conditions are treated by the craniofacial team:[1] congenital anomalies; tumours involving the orbit, cranium and upper face where reconstruction is possible; and major craniofacial trauma. Approximately 50% of the work of the craniofacial team is involved with the correction of congenital abnormalities. These have been classified by Stewart[2] into six major groups:

1. Otocranialfacial syndromes with bilateral symmetric involvement (e.g. Treacher Collins syndrome);

2. Otocranialfacial syndromes with asymmetric involvement (e.g. Goldenhar's syndrome; hemifacial microsomia);

3. Craniosynostosis and craniofacial synostosis;

4. Midface abnormalities (e.g. cleft lip and palate — this is the most common anomality seen, with an incidence of 1 in 800 live births Pierre Robin syndrome);

5. Frontonasal dysplasia (e.g. hypertelorism); and

6. Craniofacial clefts which may be associated with an encephalocoele.

Groups 1, 2 and 4 may be associated with serious airway problems including intubation difficulties. General anesthesia may be required for X-ray investigations, investigation and treatment of associated deafness as well as for facial remodelling.

Premature fusion of one or more of the cranial sutures results in craniosynostosis. Approximately 1/2000 children suffer from some degree of premature fusion of the cranial bones. If only one suture is involved, then compensatory growth will occur at other unfused sutures, this may cause some degree of cranial deformity. Some cases do not require surgery, others many be corrected by early craniectomy. Only the more severe cases require formal remodelling of the skull, which is usually performed at around 6 months of age.

Involvement of multiple sutures may reduce intracranial volume. This may result in an increase in intracranial pressure with retardation of brain growth and development. Intracranial hypertension may be difficult to diagnose in infancy, and continuous monitoring of the intracranial pressure may be required over 24 hours. Premature fusion may also affect the bones of the base of the skull and face (craniofacial synostosis) producing maxillary hypoplasia with partial airway obstruction and exophthalmos. If these conditions are left untreated, as well as the risk of intracranial hypertension, corneal ulceration and damage may occur, and in later childhood malocclusion of the teeth will add to the list of complications. Specific syndromes can be recognised, of which Crouzon's syndrome is one of more frequently occuring craniofacial dysostosis. In this condition, there is premature fusion of both coronal sutures, with hypoplasia and retrusion of the maxilla. The shallow orbits lead to proptosis of the eyes and these may be set widely apart (hypertelorism). A similar cranial deformity is seen in infants with Apert's syndrome but, in addition, symmetrical syndactyly affects both the hands and feet. These children may also suffer from a cleft palate and primary mental retardation is common. Less frequently occuring syndromes include Pfeiffers, Saethre Chotzens and Carpenters.

When multiple sutures are involved or there is intracranial hypertension, early surgery is required. A bifrontal craniotomy is performed; this allows access to the base of the skull and the roof of the orbit. The supraorbital margin is removed and enlarged by bone grafts; allowing it to be slid forward. The frontal bones are then reattached to the supraorbital ridge as a floating segment, leaving a wide artificial suture (Fig. 8.1). This procedure increases the intracranial volume, as well as allowing any asymmetry of the cranium and upper orbits to be corrected. The orbits are also deepened, providing protection for the protruberant eyes. Ideally, this surgery should be performed as soon as possible; however, in practice, surgery is usually performed between 3–6 months of age. Fronto-orbital advancement does not improve the airway, if airway problems exist because of craniofacial synostosis, a mid-facial advancement is required. This is usually delayed until the child is older; although occasionally advancement of the maxilla will be undertaken during infancy to relieve severe upper airway obstruction. Total correction of both cranial and facial deformity is rarely performed together because of the high risk of infection.

The surgical correction of hypertelorism is usually delayed until later childhood since early surgery may have to be repeated as the child grows. An intracranial approach may be used, to allow a block of bone to be removed from the midface so that the orbits can be repositioned. Midline clefts associated with an encephalocoele will, of course, require earlier surgery.

In summary, for the congenital defects, the main indications for surgery are intracranial hypertension, corneal exposure and ulceration, airway difficulties and dental malocclusion.[3] However, in some cases, the major indication for surgery is cosmetic.

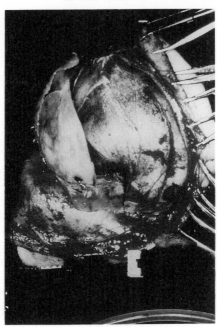

Fig. 8.1   Frontal advancement showing the supraorbital ridge and frontal bones wired into position leaving a wide artificial coronal suture.

Malignant tumours involving the facial bones and sinuses require a wide removal this may include the base of the skull, dura and occasionally brain tissue. The craniofacial approach using a bicoronal incision allows excellent exposure that aids surgical clearance of malignant tissue. Cosmetic reconstruction may be performed either as a primary procedure, or delayed until there is histological evidence of tumour clearance. Some benign tumours and tumour-like conditions of the craniofacial skeleton may be relatively inaccessible and therefore benefit from this type of approach.

Craniofacial trauma remains a serious problem, despite the compulsory use of seat belts. Fractures that involve the maxilla and naso-ethmoidal bones may cause long-term complications; these include c.f.s. leaks with the constant risk of meningitis, nasal deformity and diplopia. Major surgery is delayed until the patients neurological condition has stabilized, then a primary reconstructive procedure is performed. There is evidence that this combined approach reduces both the duration of patient stay in hospital and the frequency of late complications.

PRE-ANAESTHETIC ASSESSMENT

Assessment of the patient prior to major surgery is extremely important and must include a detailed evaluation of the airway. Facial trauma may cause airway obstruction, which must be quickly recognized and the airway promptly secured, if necessary by a tracheostomy.

Partial obstruction of the airway is common in patients with craniofacial anomalies and may be caused by micrognathia, mandibulo-facial dysostosis and maxillary hypoplasia. Symptoms include noisy breathing, often during sleep, with paradoxical movements of the chest wall. Total obstruction of the airway may occur during sleep, resulting in sleep apnoea. This may be recognised from the history of noisy, disturbed sleep, day-time somnolence and failure to thrive. Left untreated, pulmonary hypertension may occur.[4] Various arrhythmias have been recorded during apnoeic periods. These include bradycardia, tachycardia and ventricular extrasystoles, and may be responsible for sudden death occuring during sleep.[5]

In addition to the sleep apnoea produced by upper airway obstruction, there may also be an element of central apnoea. If this is the case, the patient may be extremely sensitive to respiratory depressants and may require prolonged postoperative ventilation. Enlarged tonsils and adenoids may contribute to the obstruction, if this is the case they should be removed. Any patient who shows signs of airway obstruction pre-operatively is likely to have significant postoperative problems. Some surgeons consider that early tracheostomy is beneficial,[6] but this view is not universally accepted. Decannulation of the tracheostome may prove extremely difficult, hence the reluctance of many surgeons to resort to a tracheostomy.

It may be difficult to obtain an airtight seal with the face mask, making mask ventilation impossible. (Fig. 8.2) This problem may be overcome by using either a large mask to cover the entire face, or the clear plastic 'puff' mask (vital signs anaesthesia mask). This mask has a large air-filled rim, which conforms to some facial irregularities.

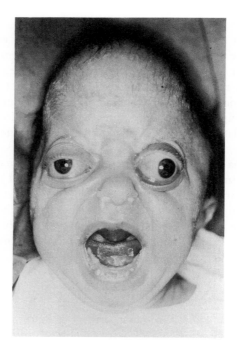

Fig. 8.2 Infant with severe craniofacial abnormalities in whom mask ventilation proved difficult. (Reproduced with permission.)

A difficult intubation must be anticipated in all patients where there is either limited mouth opening, or restricted movement at the atlanto-occipital joint or the cervical spine. Inspection of the fauces is a useful simple way to assess ease of intubation. In the seated position with the tongue maximally protruded, visualization of the uvula and faucial pillars suggests that direct laryngoscopy will expose the glottis.[7] The cervical spine of all patients presenting with major craniofacial trauma should be regarded as unstable until proven otherwise.

There may be other congenital abnormalities present, including syndactyly, congenital cardiac defects, cleft palate, choanal atresia and fusion of the cervical spine.[8] The latter will add to difficulties with intubation. Metabolic problems although uncommon, may be encountered.

The anaesthetic history is important as multiple anaesthetics are frequently required. Where there have been difficulties with the anaesthetic, the patient or parents should be informed about the problem so that they are in a position to alert future anaesthetists.

Repeated chest infections are common and these must be agressively treated before surgery. Most centres use prophylactic broad-spectrum antibiotics to reduce the risk of perioperative infection and, in Oxford, anticonvulsants are started 5 days before surgery and continued for a minimum of 6 months. Since this regimen was adopted there have been no cases of post operative convulsions.

The patient, or parents, in the case of children, should receive a detailed explanation of the anaesthetic and surgical procedures. Potential postoperative problems including postoperative ventilation must be discussed. The patient should also be warned of the presence of vascular lines, drains, urinary catheter and monitoring in the recovery period, and should be reassured that he will be kept comfortable and pain-free following surgery. Swelling around the eyes retricts eye opening, and if not anticipated may cause considerable distress.

Routine investigations should include full blood count, electrolytes, clotting screen, e.c.g. and chest X-ray. Adequate blood must be cross-matched, using fresh whole blood wherever possible. In Oxford, blood is cross-matched on a weight basis, a minimum of 3 adult units for infants under 10 kg, to a maximum of 6 units for adults. Two of the units are provided in split packs for the paediatric cases. These are reserved for the postoperative period when blood is required intermittently for the first 24 hours. This minimizes the number of donors to whom the patients are exposed.

ANAESTHESIA

Heavy premedication should be avoided in the presence of intracranial hypertension or airway obstruction. Atropine premedication ensures drying of the oral secretions and prevents vagal stimulation during laryngoscopy. Some sedation may be required for older children and adults; oral diazepam 0.15 mg/kg given 2 hours before the induction of anaesthesia is a useful anxiolytic. It is important during the induction of anaesthesia that the 'point of no return' is not passed until it is certain that assisted ventilation is possible. The airway must take priority. In most cases, intubation is not a problem and an intravenous induction is appropriate. If intubation difficulties are anticipated, a gaseous induction with halothane is my technique of choice. A range of intubation aids and tubes should be available, and the patient must not be paralysed

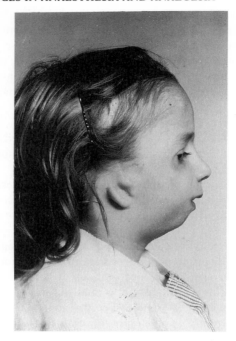

Fig. 8.3   Treacher Collins syndrome. Previous attempts at intubation had failed. (Reproduced with permission.)

until ventilation has been successfully controlled. While an inhalational induction with halothane may cause intracranial pressure to rise, this is usually reversible. Hypoxia following a failed intubation may cause permanent brain damage.

An alternative technique suitable for adults with potential intubation problems, is to perform an awake intubation under local anaesthesia. This is obviously inappropriate in children, although awake intubation is possible in the small infant. Delays during intubation and breath holding may result in cyanosis. This can be avoided by pre-oxygenation and by administering oxygen via a fine nasal catheter, during attempts at laryngoscopy and intubation.

Where intubation has previously failed or pre-operative assessment suggests serious difficulties, (Fig. 8.3) transtracheal jet ventilation is the method of choice in Oxford. A transcricothyrotomy device (Fig. 8.4) is inserted under local anaesthesia into the upper trachea. (Fig. 8.5) Once its correct placement has been confirmed by the free aspiration of air, the patient is anaesthesized and paralysed, and ventilation controlled using a Sanders injector. This technique has been successfully used both in paediatric patients[9,10] and adults. It is important that barotrauma is avoided by allowing free exhalation of the inspired gases, and that the maximum pressure of the injector is reduced to a level appropriate to the size of the patient. Intubation can then be attempted, un-hurried and under optimal conditions, when it is usually successful. A fibreoptic laryngoscope may be a useful aid to intubation provided the operator is experienced in its use. The smallest fibreoptic scope available will pass through a 4.5 mm tube. If in-tubation proves impossible, a trachestomy can be performed below the level of the transtracheal cannulation.

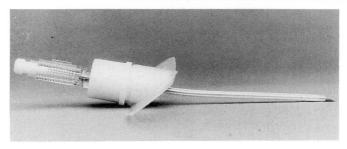

Fig. 8.4 Transcricothyrotomy cannula.

Other methods of dealing with a difficult intubation have been described. They include the use of bougies, blind nasal and oral intubation and retrograde catheterization through a cricothyroid puncture.[11] Nasal intubation may be required for surgery involving the maxilla to allow access to the oropharynx and to permit jaw fixation at the completion of surgery.

Accidental extubation is a well recognized hazard. The position of the head may be changed by the surgeons, and it is easy for uncuffed tubes to flip out of the larynx. Facial advancement may result in the advancement of the nasotracheal tube by 3–4 cm. Davies and Munro[12] described a simple method for tube placement; with the head in the position required for surgery, the endotracheal tube is deliberately advanced until it is endobronchial. The tube is then slowly withdrawn until both lungs inflate equally, at which time it is marked and fixed securely either to the lower lip or the

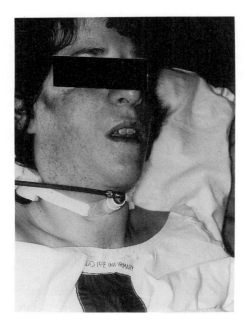

Fig. 8.5 Cannula in place allowing jet ventilation.

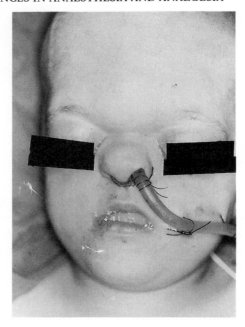

Fig. 8.6   Facial advancement, use of a long, reinforced nasal tube.

nares — its tip should then be sitting just above the carina. It is important to check ventilation of both lungs after the patient has been positioned on the operating table, as a slight change in the position of the head may result in endobronchial intubation with one-lung ventilation. The use of armoured tubes is advisable when access to the airway is limited. Long reinforced tubes can be used for nasal intubation, so that the connections can be removed from the surgical field (Fig. 8.6).

It is important that the correct size of tube is selected for children. There should be an air leak during controlled ventilation, demonstrating the presence of a gap between the tube and the tracheal mucosa, thus reducing the risk of postoperative subglottic oedema.

The number of connections used in the breathing system should be kept to a minimum to reduce the risk of accidental disconnection. Essential joints should be firmly taped together and a disconnection alarm used. Lightweight coaxial circuits are useful since there is less drag exerted on the endotracheal tube, and when used with a condenser humidifier help to conserve both heat and moisture.

The endotracheal tube may be inadvertently sabotaged during the procedure. In addition to accidental extubation, there have been reports of transection of the tube[13] transfixion of the tube to facial bones by a Kirshner wire[14] and obstruction. The anaesthetist must be vigilant, anticipate these problems, and have a suitable replacement tube immediately available.

Anaesthetic access to the patient may be extremely limited with multiple teams of surgeons around the patient. It is important to discuss surgical requirements beforehand, so that the anaesthetic tubing can be removed as far as possible from the surgical field.

An anaesthetic technique should be chosen to reduce intracranial volume and also allow a rapid return of reflexes at the conclusion of surgery. Reduction of intracranial volume is important, since this will allow surgical access to the anterior cranial fossa with the minimum of surgical retraction of the frontal lobes. Retraction of brain tissue may impede local blood supply resulting in intra-operative ischaemia and postoperative swelling. Intracranial volume can be reduced by decreasing the volume of one of the three components within the skull; the blood, cerebrospinal fluid (c.s.f.) and brain tissue.

The volume of blood within the cranium can be reduced by hyperventilation. Cerebral blood vessels are extremely sensitive to the tension of carbon dioxide in the arterial blood, for each 1 kPa reduction in $PaCO_2$ there is a 15% decrease in cerebral blood flow. Changes in arterial blood pressure have little effect upon cerebral blood flow, unless they are outside the levels for autoregulation (mean arterial pressure 60–130 mmHg). Hypertension must be avoided. All volatile anaesthetic agents increase cerebral blood flow by causing direct vasodilation of the cerebral vessels. This can be minimized by using low concentrations of the volatile agents and by employing hyperventilation. Isoflurane causes the least increase in cerebral blood flow and would appear to be the volatile agent of choice for intracranial procedures. Some anaesthetists prefer to avoid volatile agents altogether, but it is important to minimize sympathetic overactivity by adequate analgesia and anaesthesia.

Opioids and neuroleptic drugs reduce intracranial pressure so long as ventilation is controlled. A reduction in cerebral metabolism is accompanied by a reduction in cerebral blood flow. Infusions of thiopentone and propofol have a similar effect upon cerebral metabolism and cerebral blood flow.

Cerebral venous drainage can be enhanced by using a head-up tilt, taking care that the head is placed in the neutral position with no obstruction of the jugular veins. It is also important to reduce mean airway presure, the compliance of the chest wall can be reduced by using muscle relaxants, facilitating hyperventilation using low airway pressures.

Intracranial volume can also be reduced by decreasing the volume of c.s.f. within the cranium. In adults, spinal drainage can be employed, using an extradural catheter placed within the lumbar subarachnoid space. Once a burr hole has been made, c.s.f. is allowed to drain into a closed system. The rate of drainage must be carefully controlled, since if it is allowed to proceed too rapidly, distortion of the brain stem may produce hypertension and tachycardia.[15] This technique is inappropriate in small children because of the size of the subarachnoid space, instead a lumbar puncture is performed, and the needle is removed; this leaves a tract along which c.s.f. can drain during surgery.

Diuretics reduce brain bulk and are used routinely in some centres. Loop diuretics are effective in reducing brain water and lack the rebound effect occasionally seen with mannitol. If loop diuretics are used, the serum potassium must be carefully monitored and replacements given when necessary. Dexamethazone reduces cerebral and facial swelling and is given peri-operatively.

BLOOD LOSS

Blood loss is one of the major intra-operative problems. It starts with the first incision and continues throughout the procedure into the postoperative period. Various methods for the measurement of blood loss have been described. They include intra-operative weighing of blood-stained swabs and measurement of the volume of blood draining into the suction bottles. It is difficult to measure the ongoing loss in these procedures, as spilt blood often remains concealed until the drapes are removed at the completion of surgery. The surgical practice of flushing the wound with Ringer's lactate solution also complicates the picture. However, postoperative estimates of blood loss are possible using various markers, including haemoglobin, cell counts or potassium. These measurements are of little use to the anaesthetist in theatre. The rate of blood loss appears directly proportional to the number of surgeons operating, and the complexity of the procedure. Losses in excess of the patients total blood volume are common, and blood loss in excess of 2–4 times the patient's blood volume have been reported in some paediatric cases.[16,17] Blood loss can be reduced by the use of hae-mostatic sutures, infiltration with vasoconstrictors and induced hypotension.[18] As the craniofacial team becomes more experienced the operative time and blood loss is reduced.

There must be adequate access to the circulation for transfusion. The author prefers to have two peripheral drips sited in all patients, as large as is technically possible; one is reserved for maintenance crystalloids, the other for colloid replacement. Dextrose NaCl solution is used as a maintenance crystalloid according to the guidelines of Holliday and Segar:[19]

1. Children weighing between 0 and 10 kg are given 4 ml/kg.h^{-1}
2. Children weighing between 10 and 20 kg are given 40 ml/h plus 2ml/kg.h^{-1} for each kg over 10 kg.
3. Children weighing over 20 kg are given 60 ml/h plus 1 ml/kg.h^{-1} for each kg over 20 kg.

Colloid replacement should be commenced as early as possible. Massive blood loss may occur during scalp dissection, and early replacement prevents gross haemodyna-mic changes. The author preloads children with 10% of their calculated blood volume, using warmed 4.5% human albumen solution. Filtered warmed blood is then given and its rate of administration adjusted to maintain the arterial blood pressure and the pulse rate within normal limits. At the completion of surgery, the anaesthetist should ensure that the patient is in blood balance on clinical grounds, postoperative blood loss is then measured and replaced once drainage exceeds 10% of the calculated blood volume. It is important to check the platelet count and clotting profile regularly throughout surgery for dilutional coagulopathy and thrombocytopenia. In practice these are uncommon,[16] but fresh frozen plasma and platelets should be available. Calcium is not given routinely, but is considered when the rate of transfusion exceeds 2 ml/kg.min.

It is easier to monitor the adequacy of blood replacement than to measure the volume of blood loss. Wherever possible, arterial blood pressure is measured directly. As well as providing a beat-by-beat measurement of the systolic, diastolic and mean pressures, analysis of the shape of the waveform may provide additional information about the circulation. Normal myocardial contractility produces a rapid upstroke of the arterial pressure wave. This is depressed when there is either myocardial dysfunction or hypovolaemia; in addition, the waveform of the latter has a steep downstroke, and the dicrotic notch may be absent.[20] The variation of systolic blood pressure produced by controlled ventilation is exaggerated in the presence of a decreased circulating blood volume,[21] and is an early indicator of hypovolaemia. Other parameters may help to assess the adequacy of blood replacement; these include the core-peripheral temperture difference, hourly urine output, and the metabolic status of the patient. Experience obtained from previous procedures is also important.

Hypotensive anaesthesia has its advocates and can be used to reduce blood loss, even in small infants. Tachycardia is likely to occur, but can be prevented by the administration of beta-blocking agents.[22] Reduction of the mean arterial blood pressure to 60 mmHg is generally considered safe and significantly reduces blood loss.[23] The patient must be carefully monitored, and ganglion-blocking drugs avoided because of the problem of persistent pupillary dilatation.

It is preferable to use directly acting vasodilating agents to lower the blood pressure. These drugs will dilate cerebral blood vessels, allowing lower mean pressures to be tolerated before flow is reduced. Initially, there will be an increase in intracranial volume, but as the arterial blood pressure is reduced the cerebral blood flow will also start to fall.

Tachycardia is an early indicator of hypovolaemia in children. This valuable sign will be lost during deliberate hypotension, because of this, many anaesthetists (myself included) avoid lowering the blood pressure in small infants. Infiltration with vasoconstrictors, such as adrenaline has been used to reduce blood loss.[18] The total dose of adrenaline used should be limited to 5–10 μg/kg and, when halogenated anaesthetics are used, the lower dose should be employed.

MONITORING

Routine monitoring should include e.c.g., arterial blood pressure, end-tidal CO_2, airway pressure and hourly urine output. Heart and breath sounds should be monitored by an oesophageal stethoscope, while rectal and limb temperatures should be continuously recorded. Arterial cannulation also permits the frequent estimation of arterial blood gases, haematocrit, blood glucose and serum electrolyte levels.

Measurement of central venous pressure may provide additional information about the circulation but it is important to consider the potential hazards associated with the cannulation of central veins — especially in young children. Access to the patient is very restricted during surgery, this may make it difficult to detect and treat a pneumothorax. Some workers feel that in the presence of a normal heart, most of the information is already available from the arterial pressure, the pulse wave and urine output.[16,20]

Heat loss may be a major problem as surgical procedures may take several hours, thus allowing significant cooling to occur. Accidental hypothermia is seen more frequently in small infants, as their insulation is poor and many of the heat-conserving mechanisms normally at work are abolished by general anaesthesia. Hypothermia is likely to cause problems in the post-operative period. Metabolism of drugs may be depressed and recovery delayed. Also, a fall in body temperature may increase oxygen consumption as the infant shivers in an attempt to compensate.

Heat loss can be reduced by several methods, including increasing the ambient temperature to 24–28°C, the use of warming and space blankets, humidification of inspired gases and warming all fluids to body temperature. It is important that heat is conserved during the induction of anaesthesia. The use of an overhead radiant heater, allows adequate observation and access to the infant, while conserving body temperature.[24]

Neuromuscular monitoring allows a constant level of neuromuscular block to be achieved, which may be altered should the surgeons wish to use a nerve stimulator to aid in the identification and preservation of the facial nerve. Free flaps may be required for facial reconstruction. This will lengthen the procedure and may require the use of alpha-blocking drugs to improve tissue perfusion. Occasionally, the surgeon requires additional bone for grafting, if there is insufficient available from the skull, then ribs or iliac crest bone may be used. This will reduce anaesthetic access even further and, if rib grafts are taken, the possibility of a pneumothorax must be considered.

During surgical manipulation of the orbits, severe bradycardia occurs in a significant number of patients. This is usually terminated by stopping the surgical stimulus; if this fails then a small dose of atropine should be administered.

Air embolism is a potential hazard; early signs of air embolism include a sudden reduction in the end-tidal carbon dioxide tension, and a mill-wheel murmur heard over the right atrium.

POSTOPERATIVE MANAGEMENT

Postoperatively, the airway may be compromised by swelling around the upper airway and larynx, and persistant bleeding from the nose and mid face. It is prudent to delay extubation until the patient is fully awake — especially if there has been a difficult intubation, or if the jaws have been wired together. Fronto-orbital advancement does not improve the airway, and pre-existing problems will be exacerbated by prolonged anaesthesia and surgery. If there is any doubt about the adequacy of the airway postoperatively, the patient should remain intubated and ventilated. It is advisable to replace the long re-inforced tube with a shorter one made of polyvinyl chloride (PVC). This permits optimal tracheobronchial toilet, and reduces airway resistance and dead space. However, despite these problems, most patients are extubated as soon as they are fully awake and making purposeful movements.[16,18,20] Many of these operations increase the size of the cranium and so the extra space created may delay the detection of an extradural haematoma. Diagnosis of this life-threatening complication may be further delayed if the patient has been sedated to permit ventilation; thus the benefits of sedation and controlled ventilation must be weighed against the possibility of missing intracranial bleeding.

The surgeons usually request that the patients are nursed supine for the first 24 hours to avoid distortion of the remodelled skull. Intensive physiotherapy is important to reduce the incidence of postoperative chest infections. Postoperative pain, as in most intracranial procedures is not severe, and can be controlled by codeine phosphate 0.5–1 mg/kg. Donor sites for skin and bone may cause more pain and necessitate the use of more potent opioids. Neurological assessment is essential because of the increased risks and difficulties experienced in the early diagnosis of intracranial haematoma; any deterioration in the conscious level of the patient postoperatively justifies an immediate computerized tomography scan. Visual disturbances may arise because of local damage to the optic nerves. If the patient is unable to co-operate with clinical testing, then visually evoked responses can be elicited. Postoperative recovery is usually very rapid, most infants are accepting normal feeds within 24 hours.

Several surgical firms will be involved in the management of the patient, and it is important that one team is in overall charge. In Oxford, the craniofacial patients are admitted under the joint care of the consultant plastic surgeon and consultant neurosurgeon. The junior staff of the plastic surgeon are responsible for the immediate pre-operative workup and postoperative care. A detailed checklist has been drawn up to prevent important omissions. Postoperatively, the junior staff are closely supported by the anaesthetist, who prescribes all postoperative fluids including blood and is also responsible for postoperative analgesia. If controlled ventilation is required, this is performed in either the adult or paediatric intensive therapy unit under the close supervision of the anaesthetic department.

Three of the more common craniofacial procedures will be briefly discussed with special reference to the anaesthetic problems.

Cleft lip and palate

This is the most common of the craniofacial abnormalities. In most cases, it occurs as an isolated defect but it may be associated with other congenital disorders, including other craniofacial problems. In most centres, the lip is repaired at about 3 months of age, the palate being left until 6–12 months. Pre-operative fasting should be kept to a minimum, and it is usually unnecessary to use sedative premedication, although an antisialogue may be helpful. If those children with multiple congenital disorders are excluded, intubation is rarely a problem; although laryngoscopy may be made difficult by the laryngoscope blade lodging in the cleft. This can be prevented either by packing the cleft before laryngoscopy or by using a Bryce-Smith blade. Pre-formed tubes are usually employed, and it is important to check that they are not obstructed when the mouth gag is opened. A split blade should be used to minimize the risk of this occuring during surgery. Blood loss may be heavy, so for all infants blood must be available before surgery. Extubation may be a problem, as the child may take some time to adapt to the new airway. It is prudent to wait until the child is fully recovered from the anaesthetic before he is extubated and a tongue suture may be needed to pull the tongue forward in the postoperative period.

Craniectomy

Strip craniectomy is performed usually for premature fusion of the saggital suture to decompress the brain and to allow normal brain growth. The procedure is performed as early as possible and is not without hazard. Shillito and Matson[25] reported a mortality of 0.4% with a morbidity of 14% in a large series of patients. Massive bleeding from dural venous sinuses and exposed bone is the biggest problem, requiring adequate venous access and blood replacement. This may exceed 50% of the infants blood volume. Again, measurement of blood loss may be very difficult. Blood loss can be reduced by hypotensive anaesthesia[26] meticulous surgery and the use of vasoconstrictors. Care must be taken to limit the total dose of vasoconstrictor used.

Major oral and maxillofacial surgery

Major oral and maxillofacial surgery is performed for three major reasons, congenital abnormalities, the removal of tumours and trauma; the latter group is possibly the largest and frequently involves young motorcyclists.

Fractures of the maxilla and mandible are often associated with a primary head injury as well as fractures of the cervical spine. In addition, there may be injuries of the chest and abdomen and these must be excluded before maxillofacial surgery is undertaken. Bilateral fracture of the mandible may cause acute obstruction of the airway. In the concious individual this may be relieved by placing the patient into the prone position, but in the unconscious patient may require emergency intubation. Swallowed blood and loose teeth are potential hazards, the cervical spine must be considered unstable until proven otherwise, and the loss of normal facial contours may make mask anaesthesia difficult. All these factors must be considered when choosing the technique for induction of anaesthesia. Occasionally, a preliminary tracheostomy may be required. The risk of airway problems occuring during anaesthesia for major oral and maxillofacial surgery is high. Apart from problems with intubation, accidental extubation is a real risk during surgery. During surgical advancement of the maxilla, the nasotracheal tube will also be advanced by up to 3–4 cm, so it is essential that the tip of the tube is sited just above the carina at the start of surgery.

Occasionally, the surgeon will require the oral tube to be replaced by a nasal one. This is usually requested once the maxilla has been mobilized, to allow intra oral work and to permit occlusion of the teeth at the end of the surgery. The tube should be changed under direct vision after deepening anaesthesia, giving additional muscle relaxants, if required, and ventilating the patient with high concentrations of oxygen. Flexion of the neck may facilitate passage of the nasal tube through the larynx.[27] Some workers consider that c.s.f. rhinorrhoea is a contra-indication to nasal intubation because of the potential risk of infection.[28] Obstruction of the tube, fixation by sutures, and transection of the tube and its pilot balloon have all been reported. The anaesthetist and surgeon must work together and both be aware of the additional hazards of a shared airway.

Postoperatively, the surgeon may wire the jaws together, and the nasotracheal tube should be left in situ until the patient is fully conscious. An anti-emetic should be given routinely to prevent postoperative vomiting, low-dose droperidol may be useful. Wire cutters must be immediately available and the nursing staff aware of the sutures to be cut. Postoperative oedema may compromise the airway and, when this is anticipated, the tube should be left for 24–48 hours. Prophylactic antibiotics are given routinely and dexamethazone may be used to reduce postoperative swelling. Analgesics should be used sparingly because of the risk of respiratory depression and the patient should be closely monitored in a high-dependency nursing area. An elective tracheostomy should be performed if airway obstruction is present, or if there is any associated chest or head injury.

Craniofacial surgery presents many challenges to the anaesthetist, there may be a major airway difficulties and blood loss is heavy and continuous. It is important that the procedure is well planned and that the anaesthetist is experienced in this major surgery. However, the anaesthetist has the satisfaction of being an important member of the team and can, by paying meticulous attention to detail, make a valuable contribution to the surgical outcome.

REFERENCES

1. Poole M, Briggs M, Rayne J, Cheng H 1985. Craniofacial surgery. British Medical Journal 290 (1): 693–695

2. Stewart R E 1978 Craniofacial malformations: Clinical and genetic considerations. Pediatric Clinics of North America 25: 485–515
3. Matthews D 1979 Craniofacial surgery — indications, assessment and complications. British Journal of Plastic Surgery 32: 96–105
4. Freeman M K, Manners J M 1980 Cor pulmonale and the Pierre Robin anomaly. Anaesthesia 35: 282–286
5. Chung F, Crago R R, 1982 Sleep apnoea syndrome and anaesthesia. Canadian Anaesthetist's Society Journal 29: 439–444
6. Lauritzen C, Liljio J, Jarlstedt J, 1986 Airway obstruction and sleep apnoea in children with craniofacial anomalies. Plastic and Reconstructive Surgery 77: 1–6
7. Mallampati S R, Gatt S P, Gugino L D, Desai S P, Waraksa B, Freiberger D 1985 A new sign for predicting difficult intubation. Canadian Anaesthetists' Society Journal 32: 429–434
8. Berryhill R E 1981 Skin and bone disorders. In: Katz J, Benumof J, Kadis L B (eds.) Anaesthesia and uncommon diseases. Saunders, Philadephia
9. Smith B R, Myers E N, Sherman H 1974 Transtracheal ventilation in paediatric patients. British Journal of Anaesthesia 46: 313–314
10. Ward M E, Goat V A 1986 Use of transtracheal jet ventilation for patients with difficult intubation. Todays Anaesthetist (4): 22
11. Barham C J 1987 Difficult intubation. In: Judkins K C (ed.) Clinical anaesthesiology: burns and plastic surgery. Bailliere Tindall, London
12. Davies D W, Munro I R 1975 The anaesthetic management and intra-operative care of patients undergoing major facial osteotomies. Plastic and Reconstructive surgery 55: 50–55
13. Fragraeus L, Angelillo J G, Donlan E A 1980. A serious anesthetic hazard during orthognathic surgery. Anesthesia and Analgesia 59: 150–153
14. Lee C, Schwartz S, Mok M S 1977 Difficult extubation due to transfixation of a nasotracheal tube by a Kirshner wire. Anesthesiology 46: 422
15. Barker J 1975 An anaesthetic technique for intracranial aneurysms. Anaesthesia 30: 557
16. Uppington J, Goat V A 1987 Anaesthesia for major craniofacial surgery: a report of 23 cases in children under 4 years of age. Annals of The Royal College of Surgeons of England 69: 175–178
17. Scholtes J L, Thauvery C L, Moulin D, Gribomont B F 1985 Craniofaciosynostosis: anaesthetic and peri-operative management: report of 71 operations. Acta Anaesthesia Belge 36: 176–185
18. Broennle A M, Teller L, 1987 Anaesthesia for craniofacial procedures. In: Whitaker (ed.) Clinics in plastic surgery: craniofacial surgery. Saunders, Philadephia
19. Holliday M A, Segar W S 1957 The maintenance need for water in parenteral fluid therapy. Pediatrics 19: 823–832
20. Christianson L 1985 Anaesthesia for major craniofacial operations. In: Godinez R I (ed.) International anesthesiology clinics: special problems in paediatric anesthesia. Little and Brown, Boston
21. Parel A, Pizov R, Colev S 1987 Systolic blood pressure variation is a sensitive indicator of hypovolemia in ventilated dogs subjected to graded haemorrhage. Anesthesiology 69: 498–502
22. Salem M R, Toyama T, Wong A Y, Jacobs H K, Bennet E J 1978 Haemodynamic responses to induced arterial hypotension in children. British Journal of Anaesthesia 50: 489–493
23. Schaberg S J, Kelly J F, Terry B C, Posner M A, Anderson E F 1976 Blood loss and hypotensive anaesthesia in oral-facial corrective surgery. Journal of Oral Surgery 34: 147–156
24. Gauntlett I, Barnes J, Brown T C K, Bell B J 1985 Temperature maintenance in infants undergoing anaesthesia and surgery. Anaesthesia and Intensive Care 13: 300–304
25. Shillito J, Matson D D 1968 Craniosynostosis: a review of 519 surgical patients. Pediatrics 41: 829–853
26. Diaz J H, Lockhart C H, 1972 Hypotensive anaesthesia for craniectomy in infancy. British Journal of Anaesthesia 51: 233–235
27. Fergusson D J M, Barker J, Jackson I T 1983 Anaesthesia for craniofacial osteotomies. Annals Plastic Surgery 10: 333–336
28. Davies R M, Scott J G 1968 Anaesthesia for major oral and maxillofacial surgery. British Journal of Anaesthesia 40: 202–288

9. Capnography and pulse oximetry

A.P. Adams

CAPNOGRAPHY

Luft developed the principle of capnography in 1943 from the knowledge that CO_2 is one of the gases that absorbs infra-red (IR) radiation of a particular wavelength. Infra-red radiation is absorbed by all gases with more than two atoms in the molecule. If there are only two atoms, absorption only occurs if the two atoms are dissimilar. A capnometer is an instrument that measures the numerical concentration of CO_2. A device that continuously records and displays CO_2 concentration in the form of a tracing of waveform is called a capnograph — the tracing on recording paper being called a capnogram. The accuracy of rapid IR CO_2 analysis in determining alveolar carbon dioxide concentration ($FACO_2$) was established by Collier and his colleagues[1] and the value of the end-tidal (ET) sample established by Ramwell.[2] The introduction of capnography into routine clinical practice was pioneered by Smalhout and Kalenda in The Netherlands.[3]

The presentation of the CO_2 waveform obtained from breathing systems used in anaesthesia and intensive care in the analogue (waveform) format, i.e. the capnograph or capnogram, is vastly preferable to a meter or even a fast digital display. Indeed, both the latter are useless in anaesthetic practice where the breath-by-breath waveform needs to be displayed to permit continuous monitoring and analysis. Moreover, it is essential where fractional rebreathing techniques are employed, as with the Mapleson D/E/F and Bain breathing systems, because a meter or digital display cannot indicate the CO_2 concentration of the end-tidal CO_2 plateau as CO_2 also appears in the inspiratory part of the respiratory cycle.

Capnography is the study of the shape or design of the changing concentrations of CO_2 in respired gas. A high-speed capnogram gives detailed information about each breath, while overall changes in CO_2 may be followed at a slower paper speed. The capnograph may now be regarded as the most useful monitor for use in anaesthesia and intensive care, and it is an excellent early warning system. Capnography has wide application in a variety of circumstances including teaching and research, although many are unaware of its full clinical value. The association of certain patterns with specific circumstances is now recognized and the curves are often diagnostic; indeed, the effect of various drugs (e.g. pethidine and fentanyl) and different breathing systems and malfunctions produce their own individual 'signature' capnograms.[3]

General principles

The quantity of CO_2 reaching the alveoli depends upon the amount produced by the cells of the body, which varies with metabolism and on the adequacy of transport to and through the lungs.[4] Changes in metabolic rate will produce proportionate changes in alveolar CO_2 concentration unless a change in alveolar ventilation occurs. The concentration of CO_2 in the alveoli is a dynamic result of the rate of CO_2 production ($\dot{V}CO_2$) and alveolar ventilation ($\dot{V}A$). The elimination of CO_2 relies on the state of the lungs and airways, and the functioning of an integrated respiratory system, both centrally and peripherally. Blood leaving ventilated alveoli mixes with blood from parenchymal lung tissue and also with blood passing through non-ventilated alveoli (venous admixture). This produces the normal alveolar-arterial CO_2 tension difference (a–AΔPCO_2) of less than 5 mmHg but which is much greater in pathological states. End-tidal (ET) gas originates mainly from the alveoli and for many practical purposes $PET,CO_2 = PaCO_2$. If the alveoli from all parts of the lung are emptying synchronously PET,CO_2 (i.e. $PE'CO_2$) will be synonymous with $PACO_2$ and a *nearly* horizontal plateau, i.e. the characteristic normal pattern of the capnogram, is obtained. Thus, the measurement of changing CO_2 concentrations is of value in recognizing abnormalities of metabolism, ventilation and circulation. In the normal state alveolar CO_2 concentration is maintained within rather narrow limits independent of the metabolic state or the size of the physiological dead space. Thus alveolar CO_2 concentration can serve as a valuable guide to CO_2 homeostasis during prolonged periods of mechanical ventilation of the lungs that is required in anaesthesia, intensive care or other conditions associated with altered breathing.

Carbon dioxide in respired gas may be continuously measured by mass spectrometry or IR analysis. Both methods are examples of yesterday's research becoming today's clinical tool. The IR method is the most widely used and most cost-effective and is generally taken as synonymous with 'capnography'. Infra-red rays are given off by all warm objects and are absorbed by non-elementary gases (i.e. those composed of dissimilar atoms), while certain gases absorb particular wavelengths producing absorption bands on the IR electromagnetic spectrum. The intensity of IR radiation projected through a gas mixture containing CO_2 is diminished by absorption; this allows the CO_2 absorption band to be identified and is proportional to the amount of CO_2 in the mixture.

Infra-red rays have a wavelength greater than 1 μm and thus lie beyond the visible spectrum (0.4–0.8 μm); CO_2 shows strong absorption in the far IR at 4.3 μm and so this wavelength in the far IR range is used. A narrow-band IR filter prevents the passage of light, which would otherwise be absorbed by gases other than CO_2. There is some overlap in the absorption bands of other gases (e.g. N_2O distorts the absorption bands for CO_2). Hence, allowance must be made for any interfering gases; N_2O molecules also interact with CO_2 molecules to produce a collision broadening effect, which affects the sensitivity of the IR CO_2 analyzer.

An IR analyzer basically consists of a source of IR radiation, an analysis cell, a reference cell and a detection cell. In the Luft system, rays of light from the source are filtered to obtain the required wavelengths and then pass through the analysis cell to fall on the detector, which contains pure CO_2. Any IR radiation that is not absorbed by the gases in the analysis cell is absorbed in the detector and heats the CO_2. The pressure in the detector (which is, in effect, a differential micromanometer as opposite sides are subjected to the light transmitted through the measuring and reference cells respectively) will vary according to the heating effect from the IR radiation. These alinear changes are suitably detected, amplified and displayed, and modern instruments use a linearizing circuit. Drift is reduced by interrupting or chopping the IR beam with a rotating shutter at 25–100 Hz; the pulses of IR radiation thus produce pulses of pressure in the detector cell.

The modern alternative to the classical Luft system uses a light-emitting diode (LED) to produce light of the required wavelength, together with a solid-state photodetector (instead of relying on a micromanometer) to measure the amount of light reaching it alternatively via the measuring and reference cells, with the beam chopped 4000 times/min. In some designs, the chopper is omitted and the infra-red LED is switched on and off by a microprocessor. Some instruments dispense with the need for a reference cell and instead obtain a CO_2 zero for reference from the sample cell itself at a time when the cell is known not to contain CO_2. Thus, in both types of capnograph, the electrical output consists of a series of pulses whose height varies with the CO_2 concentration in the analysis cell. The IR cell is the most critical part of the system and must be protected from contamination by liquids or particulate matter as these invariably cause high erroneous readings because of their high IR absorbance.

It has been common for capnographs to be provided with an automatic zeroing device, which returns the trace to the baseline just as the next inspiration is sensed. This was helpful in the past because of the drift arising from electrical components. However, today this facility is somewhat limiting because it does not permit the instrument to be used in the presence of breathing systems where it may be normal to have some CO_2 in the inspired mixture, such as controlled fractional rebreathing during intermittent positive ventilation of the lungs with circuits such as the Bain breathing system.

Sidestream and mainstream analyzers

Medical analyzers are of two types: sidestream and mainstream.[5]

Sidestream analyzers

These draw gas continuously from the sampling site via a small bore tube of about 2 m length to the measuring cell for analysis and display. The bore should be not greater than 1–2 mm to avoid mixing of gas, to resist the introduction of foreign matter and to facilitate the withdrawal of small sample volumes. The length of the sampling tube should be kept as short as possible to obtain a fast response time for greatest accuracy. The sampling tube must be impermeable to CO_2, thus polyvinylchloride (PVC) is often used but because halogen hydrocarbons react with this material a tube made of Teflon® is preferred in anaesthetic practice. Several manufacturers provide sampling tubes and T-pieces that are hydrophobic, i.e. treated with a material that resists the entry of water, while one manufacturer provides a flexible hydrophobic metallic sampling tube. The sampling rate is of the order of 50–500 ml/min and can be varied, either continuously or by preset steps. However, the flow control is often inconveniently positioned at the rear of some instruments so that the user may be unaware of the sampling rate. This may pose a hazard, for instance where excessive sampling rates are accidentally applied to childrens' breathing systems. Excessive sampling rates should generally be avoided in case loss of gas upsets the homeostasis of the breathing system. Alternatively, too low a sampling rate may produce a capnogram where the curves are raised above the baseline and are sinusoidal in form without a plateau.

A poor connection at some point along the sampling tube can cause the entrainment of air thus producing an abnormal capnogram.[6] Gas that has been sampled by the analyzer is usually discarded and not returned to the breathing circuit because of the inconvenience involved, as well as the possibility of interfering with the gaseous homogeneity of the breathing system. However, the loss of gas through sampling may pose a problem in paediatric practice or with the use of closed or low-flow circle breathing systems; in such circumstances gas may be returned to the breathing system or an extra equivalent fresh gas inflow provided to compensate.

Sampling sites

It used to be common for the tip of the sampling catheter to be positioned just above the carina to obtain a good sample of alveolar gas. However, this is inconvenient and the risk of aspiration of secretions and water into the apparatus is considerable. It is now usual to position the end of the sampling tube at the proximal end of the endo-tracheal tube using a T-piece adaptor; this is also analogous with the position of the IR measuring cell in mainstream analyzers.

Care must be taken in obtaining the correct sampling position when T-piece breathing systems on the Ayre principle are used, lest fresh gas from the anaesthetic machine is drawn into the sampling tube, along with the expired gas sample, to produce an erroneous low value for the end-tidal sample because of the dilution. The same problem occurs with the use of certain lung ventilators which produce a constant flow. The problem can be prevented by interposing a right angle adaptor (such as that used with a facepiece) between the breathing system (Ayre's T-piece or Bain system) and the endotracheal tube and interposing the sampling tube on the patient's side of the angle piece.[7,8] Where conventional twin breathing hoses are used with a Y-piece, the sampling site should be as close to the patient's mouth as possible; if a catheter mount is used, care must be taken to ensure that the sampling site is *not* at the junction of the Y-piece with the catheter mount because of the extra deadspace introduced by the mount. The same consideration should be given with the use of filters and condenser humidifiers, despite the increased risk of water getting into the sampling tube. Manufacturers produce a wide variety of adaptors for sampling and these are re-commended; special adaptors to cope with the special problems of small children are also available; the use of a hypodermic needle inserted through non-disposable breathing tubes to achieve access to the respired gas is to be deplored.

Mainstream analyzers

These do not draw gas but incorporate the analysis cell with IR source, detector and associated electronics into a specially designed airway adaptor, which is interposed into the breathing system. There is no specific reference cell. This form of 'no loss' system offers the advantages of a very fast response. The possibility of condensation of water vapour is prevented by heating the measuring chamber to about 40°C, but there remains the possibility of contamination from secretions that absorb IR radiation and lead to a spurious high value for CO_2 concentration. The added deadspace is a disadvantage in infants. In clinical practice, the sidestream system is often to be preferred, purely because of the expense involved in the repair of accidental damage sustained to the delicate components in the mainstream adaptor.

Calibration and interference

Problems occur because carbon dioxide and nitrous oxide have the same mass number of 44. Unfortunately, N_2O absorbs some light at the most convenient CO_2 wavelength of 4.3 μm. Furthermore, the absorbance properties of CO_2 molecules are affected by the presence of N_2O molecules that collide with them. The effect is to cause the absorption spectrum to become broader, with the result that the degree of overlap in the absorption bands of different gases varies according to the gas concentrations.

This collision broadening effect (sometimes also called pressure broadening) results from the fact that the IR absorption of CO_2 is based on the vibrational motion of the molecules. When the CO_2 molecule vibrates in a crowd of other molecules the collisions affect their vibrational energy states and thus the absorption of IR light. The degree of interaction depends on the ambient pressure and on the mass and nature of the neighbouring molecules. The overall effect when CO_2 is measured in gas mixtures containing N_2O is an overestimate by an amount of about 10% for a mixture containing 50% N_2O, 45% O_2 and 5% CO_2. This is overcome commercially by introducing an electronic bias of the results through compensation buttons for N_2O, and often for O_2 as well; sophisticated instruments also monitor N_2O (by another infrared LED) and O_2 concentrations simultaneously to provide a continuous and varying compensation according to the changing concentration of the interfering gases.

Other considerations include the influence of water vapour, atmospheric pressure and calibration procedures. Erroneous results will occur if water or particulate matter that have high IR absorbances enter the cell. An effective water separation system is required for continuous use but a filter may produce an undesirable sinusoidal curve because of a mixing effect. A water trap is used in sidestream analyzers to remove water in particulate form before it can enter the analysis cell. The design of the trap relies on gravitational forces to separate drops of water from the gas stream and the trap must be frequently dried out and attention directed to prevent water accumulating.

Because the principle of capnography is based on the measurement of partial pressure of CO_2 the method is affected by changes in barometric pressure. For this reason, calibration procedures with gaseous mixtures must be performed using the same type of sampling tube as will be used when the analyzer is connected to the patient system; omission of the standard, long, narrow 2 m sampling tube during such calibration procedures will thus fail to take account of the large pressure drop across the ends of the tube and a measuring error will therefore result during subsequent clinical use. Equipment suppliers now provide canisters of gas mixtures containing known amounts of CO_2 in a mixture of anaesthetic gases and vapours. Although modern instruments provide means for electronic calibration, regular checks using such gaseous calibration are recommended. Some modern capnometers sense changes of barometric pressure and automatically correct the CO_2 reading. In cases of doubt, a rough check may be made by a healthy individual making a forced vital capacity into the sampling tube and observing the peak CO_2 reading, which should be about 5.0–5.5% (mean 5.3 kPa, 40 mmHg). The presence of water vapour also affects the reading since usually the temperature of the patient is 37°C, while that of the instrument cell is, say, 25°C, i.e. a difference of 3 kPa (23 mmHg) in PH_2O resulting in an overestimate of PCO_2 by 0.15% (0.15 kPa, 1.13 mmHg).

The normal capnogram

In conditions of cardiovascular stability, PET,CO_2 bears a constant relation to $PaCO_2$ and the normal $PET,CO_2 - PaCO_2$ difference is 0.7 kPa (5 mmHg). If the alveoli from all areas of the lung are emptying synchronously, PET,CO_2 will be synonymous

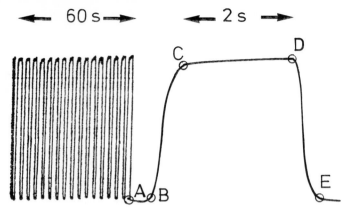

Fig. 9.1   The normal capnogram at slow and fast recording speeds. A–B denotes the expiration of gas from the anatomical deadspace (containing zero CO_2); B–C denotes the exhalation of mixed expired gas; C–D is the alveolar or end-tidal 'plateau'; D denotes the onset of inspiration and D–E denotes the return of the CO_2 trace to the baseline as fresh gas is inspired.

with $PACO_2$. The normal capnogram is shown in Figure 9.1. The fast speed (12.5 mm/s) is essential to detect changes in individual respiratory cycles. When expiration begins, the first part of the gas passing out of the patient's mouth is composed of gas from the mechanical and anatomical deadspace and since this normally contains no CO_2 the capnograph registers zero. Next, a sharply rising front is seen, which represents the mixing of deadspace gas with alveolar gas. It is important to note that the end-expiratory plateau that follows is not an isocapnic trace but that there is a very slight and steady increase in the end-tidal CO_2 concentration as the alveolar fraction is expelled from the lungs. This effect is exaggerated in patients with chronic bronchitis and emphysema. There then follows a sharp downward return of the trace towards zero as gas flow ceases during the expiratory pause until the next inspiration begins. It is common to see a ripple effect superimposed on this downward part of the trace (Fig. 9.2), the so-called cardiac oscillations, although this is now thought to result from small gas movements created largely by the pulsations of the aorta. These oscillations are especially noticeable at slow respiratory rates and where opioids such as fentanyl have been given. It is claimed that individual drugs produce their own

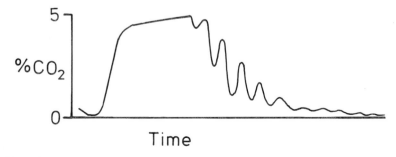

Fig. 9.2   Normal capnogram with the so-called 'cardiac' oscillations.

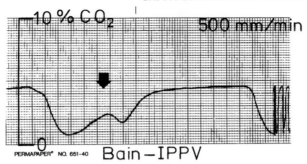

Fig. 9.3 The normal 'signature' capnogram of a patient anaesthetized using IPPV with the Bain breathing system. Note the rebreathing wave (arrow) during inspiration.

characteristic shapes or signatures and observation of this part of the capnogram is helpful in this respect.[3]

The normal capnogram seen at low (known as 'trend') speed recording (25 mm/s) is rather like looking at an open box of matches and observing the striped effect of the heads of the matches all lined up next to one another. Trends are best observed at this recording speed. Reference has already been made to the often distinctive 'fingerprint' or 'signature' shapes produced in the capnogram in special circumstances. Such pattern recognition (as with the electrocardiogram (e.c.g.)) enables instant detection of problems with the patient or breathing apparatus. Figure 9.3 shows the normal characteristic capnogram 'signature' of a healthy patient undergoing uneventful IPPV of the lungs with a Bain breathing system. The small amount of CO_2 appearing during inspiration (the rebreathing wave) represents the controlled fractional rebreathing, which enables a predetermined $PaCO_2$ to be achieved in the face of large tidal volumes (thus avoiding excessive hypocapnia with all its attendant disadvantages) and hence the maintenance of good oxygenation. The exact position and shape of this rebreathing wave depends on the magnitude of the fresh gas flow from the anaesthetic machine.

The abnormal capnogram
Abnormalities should be sought by analyzing the various phases of the capnogram for individual breaths as well as observing the trends occurring over a period of time. Five characteristics should be inspected, namely height, frequency, rhythm, baseline and shape. Rebreathing may be observed by the appearance of carbon dioxide in the inspired gas; this may or not be abnormal depending on the type of breathing system used. Blunting of the normal sharp upward deflection as expiration proceeds (mixed alveolar gas) occurs with atelectasis or with a leak in the breathing circuit. A second alveolar plateau superimposed on the first (the so-called 'camel' capnogram) represents one lung emptying slightly before the other and may be seen in patients in the lateral position. Small indentations or dips in the final portion of the alveolar plateau may represent gas movement caused by someone leaning on the chest, or the patient making a very small movement of the diaphragm as a muscle relaxant is wearing off (the so-called 'curare cleft'). Complete disconnection or total obstruction of the breathing system shows a sudden return to a zero trace, but torsion or kinking of the endotracheal tube or breathing circuit with some gas passage remaining shows a peaked effect in place of the normal end-tidal plateau.[9]

Unrecognized intubation of the oesophagus instead of the trachea is a common problem in anaesthetic practice and accounts for many medico-legal actions.[10] It is often thought that intubation of the oesophagus by mistake for the trachea is associated with a zero CO_2 signal. However, this is not necessarily the case because previous attempts to inflate the lungs by facemask drive some expired gas into the oesophagus and stomach so that when oesophageal intubation unknowingly occurs some of this CO_2 returns to the breathing system to appear on the capnograph when IPPV is attempted.[10] Such a tracing has a peaked effect and does not resemble the normal end-tidal plateau; the concentration of CO_2 is low and gastric CO_2 decreases to zero after about a minute. A spin-off from this work is the observation that intubation of the oesophagus followed by intermittent compression of the reservoir breathing bag, or use of a ventilator, ventilates the oesophagus and stomach to an extent that produces some gas movement in and out of the lungs as they are compressed by the movements of the mediastinum.[10] This accounts for the fact that accidental oesophageal intubation can go undetected for a considerable period of time, which is extended when valiant attempts have previously been made at pre-oxygenation by facemask. The golden rule to remember with capnography is that any trace other than the normal pattern with a smooth distinct end-tidal plateau should immediately suggest that something is wrong somewhere.

Clinical applications
There are very many applications for the use of capnography and these are summarized below. This form of non-invasive monitoring, especially in conjunction with others, e.g. pulse oximetry, has obvious advantages.

Establishing mechanical ventilation
Selection of optimal ventilator settings is greatly facilitated by the use of ET,CO_2 monitoring and reduces the need for invasive blood-gas analysis.

Monitoring mechanical ventilation
End-tidal CO_2 monitoring warns of sudden changes in the breathing system due to disconnection, leaks, obstruction, twisting or torsion of tubes, or ventilator or valve malfunction.[11] The exhaustion of soda-lime is also quickly detected by capnography.

Weaning from mechanical ventilation
Continuous ET carbon dioxide monitoring warns of recurrent respiratory failure: patients who maintain a steady PET,CO_2 during weaning usually progress well, whereas those with a progressive rise or fall often have difficulty.

Monitoring patterns of breathing
End-tidal CO_2 monitoring provides information about hypo- and hyper-ventilation, apnoea, and periodic breathing.

Monitoring of anaesthetic breathing systems
In a few countries, CO_2 is still used by some anaesthetists as part of the anaesthetic technique to stimulate breathing, to aid blind nasal intubation, or to prevent hypocapnia in paediatric anaesthesia; in such circumstances, the capnograph should

be mandatory to warn of an excess of PCO_2 or its accidental administration. In the UK such incidents of inadvertent CO_2 administration continue to occur with tragic results. In Holland, capnography in anaesthetic practice has been mandatory by law since 1978.[12] During spontaneous breathing, it should be borne in mind that return of the CO_2 trace to the zero level between each breath does not necessarily imply that rebreathing is not occurring because the retention of CO_2 stimulates breathing; simultaneous measurement of expired volume should indicate whether or not this is the case. However, failure of the CO_2 trace to return to zero during spontaneous breathing with any breathing system indicates the presence of gross rebreathing of carbon dioxide.

Measurement of CO_2 elimination

The measurement of CO_2 fraction of mixed expired gas ($F\bar{E}CO_2$) to permit the calculation of physiological deadspace and the rate of elimination of CO_2 ($\dot{V}CO_2$) is usually performed by analyzing mixed expired gas over a period of time by collection into a Douglas bag. However, a more convenient method for obtaining $F\bar{E}CO_2$ is to measure the instantaneous expiratory flow ($\dot{V}E$) and expiratory carbon dioxide fraction ($FE'CO_2$ or ET,CO_2). The product of these two signals gives carbon dioxide flux, and integration with time yields expiratory carbon dioxide volume. Processing of these signals is achieved on-line electronically and provides particularly useful information for patients in intensive care who are receiving IPPV. Because it is not practicable for commercial systems to measure both flow and ET,CO_2 at the same point in the system the CO_2 production is overestimated. The error occurs in the measurement of the instantaneous flow of CO_2 to and from the patient as a result of rebreathing, and corresponds to about 24 ml of end-expiratory gas per breath using the standard Y-piece and tubing of the Siemens-Elema Servo ventilator with the Siemens-Elema CO_2 analyzer.[13] This problem can be largely decreased by the use of non-return valves in the Y-piece.

Monitoring metabolic activity

Continuous monitoring of ET,CO_2 is of value for the early detection of the malignant hyperthermia syndrome (MHS) and dramatic rises in PCO_2 occur before body temperature has much increased.[14,15] Continuous CO_2 monitoring is also useful in other conditions associated with increases in metabolism such as shivering, pain and seizures.

Monitoring the circulation

Reductions in cardiac output are accompanied by reductions in carbon dioxide output and ET,CO_2 monitoring is quite a useful adjunct in monitoring cardiogenic or hypovolaemic shock. A gradually diminishing ET,CO_2 concentration should alert the anaesthetist to the possibility that blood loss has been more than is realized. When a sudden interruption in pulmonary perfusion occurs, such as with cardiac arrest (or cardiac failure or gross arrhythmias), the transport of CO_2 to the lungs ceases and the capnograph tracing quickly and exponentially decays towards zero. The capnograph is also a very sensitive monitor of venous air embolism and is second only in sensitivity to the Doppler ultrasonic technique[16] without the disadvantage of interference by surgical diathermy. The blockage in the lung capillaries caused by emboli disturbs the existing ventilation/perfusion ratio so that gas exchange in affected units is either grossly impaired or ceases. The overall effect is thus one of an increased physiological deadspace with gas returning from affected alveolar units (having the same composition of fresh gas, i.e. not containing CO_2) hence diluting the mixed expired gas containing CO_2 from unaffected regions of the lung to produce a lowering of the ET,CO_2 concentration. This monitor is of particular value in neurosurgical operations and continuous monitoring of the carbon dioxide trace is important.[17] In such circumstances, even the slightest reduction in the ET,CO_2 concentration should raise the possibility that an air embolus has occurred.

Single-breath CO_2 analysis
Indirect use of PET,CO_2 permits the calculation of deadspace using the Bohr equation.[18,19] Mixed venous PCO_2 ($P\bar{v}CO_2$) is more dependent on changes in alveolar ventilation than on changes in cardiac output. If a difference between arterial and mixed venous CO_2 concentrations occurs, a low cardiac output is likely. Tissue hypoxia can be assumed when this difference exceeds 10 ml/dl. Variation in $P\bar{v}CO_2$ may also lead to the detection of abnormally low saturation of the arterial blood (SaO_2); single-breath CO_2 analysis also allows the calculation of a-AΔPCO_2. The most common causes of an increased a-AΔPCO_2 are $\dot{V}/\dot{Q}$ maldistribution and poor sampling of gas from the patient.

Monitoring the extracorporeal circulation
Carbon dioxide monitoring is of value in monitoring during cardiopulmonary bypass because hypocapnia is an invariable consequence when pure oxygen is used in the oxygenator. Capnography based on airway sampling is invalid during the period of cardiopulmonary bypass but monitoring of the heart-lung machine and oxygenator may be achieved by sampling the gas being vented from the oxygenator. Thus the per-fusionist has a guide to the amount of CO_2 required to be added to the gases used for equilibration of the blood in the oxygenator.

Paediatrics
Carbon dioxide measurements are inaccurate, especially in children, if the response time of the CO_2 analyzer is too slow and its output fails to reach the actual CO_2 concentration at the end of each breath. An accurate, high-frequency response is essential when end-tidal PCO_2 is monitored during paediatric anaesthesia. In a laboratory study, 6 infra-red capnometers and 1 multiplexed mass spectrometer were assessed in the face of increasing respiratory rates from 8–101 cycles/min.[67] At or below frequencies of 31 cycles/min, 4 capnometers overestimated and 3 underestimated the true PET,CO_2. At frequencies above 31 cycles/min, 6 capnometers underestimated and 1 overestimated PET,CO_2. The differences in displayed CO_2 from known CO_2 over the entire range of frequencies studies was between -16.4 mmHg and $+6.6$ mmHg, although if two suspect values obtained from 1 capnograph are removed from the reported results the range narrows to between $+6.6$ mmHg and -11.4 mmHg (and is $+6.6$ mmHg to -7.4 mmHg if the mass spectrometer results are also discarded (see below). The cause of the underestimation in PET,CO_2 is thought to be the mixing of adjacent breaths during transport down the sampling catheters and in

the analysis chamber; the long sampling line (50 m) of the multiplexed mass spectrometer system presumably contributes to this error. The Hewlett-Packard 47210A capnometer was the instrument least affected, presumably because there is a mainstream analysis cell and no sampling tube. The rise time of a capnograph is the time taken for the analyzer output to respond to a sudden step change in CO_2 concentration, i.e. the time (T_{90}) it takes for the analyzer to change from 10% of the final value to 90% of the final value. Alternatively, the response time (T_{70}) is used in place of T_{90} because the 70% point is a steeper part of the response curve; for all practical purposes, T_{90} is twice the value of T_{70}. The rise times of capnographs for clinical use range from 50–600 ms. The distortion of the CO_2 waveform is a function of the rise time of the analyzer. The rise times of 11 commercially available CO_2 analyzers were measured in a laboratory study:[20] only 6 instruments responded quickly enough to be accurate for rates up to 100 breaths/min. All 11 responded rapidly enough to measure end-tidal CO_2 concentration with 5% accuracy when ventilatory rates were less than 30 breaths/min. To measure CO_2 output ($\dot{V}CO_2$ with 5% accuracy, an analyzer should have a rise time of 20 ms; the analyzer rise time (for analyzers with T_{70} rise times less than 200 ms) can be estimated clinically to within 10 ms (± 8 ms S.D.) by a simple breath hold and forced exhalation, thus providing an estimate of the accuracy of CO_2 measurements in adults or children.[20] Hence, the limitations of capnography should be appreciated in special situations such as paediatric anaesthesia as some capnographs show a better performance than others. It has been recommended that a CO_2 analyzer should have a T_{90} of less than 100 ms to measure ET,CO_2 accurately in adults; when the ventilatory rate is high, as in children, even faster rise times are recommended. A sidestream capnometer should only be considered reliable if the total delay time is less than the respiratory cycle time;[21] total delay time can be reduced by increasing the rate of gas sampling, or by reducing the length of the sampling tube, or both, although other factors are involved.

CONCLUSIONS

Capnography is not solely a measurement of respiratory function, thus capnograms must be interpreted in conjunction with other clinical findings. The capnogram like the electrocardiogram (e.c.g.) requires systematic analysis to obtain the best information (i.e. baseline, height, frequency, rhythm, shape). Various monographs[3,22-25] detail numerous such examples.

OXIMETRY

Transient hypoxaemia is common during anaesthesia and often results from hypoventilation during induction and recovery, or from minor degrees of obstruction. Measures can be taken to avoid its occurrence when hypoxia may be anticipated such as during endoscopy, one-lung anaesthesia or possible difficult intubation. At other times it is unexpected, may be unrecognized and may be lethal.[26] For decades, attempts have been made to find a convenient and reliable means of monitoring the delivery of oxygen to the tissues. Pulse oximetry has now emerged as the most useful method as it is simple, non-invasive and accurate under most circumstances. The various types of oxygen monitoring in the operating theatre have been reviewed by Brodsky.[27]

Matthes published at least 20 papers on oximetry between 1934 and 1944 and may safely be regarded as the father of oximetry.[28] In the mid-1930s, Professor Robert Brinkman used the newly invented barrier layer photocell to measure oxygen saturation of blood. During World War II non-invasive ear oximeters were developed for use in aviation research; this led to the introduction of the classic Atlas® and Cyclops® oximeters but, although the benefits of continuous oximetry were appreciated, technical problems prevented their routine clinical use. In 1948, Brinkman substituted the conventional technique of light transmission for a reflection measurement. This led to the introduction of the Haemoreflector®, the CC-Oximeter®, and the American Optical Oximeter®. These instruments are in-vitro devices although the CC-Oximeter® is connected to the patient through an intravascular catheter for determination of the oxygen saturation of the blood in the chambers of the heart. In the late 1960s Shaw developed a self-calibrating 8-wavelength ear oximeter, which eventually became the Hewlett-Packard ear oximeter.[28] However, the introduction of the Clark oxygen electrode in 1956 directed clinical thinking and technology for the ensuing 30 years away from the concept of saturation and instead focussed upon the tension of oxygen in the blood. This led to the concept of tension as the driving gradient for oxygen between the inspired air and the mitochondria of tissue cells through the various intermediate steps of alveolar gas, pulmonary capillary blood, and so on.

Many devices have been used as pulse meters, e.g. mercury-in-rubber strain gauges, microphones, piezo-electric crystals, Doppler devices and photo-electric cells. Although Hertzman[29] reported the use of photo-electric finger plethysmography in 1937, it was not until 1975 that the concept of pulse oximetry was reported from Japan, developed by Minolta and tested by Japanese researchers.[30] The introduction of the Nellcor pulse oximeter into clinical practice by Yelderman and New in 1983 to measure arterial oxygen saturation easily by non-invasive means, has opened up the prospect of reliable and continuous monitoring of oxygen saturation in every patient.[31-34]

Cyanosis is notoriously difficult to detect clinically owing to lighting conditions and variability among individual observers;[35-37] it is even more difficult to detect where the epidermis is thickened, the skin is pigmented or there is pigment associated with jaundice or Addison's disease. Cyanosis and bradycardia are late signs of hypoxaemia and pulse oximetry represents a very significant advance in patient safety because even astute clinicians do fail to detect cases of severe arterial desaturation. It is worth remembering that SaO_2 will not decrease until the PaO_2 is below 11.3 kPa (85 mmHg) because of the shape of the oxyhaemoglobin dissociation curve; a useful guide in the clinical range of oxygen saturation between 90% and 75%, is that the relationship is roughly $PaO_2 \cong SaO_2 - 30$.

General principles

The basis of oximetry is to shine light of known intensity and given wavelength through a substance in solution and to measure the amount of light that is transmitted through it. The chosen wavelength depends on the absorption spectrum of the substance under investigation. The fundamental law (Lambert-Beer Law) governing the transmission, or the absorption, of the light is $I_t = I_0 e^{-Ecd}$ (where I_0 is the intensity of the incident light, and I_t is the intensity of the light after transmission through a

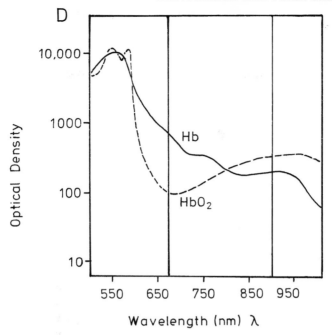

Fig. 9.4 Absorption spectrum of reduced (Hb) haemoglobin (————) and oxygenated (HbO_2) haemoglobin (- - - - -). D is the optical density (an index of the opaqueness of the medium) and λ is the wavelength in nanometres. 810 nm is one of the isobestic points where the absorbance of the two forms of haemoglobin is the same. The two vertical lines denote wavelengths in the red and infra-red parts of the spectrum used by the light-emitting diodes of pulse oximeters.

solution of a substance of concentration, c; d is the distance that the light has to travel through the substance, e is the base of natural logarithms, and E is a proportionality constant known as the extinction coefficient). The term Ecd is called the absorbance or optical density, D, of the solution.

It can be shown that $D = 2.303 \log_{10}(I_0/I_t)$. In the red region of the spectrum, at a wavelength of 650 nm, there is a large difference in optical absorption between reduced haemoglobin and oxyhaemoglobin (Fig. 9.4). When haemoglobin is oxygenated the transmission of light is increased. In the near infra-red region of the spectrum, at 805 nm, there is an isobestic point. There are several of these points and they represent wavelengths at which the optical absorption of fully reduced and fully oxygenated haemoglobin are equal. Hence, a measurement at this wavelength determines the total amount of haemoglobin present, and the difference in output between the measurements at the two wavelengths (650 nm and 805 nm) is an index of the oxygen saturation of the blood. However, when light is shone through a substance or tissue it is reflected and scattered as well as being transmitted and the Lambert-Beer law is to be regarded as entirely empirical.

A pulse oximeter analyses the changes in the transmission of light through any pulsating arterial vascular bed. The amount of light transmitted, such as through the nail bed of the finger or the lobe or pinna of the ear, depends on the amount absorbed by the various structures present, such as skin, muscle, bone, venous and capillary blood,

I_t

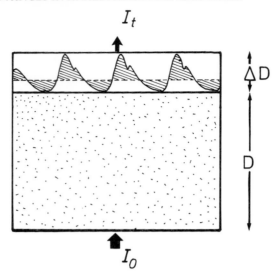

ΔD

D

I_0

Fig. 9.5   Principle of pulse oximetry. D is the fixed absorbance of light shone through the non-pulsating structures (e.g. bone, muscle, skin, veins) of a tissue; ΔD is the 'pulse added' component, or variable absorbance, of light as a result of the pulsating arterial system in the tissue. I_o is the intensity of the incident light and I_t is the intensity of the transmitted light emerging from the tissue.

and so on. The path length that the light has to travel through the finger is constant until it is changed (increased and decreased) owing to expansion and relaxation from the entry and exit of pulsing arterial blood into the system to produce the familiar plethysmographic waveform. The amount of light absorbed and transmitted will then alter. This 'pulse added' signal (Fig. 9.5) is subtracted from the background transmission signal by a microprocessor-controlled empirical algorithm, which is computed hundreds of times per second; the saturation is averaged over a short time interval of 3–6 seconds to produce a rapid response. The algorithm is created by measuring pulse-added absorbances in healthy, awake volunteers breathing various gas mixtures. These absorbances are then correlated with actual oxygen saturations obtained by arterial sampling and a CO-oximeter.[33] The differing light absorption characteristics of oxygenated and non-oxygenated blood are thus used to continuously compute the oxygen saturation of the arterial blood.

Two narrow-band light-emitting diodes (LEDs) are used at wavelengths of 660 nm in the red and 910 nm in the infra-red (IR) part of the spectrum; some manufacturers use an LED at 940 nm instead of the latter wavelength but, as either value corresponds to a plateau on the curve, the isobestic point of 810 nm is in effect mimicked (it is not technically possible to produce a reliable LED for 810 nm). Because only two wavelengths are used the pulse oximeter cannot distinguish between more than two forms of pigment, i.e. reduced and oxyhaemoglobin. If a third form is present such as carboxyhaemoglobin (COHb) it is not clear what the pulse oximeter will actually measure. Each LED switches on and off at about 720 Hz (red on, red off and IR on, both off, etc.) and a single broad-band photodiode detects the amount of light transmitted. The photodetector produces outputs for the transmitted light from each of the diodes and also for any ambient light detected during the off periods in the 720 Hz cycle. The LEDs and photodetector are housed in a probe, which is attached to a digit, pinna or lobe of the ear, or across the foot, heel or hand in the case of infants. Skin, flesh, bone and venous blood reflect and absorb a constant amount of light; arterial blood, by contrast, absorbs varying amounts of light because of the pulsatile blood flow. Until recently, all commercially available LEDs were homostructures, i.e. they consisted of *pn* junctions formed in one type of material. Over the past few years, new types of LEDs (hetereostructures) such as those based on the aluminium gallium arsenide (AlGaAs) system have appeared with significant improvements in light output efficiency, and even further advancements in LED technology are due to appear.

Conventions and symbols

The plethora of symbols used in connection with pulse oximetry can be confusing.[38] The symbol SaO_2 for arterial oxygen saturation is that best known and used by the American Physiological Society. The symbol $sO_2(aB)$ is used by the International Federation of Clinical Chemistry and by the International Union of Pure and Applied Chemistry, while the symbol SpO_2 for the pulse oximeter method of oxygen saturation is under consideration for adoption by the American Society for Testing Materials and by the International Standards Organization (ISO).

Calibration and performance

The calibration of the instrument is pre-set during manufacture and cannot be altered by the user; it is unfortunate that no external standards have so far been developed. Most instruments are programmed to check their internal calibration and sensor function when switched on and intermittently thereafter. Most pulse oximeters are tested down to saturation values of 70%, the lower limit of tolerable hypoxaemia,[34] the error above this value is about $\pm 2\%$, and $\pm 3\%$ in the range of 70–50% saturation. The PaO_2 corresponding to a saturation of 70% on the standard oxygen dissociation curve is 5 kPa (37 mmHg). Below this point on the dissociation curve, the calibration is generally achieved by extrapolation and, in this region, the detection of very small optical signals together with the need to reject artefacts requires the averaging of the data over several seconds, and this procedure can affect the response to rapid changes in saturation.

In a study of 6 different makes of pulse oximeter, it was found that some instruments continued to show nearly normal saturation when the true saturation was down to 40–70%, and some routinely failed to indicate any saturation at all during the critical period of falling saturation.[27] Responses times tend to be longer for desaturation than for increasing saturation perhaps as a result of an increase in finger and ear blood flow when hypoxic blood reaches the tissue. Other studies have explored the range of saturation 95.5% down to 56% and have found good correlation with arterial blood samples.[39-42] Studies of oxygen saturation in volunteers submitted to hypoxic gas mixtures have shown several differences between the various instruments available; however, improved models are continually appearing.[31] The arterial oxygen saturation is usually displayed digitally with the provision of an audible tone accompanying each pulse so that the pitch falls as saturation falls. The magnitude of the pulse waveform is indicated either by a bar graph or else by display of the pulse waveform; however, in some instruments, this form of waveform presentation can be rather misleading because decreases in signal produced, for example by vasoconstriction, are compensated by an increase in gain of the amplifier.

The pulse oximeter is designed to be insensitive to changes in haemodynamics although situations where the pulse is diminished, such as in peripheral vascular disease, hypothermia, extreme hypotension or vasoconstriction, may produce too weak a signal. However, from Lawson and his colleagues' study it appears that a pulse oximeter is able to estimate saturation even in states of severely reduced peripheral blood flow.[43] They found that when the arm was progressively occluded using a blood pressure cuff, the flow rate (which was measured with a laser Doppler flow probe) decreased to approximately 9% of the control value before the pulse oximeter (Nellcor N-100®) was unable to estimate the saturation. When the cuff was released from total occlusion, the pulse oximeter regained a measured pulse and an estimation of saturation at only 4% of the original blood flow. In this study, no attempt was made to compare the saturations obtained with an independent method, but another study addressed this problem that venous congestion may cause low readings of saturation. In this study,[44] on the effect of venous congestion, the average value of SaO_2 measured by pulse oximetry in the finger tip and finger base was found to be between 1.5 and 7.8% lower, respectively, than when the digit was elevated. This effect is thought to be a result of venous pulsations associated with the shunting of arterial blood through open arteriovenous anastomoses in the cutaneous circulation. The ear appears to be a more consistent site for the probe than the finger.[31] Movement artefacts cause problems, although this is only a problem in non-anaesthetized patients. The Nellcor N-200® model has the facility to synchronize the determinations of arterial saturation with the patient's e.c.g. and thus is particularly useful in monitoring awake patients.

Forms of haemoglobin such as methaemoglobin (MetHb) and carboxyhaemoglobin (COHb) cannot be distinguished from oxyhaemoglobin by pulse oximetry. Because COHb is red it is seen by the pulse oximeter as oxyhaemoglobin, therefore, in the presence of COHb, the oximeter reads the sum of the O_2Hb and the COHb. A heavy smoker with 10% of his haemoglobin combined as COHb shows a 2–3% overestimate of haemoglobin saturation when actually 90% of the available haemoglobin is saturated. Alternatively, transcutaneous PO_2 ($PtcO_2$) falls as COHb increases.[45] The effective acute 'anaemia' of carbon monoxide poisoning does not alter the oximeter reading, thus the instrument does not alert to the low arterial oxygen content under these circumstances. It appears that a pulse oximeter sees COHb as 90% O_2Hb and 10% reduced Hb.

Methaemoglobinaemia has a more complex effect because the ability of the pulse oximeter to register desaturation is impaired and no indication of the functional haemoglobin is given. Methaemoglobin is seen as a large absorbance in both the red and infra-red wavelengths of the pulse oximeter; this large pulsatile absorbance seen in both wavelengths forces the ratio of the added pulse absorbance towards unity, which is interpreted by the pulse oximeter as a saturation of 85% O_2Hb and 15% reduced Hb.[26] Therefore, in the presence of significant amounts of methaemoglobin, the pulse oximeter will tend towards a reading of 85%, regardless of the saturation. The Radiometer 'OXImeter®' has provision for adjusting the read-out from the instrument according to known amounts of abnormal forms of haemoglobin determined separately from the Radiometer OSM3 hemoximeter.® This approach has obvious value when dealing with victims of smoke inhalation where high concentration of COHb are common.

Dyes that absorb light in the region of 660 nm, such as indocyanine green, indigo carmine and especially methylene blue, may also cause sudden false low readings for a time after intravenous injection.[46,47] The time course for these changes is about 1–2 circulation times and recovery to baseline values occurs within 3 minutes of bolus dye injection in young healthy subjects breathing room air.

Artefacts may result from interference from radiofrequency diathermy apparatus, light of high intensity and some infra-red heat lamps.[48] Because the photodetector can measure weak signals, oximeters are designed to reject ambient light. When the intensity of ambient light is high the photodetector cannot sense light transmitted through tissue or calculate SaO_2. Certain operating theatre lights may cause interference and cause erroneous high saturation readings. It is recommended that the probe be shielded by wrapping in a thin opaque metal foil. The junction box on the cable of the Nellcor® oximeter should be positioned as far away from the electrocautery apparatus as possible and interference minimized by screening with metal foil. Nail polish was reported not to affect the pulse oximeter saturation in volunteers, unlike synthetic finger nails, although the response to oxygen and not hypoxia was tested.[49] However, a better study considered the effects of nail polishes of different colours;[50] black, blue and green nail polish lower pulse oximeter readings of SaO_2. Blue and green produced greater decreases than purple and red; black produced an intermediate decrease. Nail polish should therefore be routinely removed before pulse oximetry.

Clinical applications

Pulse oximetry is becoming a valuable routine monitor in anaesthesia and is especially valuable in patients with skin pigmentation, and those with poor physical status with a low arterial oxygen tension, i.e. below 13 kPa (95 mmHg). Pulse oximetry is also of value in patients undergoing regional anaesthesia, sedation, endoscopies, and also procedures of brief duration as severe hypoxaemia is far commoner than hitherto realized. The clinical use of pulse oximetry has lead to many interesting observations such as the high incidence of hypoxaemia during manual ventilation (compared with ventilator controlled or spontaneous ventilation), and in patients in the lithotomy position. It also reveals the hypoxaemia of inadvertent bronchial intubation. Although pulse oximetry provides rapid non-invasive evaluation of total blood oxygenation and displays information about pulse amplitude, the conclusion that pulse oximeters monitor tissue perfusion and tissue oxygen delivery must be approached with caution.[43]

Insertion of monitoring lines

A study of 20 unpremedicated cardiac patients breathing room air showed hypoxaemia (SaO_2 less than 90%) during the insertion of monitoring lines prior to undergoing anaesthesia and surgery for coronary artery bypass.[51] These findings are of considerable interest given that it has already been shown that patients scheduled for coronary artery grafting manifest an 18% incidence of new ischaemia on arrival in the operating theatre.[52]

One-lung ventilation

The hypoxaemia that can occur during selective one-lung ventilation despite an inspired oxygen concentration of 100% makes rapid assessment of oxygenation extremely important.[53] Pulse oximetry is also a valuable tool during surgical manipulation of the pulmonary artery, such as banding or clamping where pulmonary artery flow is reduced.[54]

Postoperative care

Pulse oximetry is a valuable monitor of oxygenation in the recovery room, intensive care unit and ward; also during transfer of patients.[36] Hypoxaemia (defined as a SaO_2 of 90% or less ($\cong PaO_2$ 7.7 kPa, 58 mmHg) occurred in 35%, and severe hypoxaemia (defined as a SaO_2 of 85% or less ($\cong PAO_2$ 6.7 kPa, 50 mmHg)) occurred in 12%, of ASA Class 1 or 2 patients breathing room air during their transfer from the operating theatre to the recovery room.[37] Postoperative hypoxaemia did not correlate with anaesthetic agent, age, duration of anaesthesia or level of consciousness. Smith and Crul also recently demonstrated early profound decreases in SaO_2 in healthy patients' during transfer to the recovery room in spite of the administration of 100% oxygen for 5 minutes at the end of the anaesthetic.[55] They suggest that ventilation-perfusion mismatch is most likely to be responsible; no patient given 2 l/min by nasopharyngeal catheter during transport had a SaO_2 below 90%.

Children are potentially more susceptible than adults to airway closure and disturbances in pulmonary gas exchange. In children 21% oxygen (room air) is a potentially hypoxic mixture in the early recovery period.[56] No difference was shown between those children who received inhalational anaesthesia and those who receive narcotics, neither was there a correlation between the reduction in saturation and patient age or duration of anaesthesia. Substantial desaturation has been observed in patients receiving either traditional parenteral analgesia or epidural morphine following caesarean section.[57] Because oxygen is innocuous under most circumstances, the safe course is to provide air enriched with oxygen during postoperative transfer and in the early recovery period. In the intensive care unit, pulse oximetry is also valuable as an on-line non-invasive indicator of the benefits or otherwise of therapy; it is a particularly useful monitor during chest physiotherapy and airway suctioning.

Other applications

Several other ingenious applications have been described for the use of pulse oximetry apart from clinical monitoring, e.g. the assessment of adequacy of cardiopulmonary resuscitation, the assessment of collateral flow in the hand (Allen's test), the prevention of compression of the axillary artery during anaesthesia and testing the viability of microvascular grafts.

Safety

A heated probe used to be incorporated in some pulse oximeters in order to promote good circulation through the tissues. These may rarely cause patient injury, which is usually caused by overheating as a result of damage to the probe.[58] The probe should always be carefully placed on the finger so that no undue pressure or torque is applied and careful inspection made of both digit and probe. Other problems appear to be few, such as minor burns, abrasions and a sun-tanning effect.[59]

CONCLUSIONS

Continuous observation of the cardiovascular and respiratory systems of anaesthetized patients has been considered vital for patient safety since the earliest days of anaesthesia.[60] There are now sufficient reports to indicate that dedicated monitoring instruments can benefit the patient as an extension of the anaesthetist's human senses.[61-65] Indeed, in several countries, standards of monitoring have now been laid down by professional anaesthetic organisations[66-69] or even by law.[12] To a great extent this has come about because of the escalating rise in medical malpractice insurance premiums. Monitoring instruments are not a substitute for careful clinical observation. However, good monitoring benefits not only the patient by constant and close presentation of many vital signs and other parameters but also the anaesthetist by freeing them from many manual tasks, thus helping to relieve fatigue and tension and so concentrate his or her attention on the overall care of the patient.

Capnography and pulse oximetry can provide non-invasive, continuous information that would not otherwise be available and the use of reliable, audible and visual alarms increases patient safety, particularly when access is restricted or room lighting is reduced. There is a strong analogy between the anaesthetist and the civil airline pilot. Both must rely heavily on instruments for information and the fallacies of human error are well-known to both professions. In some operations, the anaesthetist cannot get near to his patient — rather like flying in cloud; however, with the use of adequate instruments (monitors) everything should be perfectly safe. Cooper and his colleagues have shown that human error, rather than equipment failure, is overwhelmingly responsible for anaesthetic mishaps.[65] Attention must nevertheless be directed towards combining the various monitors used in anaesthesia into a common system to simplify and reduce the number of controls and switches. It is imperative that sufficient reliable equipment is purchased and great attention must be paid to the training of anaesthetists in its use and to proper maintenance and checking. There is a powerful argument for the use of routine capnography and pulse oximetry in all patients in addition to traditional measurements such as the e.c.g., blood pressure, and so on, which may be expected to make a considerable contribution to patient safety.

REFERENCES

1. Collier C R, Affeldt J E, Farr A F 1955 Continuous rapid infrared CO_2 analysis: fractional sampling and accuracy in determining alveolar CO_2. Journal of Laboratory and Clinical Medicine 25: 526–39
2. Ramwell P W 1959 The value of the end-tidal sample. In: Woolmer R E, Parkinson J (eds) A symposium on pH and blood gas analysis: methods of interpretation. Churchill, London
3. Smallout B, Kalenda Z 1981 An atlas of capnography, 2nd edn. Kerckebosch, Zeist, Holland
4. Adams A P, Hahn C E W 1982 Principles and practice of blood-gas analysis, 2nd edn. Churchill Livingstone, London
5. Kalenda Z 1980 Equipment for capnography. British Journal of Clinical Equipment 5(5): 180–93
6. Martin M, Zupan J, Benumof J L 1988 Unusual end-tidal CO_2 waveform. Anesthesiology 67: 712–3
7. Gravenstein N, Lampotang S, Beneken J E W 1985 Factors influencing capnography in the Bain circuit. Journal of Clinical Monitoring 1: 6–10
8. Beneken J E W, Gravenstein N, Gravenstein J S, van der Aa J J, Lampotang S 1985 Capnography and the Bain circuit. 1. a computer model. Journal of Clinical Monitoring 1: 103–113
9. Murray I P, Modell J H 1983 Early detection of endotracheal tube accidents by monitoring carbon dioxide concentration in the respiratory gas. Anesthesiology 59: 344–6
10. Linko K, Paloheimo M, Tammisto T 1983 Capnography for detection of oesophageal intubation. Acta Anaesthesiologica Scandinavica 27: 199–202
11. Pyles S T, Berman L S, Modell J H 1984 Expiratory valve dysfunction in a semiclosed circle

anesthesia circuit — verification by analysis of carbon dioxide waveform. Anesthesia and Analgesia 63: 536–567

12. Advisory Report on Anaesthesiology, Part 1: Recent developments in anaesthesiology. Committee of the Health Council of The Netherlands, 1978

13. Fletcher R, Werner L, Nordström L, Jonson B 1983 Sources of error and their correction in the measurement of carbon dioxide elimination using the Siemens-Elema CO_2 analyzer. British Journal of Anaesthesia; 55: 177–185

14. Baudendistel L, Goudsouzian N, Coté C, Strafford M 1984 End-tidal CO_2 monitoring: its use in the diagnosis and management of malignant hyperthermia. Anaesthesia 39: 1000–1003

15. Liebenschütz F, Mai C, Pickerodt V W A 1979 Increased carbon dioxide production in two patients with malignant hyperpyrexia and its control by dantrolene. British Journal of Anaesthesia 51: 899–903

16. Edmonds-Seal J, Prys-Roberts C, Adams A P 1971 Air embolism. A comparison of various methods of detection. Anaesthesia 26: 202–208

17. Hurter D, Sebel P S 1979 Detection of venous air embolism: a clinical report using end-tidal carbon dioxide monitoring during neurosurgery. Anaesthesia 34: 578–582

18. Fletcher R 1984 Airway deadspace, end-tidal CO_2, and Christian Bohr. Acta Anaesthesiologica Scandinavica 28: 408–411

19. Fletcher R, Jonson B 1984 Deadspace and the single breath test for carbon dioxide during anaesthesia and artificial ventilation: effects of tidal volume and frequency of respiration. British Journal of Anaesthesia 56: 109–119

20. Brunner J X, Westenskow D R 1988 How the rise time of carbon dioxide analysers influences the accuracy of carbon dioxide measurements. British Journal of Anaesthesia 61: 628–638

21. Schena J, Thompson J, Crone R K 1984 Mechanical influences on the capnogram. Critical Care Medicine 12: 672–674

22. Swedlow D B 1986 Capnometry and capnography: the anesthesia early disaster warning system. In: Katz, R L (ed.) Seminars in Anesthesia 5: 194–205

23. May W S, Heavner J E, McWhorter D, Racz G 1985 Capnography in the operating room. Raven Press, New York

24. Smalhout B 1983 A quick guide to capnography and its use in differential diagnosis. Hewlett-Packard, Böblingen, West Germany

25. Paloheimo M, Valli M, Ahjopalo H 1983 A guide to CO_2 monitoring. Datex Instrumentarium, Helsinki

26. Morris R W, Torda T A 1988 Clinical pulse oximetry. In Kerr D R (ed.) Australasian anaesthesia 1988, Melbourne: Faculty of Anaesthetists of the Royal Australasian College of Surgeons pp. 154–155

27. Brodsky J B 1986 Oxygen monitoring in the operating room. In: Katz R L (ed.) Seminars in Anesthesia pp. 180–187

28. Severinghaus J W 1986 Historical development of oxygenation monitoring. In: Payne J P, Severinghaus J W (eds) Pulse Oximetry. Springer-Verlag, Berlin, pp. 1–18

29. Hertzman A B, Spealman A B 1937 Observation on the finger volume pulse recorded photo-electrically. American Journal of Physiology, 119: 334–335

30. Yoshima I, Shimada Y, Tanaka K 1980 Spectrophotometric monitoring of arterial oxygen saturation in the fingertip. Medical and Biological Engineering and Computing 18: 27–32

31. Severinghaus J W, Naifeh K H 1987 Accuracy of response of six pulse oximeters to profound hypoxia. Anesthesiology, 67: 551–558

32. Taylor M B, Whitwam J G 1986 The current status of pulse oximetry. Anaesthesia 41: 943–949

33. Yelderman M, New W Jnr 1983 Evaluation of pulse oximetry. Anesthesiology 589: 349–52

34. Tytler J A, Seeley H F 1986 The Nellcor N-101 pulse oximeter. A clinical evaluation in anaesthesia and intensive care. Anaesthesia, 41: 302–305

35. Morgan-Hughes J O 1968 Lighting and cyanosis. British Journal of Anaesthesia 40: 503–507

36. Tyler I L, Tantisira B, Winter P M, Motoyama E K 1985 Continuous monitoring of arterial oxygen saturation with pulse oximetry during transfer to the recovery room. Anesthesia and Analgesia 64: 1108–1112

37. Hanning C D 1985 'He looks a little blue down this end'. Monitoring oxygenation during anaesthesia. British Journal of Anaesthesia 57: 359–360

38. Payne J P, Severinghaus J W 1986 Definitions and symbols. In: Payne J P, Severinghaus J W (eds) Pulse oximetry. Springer-Verlag, Berlin, pp. 21–22

39. Chapman K R, D'Urzo A, Rebuck A S 1983 The accuracy and response characteristics of a simplified ear oximeter. Chest 83: 860–864

40. Mihm F G, Halperin B D 1985 Non-invasive detection of profound arterial desaturation using a pulse oximeter device. Anesthesiology 62: 85–87

41. Cecil W T, Petterson M T, Lamoonpun S, Rudolph C D 1985 Clinical evaluation of the Biox IIA ear oximeter in the critical care environment. Respiratory Care 30: 179–183

42. Shippy M B, Petterson M T, Whitman R A, Shivers C R 1984 A clinical evaluation of the BTI Biox II ear oximeter. Respiratory Care, 29: 730–735

43. Lawson D, Norley I, Korbon G, Loeb R, Ellis J 1987 Blood flow limits and pulse oximeter signal detection. Anesthesiology 67: 599–603

44. Kim J-M, Arakawa K, Benson K T, Fox D K 1986 Pulse oximetry and circulatory kinetics associated with pulse volume amplitude measured by photoelectric plethysmography, Anesthesia and Analgesia 65: 1333–1339

45. Barker S J, Tremper K K 1987 The effect of carbon monoxide inhalation on pulse oximetry and transcutaneous PO_2. Anesthesiology, 66: 677–679

46. Kessler M R, Eide T, Humayun B, Poppers P J 1986 Spurious pulse oximeter desaturation with methylene blue injection. Anesthesiology, 65: 435–436

47. Scheller M S, Unger R J, Kelner M J 1986 Effects of intravenously administered dyes on pulse oximetry readings. Anesthesiology 65: 550–552

48. Brookes T D, Paulus D A, Winkle W E 1984 Infrared heat lamps interfere with pulse oximeters. Anesthesiology 61: 630

49. Kataria B K, Lampkins R 1986 Nail polish does not affect pulse oximeter saturation. Anesthesia and Analgesia 65: 824

50. Coté C J, Goldstein E A, Fuchsman W H, Hoaglin D C 1988 The effect of nail polish on pulse oximetry. Anesthesia and Analgesia 67: 683–668

51. Hensley F A, Dodson D L, Martin D E, Stauffer R A, Larach D R 1986 Oxygen saturation during placement of invasive monitoring in the premedicated unanesthetized cardiac patient. Anesthesiology 65: A22

52. Slogoff S, Keats A S 1985 Does perioperative myocardial ischemia lead to postoperative myocardial infarction? Anesthesiology, 62: 107–114

53. Brodsky J B, Shulman M S, Swan M, Mark J B D 1985 Pulse oximetry during one-lung ventilation. Anesthesiology 63: 212–214

54. Friesen R H 1985 Pulse oximetry during pulmonary artery surgery. Anesthesia and Analgesia 64: 376

55. Smith D C, Crul J F 1988 Early postoperative hypoxia during transport. British Journal of Anaesthesia 61: 625–627

56. Motoyama E K, Glazener C H 1986 Hypoxemia after general anesthesia in children. Anesthesia and Analgesia 65: 267–272

57. Choi H J, Little M S, Fujita R A, Garber S Z, Tremper K K 1986 Pulse oximetry for monitoring during ward analgesia: epidural morphine versus parenteral narcotics. Anesthesiology 65: A371

58. Slowan T B 1988 Finger injury by an oxygen saturation monitor probe. Anesthesiology, 68: 936–8

59. Miyasaka K, Ohata J 1987 Burn, erosion, and 'sun' tan with the use of pulse oximetry in infants. Anesthesiology 67: 1008–1009

60. Griffiths D M, Ilsley A H, Runciman W B 1988 Pulse meters and pulse oximeters. Anaesthesia and Intensive Care 16: 49–53

61. Cooper J B, Newbower R S, Kitz R J 1984 An analysis of major errors and equipment failures in anesthesia management: considerations for prevention and detection. Anesthesiology 60: 34–42

62. Lunn J N, Mushin W W 1982 Mortality associated with anaesthesia. The Nuffield Provincial Hospitals Trust, London

63. Holland R 1987 Anaesthetic mortality in New South Wales. British Journal of Anaesthesia 59: 834–841

64. Buck N, Devlin H B, Lunn J N 1987 The report of a confidential enquiry into perioperative deaths. The Nuffield Provincial Hospital Trust, London

65. Cooper J B, Newbower R S, Long C D, McPeek B 1978 Preventable anaesthesia mishaps: a study of human error. Anesthesiology 49: 399–406

66. Eichhorn J H, Cooper J B, Cullen D J, Maier W R, Philip J H, Seeman R G 1986 Standards for patients monitoring during anesthesia at Harvard Medical School. Journal of the American Medical Association 256: 1017–1020

67. American Society for Anesthesiologists. 1986 Standards of basic intra-operative monitoring. Newsletter 50: 9

68. Cass N M, Crosby W M, Holland R B 1988 Minimal monitoring standards. Anaesthesia and Intensive Care 16: 110–113

69. 1988 Recommendations for standards of monitoring during anaesthesia and recovery. The Association of Anaesthetists of Great Britain and Ireland, London

70. From R P, Scamman F L 1988 Ventilatory frequency influences accuracy of end-tidal CO_2 measurements: analysis of seven capnometers. Anesthesia and Analgesia 67: 884–886

10. Neuromuscular blockade monitoring

A.C. Pearce

The use of a nerve stimulator in anaesthetic practice was described in 1958 by Christie and Churchill-Davidson.[1] The present methods of delineating the extent of neuromuscular blockade, where a peripheral nerve is stimulated and a muscle response is identified and quantified, remain essentially the same. However, over the last 30 years the degree of sophistication in the manner and pattern of nerve stimulation and recording of the muscle response has changed. There are currently several applications for neuromuscular monitoring and an individual anaesthetic department must decide on the envisaged uses before purchase of equipment. The monitoring needs can be summarized as follows:

1. Simple, clinical peri-operative;
2. Long-term paralysis in intensive care, extended peri-operative;
3. Closed loop systems for relaxant administration; and
4. Research into neuromuscular physiology and pharmacology.

Various factors concerning stimulation and the means of recording the muscle response influence the accuracy, reliability and relevance of methods of neuromuscular monitoring. These are now discussed, concentrating on developments or understanding that have occurred in the last 6–7 years. The reader is also referred to other reviews.[2-5]

STIMULUS

Waveform and duration
The stimulus should be a square wave and have a duration that is shorter than the refractory period of the neuromuscular junction. Most commercial stimulators use a pulse duration of 0.10–0.30 ms. Non-square wave stimuli of long duration can cause repetitive firing of the nerve leading to underestimation of the degree of blockade. This was first described in 1969 with the Block Aid monitor, which had been used as a standard stimulator for clinical research. Investigation[6] of the stimulus from this device showed it to the biphasic, with a peak duration of the positive signal of 0.75 ms. This gave a similar electromyographic and mechanical response to two 0.1 ms square wave impulses 5 ms apart.

Current
The current passing through the stimulating electrodes should be sufficient to activate all the nerve fibres in the underlying nerve. As the current is increased from very low values, the muscle response increases to a point at which further increases in current produce no or little further increases in response. In approximately 75% patients the

supramaximal current will be in the range of 15-40 mA when surface electrodes are used over the ulnar nerve at the wrist.[7] Some patients, especially those with obese wrists, may require 50-60 mA. The supramaximal current can only be determined with certainty if the motor response can be quantified. This cannot be done solely by tactile or visual determination. While it is not possible to predict in a particular patient the magnitude of the supramaximal current, the above study found that supramaximal stimulation could be assured if the delivered current was 2.75 times the current that first produced an identifiable twitch in that particular patient, provided that this calculated supramaximal current was at least 20 mA.

Some early stimulators (which may well still be in use today) only give a maximal output of 40 mA. The danger with these machines is that small changes in electrode impedance or position over the nerve may give rise to large changes in the number of activated nerve fibres and hence muscle response. Most commercial stimulators are of the constant current variety, and are able to supply a preset current despite small changes in electrode impedance. Usually they supply 250 V into open circuit, supplying, therefore, up to 70-80 mA into the resistance found when using surface electrodes.[8] Large changes in electrode impedance can cause a dramatic fall in stimulator output. One study,[9] in 1984, which specifically looked at stimulator design, showed how poorly some stimulators performed at different output resistances.

Stimulator/patient interface

Three means are used to apply the stimulus to the nerve; rounded tip or ball electrodes, needle electrodes and self-adhesive electrodes.

Rounded tip or ball electrodes

Rounded tip or ball electrodes that protrude from most hand held stimulators are applied to the skin. The position of the electrodes over the nerve is critical and small movements may produce large alterations in motor response. In the absence of a motor response, it is quite difficult to be certain that the electrodes have been placed correctly over, say, the ulnar nerve at the wrist. Stimulation of the facial nerve by this means is straightforward. Obviously, repeated, discrete monitoring is relatively laborious. It can be facilitated by applying paediatric e.c.g. electrodes to the skin in such a way that their contacts are the same distance apart as the stimulator electrodes.

Needle electrodes

These may be placed subcutaneously to lie near, but not in, the nerve. The current required for supramaximal stimuaestion is much reduced because the resistance of the skin is circumvented. Their use has been associated with infection, broken needles and intraneural placement. They have no place in routine clinical monitoring except, perhaps, in obese patients in whom it has proved difficult to deliver a supramaximal current with surface electrodes.

Surface, pre-gelled, self-adhesive electrodes

These are commonly used. Paediatric e.c.g. electrodes are appropriately sized and quite sufficient, although electrodes designed for neuromuscular monitoring are produced. The electrode surface area reduces current strength and delivery of a supramaximal current will be less likely if constant voltage stimulators are used.

Attachment of the stimulator unit is by leads with either crocodile or button clips attached to the e.c.g. electrode. At the stimulator end, the leads may fit over the protruding electrodes via a sleeve connection or into separate sockets. Sometimes, the forces generated by the weight of the leads and position of the clips causes the pregelled electrodes to become detached from the skin surface. A way round this is to use Hewlett-Packard e.c.g. electrodes No. 40426. These are supplied sith a 45-cm lead already attached to the e.c.g. electrode, ending in a standard connection that is placed in the stimulator socket.

Site of stimulation

Most research into neuromuscular monitoring has detailed stimulation of the ulnar nerve at the wrist and recording of the muscle response of adductor pollicis. The ulnar nerve is superficial, easy to stimulate, accessible in most anaesthetized patients and always supplies adductor pollicis; the muscle response is easily visible or quantified and gives a good correlation with required surgical levels of relaxation. Direct correlation between activity of adductor pollicis and respiratory or abdominal musculature is, however, difficult.[10] Muscle groups at different sites contain varying proportions of fast and slow mucle. Both animal[11] and human[12] work suggests that these two types of muscle are affected differently by muscle relaxants. Clinical experience, however, is that full recovery of adductor pollicis assures recovery of respiratory and airway musculature. Other sites of electrode placement have been used, the most common are the facial nerve, the common peroneal nerve and the posterior tibial nerve.

Facial nerve

Electrodes may be placed over the main trunk of the facial nerve or one of its major divisions, usually the temporal branch supplying orbicularis oculi and frontalis muscle. The response that is most readily observed is movement of the eyebrow and around the mouth. It is not generally possible to quantify the response mechanically. When a patient is recovering from profound blockade the response to facial nerve stimulation will precede that at the ulnar nerve.[13,14] Put another way, twitch responses at the eye will be present initially when no response is present at the wrist. Direct muscle activation of the frontalis may also occur; attempts to abolish eyebrow twitches in these circumstances lead to gross overdosage of relaxant.

The common peroneal nerve

This can be stimulated by electrodes placed near the nerve at the neck of the fibula. The response observed is dorsiflexion of the toe and of the foot. Published correlations between this and the ulnar nerve are scant. Clinical experience gathered at Guy's Hospital is that abolition of toe movement can only be achieved with dense blockade and movement of the foot correlates better with the ulnar nerve and thumb site.

Posterior tibial nerve

Stimulation of this nerve can be obtained by placement of electrodes over the course of the nerve posteriorly to the medial malleolus. The muscle response is from flexor hallucis brevis and abductor hallucis.

Electrode polarity

Since a nerve stimulator produces direct current, the effect of alterations of electrode polarity have been studied.[15] If the assumption is made that electrical excitation of the nerve is caused in the same manner whether needle or surface electrodes are used, the results can be summarized as follows. When one electrode is placed over the nerve it 'concentrates' the current on the nerve and is termed the active electrode. An electrode distant to the nerve is termed inactive or indifferent.

When the active electrode is negative, passage of current produces a cathodal current on the upper surface of the nerve, which facilitates nerve depolarization when the circuit is completed by the inactive electrode. For a given stimulating current, a greater twitch will result if the negative electrode (cathode) is used as the active electrode over the ulnar nerve at the wrist, provided that the inactive electrode is placed at some distance from the nerve. If both electrodes are placed within a few centimetres of each other along the nerve then alterations in polarity produce no change in twitch response, probably because the cathode is always an active electrode in these circumstances.

Pattern of stimulation

Single stimuli
These are usually at a frequency of 1 Hz or 0.1 Hz.

Train-of-four stimulation
The train-of-four (TOF) stimulation is 2 Hz for 2 seconds. The ratio of the magnitude of the fourth to the first response gives the TOF ratio. The determination of this ratio does not require a preparalysis train. It is, however, impossible to determine the TOF ratio by visual or tactile evaluation of thumb movement. It must not be used to determine adequate recovery from a muscle relaxant unless a quantitative measurement of muscle response is available. Where this is possible, a TOF ratio of 0.6–0.7 is consistent with recovery of respiratory and airway musculature to safe levels.

Tetanus at 50 Hz, 100 Hz and 200 Hz
These patterns have already been described. In some patients, it is possible to observe tetanic fade at the higher frequencies in the absence of muscle relaxants. Normal physiological firing rates associated with maximal sustained force are of the order of 50 Hz and this is the frequency that has most application in neuromuscular monitoring. It is usual for the tetanus to be applied for 5 seconds. The absence of tetanic fade under these circumstances correlates well with good reversal. Repeated use of a 5 second tetanus may influence recovery in the muscle studied, whereas a 1-second tetanus applied at 12-second intervals has been used as a standard stimulus without obvious ill effect in muscle relaxant studies.[16]

The stimulation patterns cited above are well established in clinical practice. Studies in surgical patients (as opposed to animal work) suggest that a mechanical TOF ratio of greater than 0.7 is associated with sustained tetanus for 5 seconds.[17]

Post-tetanic facilitation
With dense neuromuscular blockade there is no response to single stimuli, TOF or tetanic stimulation. Quantification of the degree of blockade can be achieved by post-

tetanic facilitated counts (PTC). In order to use the information collected by other workers with this form of stimulation, it is advisable to use the same technique as initially described.[18] Following stimulation at 1 Hz for 1 minute, a 50 Hz tetanus is applied for 5 seconds followed by an interval of 3 seconds and subsequent stimulation at 1 Hz. A count is made of the number of single twitches elicited. For each relaxant, a correlation exists between the post-tetanic count and the time before the first response of the train-of-four reappears. Using pancuronium[19] and tactile assessment of the thumb response, a PTC of 4 is associated with a mean time of 20 minutes before TOF reappearance, with 95% confidence limits of 4–36 minutes. With atracurium and a PTC of 4, the mean time is 4 minutes.[20] The application of a 5-second 50 Hz tetanus every 6–10 minutes did not appear to alter recovery in the monitored hand. This is the only pattern of stimulation that allows for the control of relaxation at the profound levels at which diaphragmatic paralysis occcurs.[21]

Double burst stimulation
This has been introduced in an effort to find a more reliable pattern of stimulation to determine adequate recovery from blockade. The problem with the TOF pattern when gauging the response by feeling, for example thumb movement, is that there is a decrement in response between each twitch. This makes it difficult to determine the response of the fourth in relation to the first. With double burst stimulation, two short trains (3 stimuli each train at 50 Hz) are given with an interval of 750 ms between trains. The origination of patterns of double bursts has only been presented in abstract form[22] and clinical results at meetings.[23] Most observers judge each response of the train-of-four to be equally strong when the true, mechanically measured, TOF ratio is only 0.3–0.5. The two responses of the double burst do not appear to be equal until the measured TOF is 0.5–0.7. Unpublished work from this department confirms these findings and further publications are awaited. This pattern of stimulation seems an advance, although it may be that another pattern of stimulation allows all observers to detect a safe TOF greater than 0.6.

RECORDING OF RESPONSE

The response to nerve stimulation is a muscle response, the magnitude of which is an indication of the degree of blockade. There are currently six ways in which the muscle response may be determined: visual observation, tactile assessment, visual observation of preloaded thumb, mechanomyography, electromyography and acceleromyography.

Visual observation
Visual observation of the movement of the foot, toe, thumb or face is an inaccurate method for determining the force of contraction and hence derived values such as TOF ratio. However, in clinical practice, the presence or absence of a response can be seen easily, the number of TOF or PTC responses determined and appropriate interventions made. During recovery from vecuronium, visual observation of the first response of the TOF in the thumb is seen when there is recovery of the mechanical single twitch to 8% of control values,[24] a level compatible with good surgical relaxation. Direct stimulation of muscles in the forearm from stimulation over the ulnar nerve at the wrist gives rise to movement solely of the ring and little fingers, with

ulnar deviation of the wrist. These movements do not indicate the need for further relaxant administration.

Tactile assessment

Tactile assessment of the force of contraction, if possible, gives more reliable information and should always be used in preference to visual observation when knowledge of the force of contraction is required. A small abducting preload should be used for the thumb. However, it is notoriously difficult, either by visual or tactile means, to judge accurately the magnitude of the train-of-four ratio.[25]

Visual observation of preloaded thumb

The reliability of visual observation can be enhanced by attaching a spring with a compliance of 400 g/cm to the thumb, producing an abducting preload. This may be performed simply by attaching an appropriate rubber band[26] or with an inexpensive device called the Myoscan.[27] These studies suggest that this method is the most accurate of the clinical methods during recovery.

Mechanomyography

This is undertaken when the force of contraction is measured with a force-displacement transducer. Movement of the thumb in response to ulnar nerve stimulation is monitored most readily. The transducer should measure isometric force in the correct vector, should give a linear output over the range of forces encountered (2 kgf and 7 kgf for single twitch and tetanus), and must hold the thumb in a constant position relative to the hand, with a constant and preferably known degree of preload of the muscle (approximately 200–400 g). This department uses the ring-pull transducer described by the Stanecs.[28]

The advantages of this method are that it measures the required parameter of muscle response, namely force of contraction, and calibration and determination of recording system linearity are easily accomplished. The disadvantages are that hand and thumb immobilization may be difficult to achieve, the system is susceptible to physical knocking that occurs during normal operating procedures, constancy of preload is vital and the systems are generally only suitable for the thumb although adaptions are possible.

Electromyography

This technique measures the compound muscle action potential in response to nerve stimulation. The events recorded are therefore the step before excitation-contraction coupling. This offers the theoretical advantages that the events are 'nearer' to the end plate, and certain phenomena like post-tetanic protentiation can be unequivocally interpreted in terms of transmitter release rather than muscle contraction. For example, post-tetanic protentiation may be seen with mechanomyography in patients who are not paralysed, but this is not observed with electromyography. This suggests that the application of tetanus to a muscle may alter events within the muscle itself. A full description of electromyography is given in the section concerned with commercially available machines. The major advantages of electromyography over mechanomyography are that it is possible to record from muscles not accessible to electromyography and that the electromyograph (e.m.g.) appears to be less dependent

Table 10.1 Options available in the method of monitoring neuromuscular blockade. The stimuli delivered must conform to the characteristics described in the text

Pattern of stimulation	Stimulator/patient interface	Nerve stimulated	Assessment of muscle response
0.1 Hz	Direct	Ulnar	Visual
1.0 Hz	Surface electrodes	Median	Tactile
50.0 Hz	Needle electrodes	Facial	Preloaded thumb
Train-of-four		Common peroneal	Mechanomyography
Post-tetanic count		Posterior tibial	Electromyography
Double burst			Acceleromyography

on accurate fixation or preload and is less susceptible to physical knocking. The primary disadvantages are in difficulties in production and analysis of the waveform and of interpretation of the relationship between the e.m.g. and the mechanomyograph (m.m.g.). This is discussed later. It is also sensitive to electrical interference.

Acceleromyography
This technique was first described in 1987. The mass of the thumb can be regarded as constant, suggesting that measurement of acceleration will give an accurate indication of force. Only one device is presently marketed and this is described in a later section.

It can be seen from Table 10.1 that several options are present when considering where and how to monitor the degree of neuromuscular blockade. Not all combinations are possible, however. For example, it is not possible presently to monitor blockade by using the facial nerve/muscles combination using acceleromyography. The following section deals with commercially available equipment.

NERVE STIMULATORS

The ideal characteristics of nerve stimulators can be summarized as follows:

1. Constant current design;
2. Adjustable currents up to 70–80 mA (into 5 K = kΩ);
3. Square wave stimulus, duration 0.1–0.3 ms;
4. Stimulator/patient interface by fixed rounded tip electrodes and availability of sockets for leads to surface electrodes;
5. Polarity of electrodes marked;
6. Display of current passing;
7. Stimulation at 1 Hz, 50 Hz, train-of-four;
8. Repeated stimulation possible at pre-set intervals;
9. Visual (and audible if desired) alert at time of stimulation;
10. Robust, inexpensive construction;
11. Battery operated with low battery alert; and
12. Conforming to BS 5724 Part 1.

Several nerve stimulators are available and the design features of some of them have been published.[8,29] Some commercially available stimulators are expensive and this has led several anaesthetists to design and produce devices semi-commercially. This department has found these smaller stimulators to be quite suitable for clinical monitoring. The latest of these incorporates suitable stimulation for both neuromuscular blockade and nerve location prior to local blocks (Duostim, Medical Marketing, P.O. Box 37, Grantham, NG 31 6AA).

Electromyography[30,31]

The compound e.m.g. from a stimulated muscle may be recorded with needle or surface electrodes. It is generally of the shape depicted in Figure 10.1. The duration is typically 20 ms from stimulation with peak voltage 0.5–5.0 mV. In order to obtain an accurate waveform, the recording system must possess a fast response time. This generally means a display of the waveform on an oscilloscope screen with a record obtained on light sensitive paper. Although work with electromyography and muscle relaxants was published as long ago as 1952 (with decamethonium), the difficulty and expense of obtaining research grade recordings limited its general application. Various systems have been described to facilitate its introduction into clinical monitoring. In 1973, Epstein et al[32] recorded the e.m.g. on FM tape with playback at a slower speed and display on an ink writing polygraph. Although the waveform recorded on the polygraph was very similar to that seen on the storage oscilloscope, the immediacy of recording/display and appropriate clinical action was lost.

A development in 1977[33] applied computer technology to the handling of the evoked e.m.g. using digitization, storage, playback with time expansion and analogue reconstruction of the waveform on a chart recorder. The record obtained faithfully reproduced the waveform and, by direct measurement of the height of the wave, changes in the e.m.g. could be quantified.

Another approach is to measure the area enclosed by the waveform, rather than the height of the peak. An early study[34] used planimetry to measure the area under the first positive deflection, utilizing photographs of oscilloscope tracings. A simple, non-invasive and compact electronic system that rectified and integrated the waveform was first described in 1981.[35] Further developments led to the production of the Relaxograph® (Datex) — a compound e.m.g. monitor that combines stimulator, analyzer, display and chart recorder. Other systems have been investigated.[36]

The Relaxograph® incorporates stimulator unit, patient leads, analysis of the waveform by integration, digital display of T1:control and the TOF ratio and a printer.

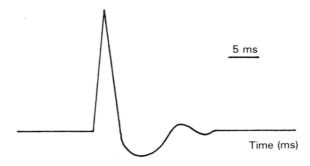

5 ms

Time (ms)

Fig. 10.1   Diagrammatic representation of the compound muscle action potential when displayed on an oscilloscope screen. Measurement can be made of the amplitude of the primary peak or of the area contained within the waveform.

The stimulator unit produces 0.1 ms square-wave pulses with routine monitoring by train-of-four. The patient is connected by 5 leads (2 stimulating, 2 recording and a ground). In normal use, the brown and white leads are attached over the ulnar nerve at the wrist, the red and green electrodes over the hypothenar muscles and the black electrode at the wrist between the pairs of stimulating and recording electrodes. Special surface electrodes are supplied for use, although in practice ordinary e.c.g. electrodes are suitable.

The leads are attached before the patient is anaesthetized. The hand should be immobilized on a board; this prevents movement of the surface electrodes in relation to the underlying muscle, which may produce artefactual changes in e.m.g. amplitude. Once the patient is anaesthetized, the machine can be switched to monitor. The initial set-up procedure is then automatic. The machine delivers 1 Hz stimuli at increasing current until the supramaximal current is found. The machine displays and prints this current. The actual stimulating current is then set approximately 20% higher than this value.

Four stimuli are then delivered and the response sets the reference or control values. A single stimulus is delivered (but the response is not displayed) in order to measure the stimulus artefact. The analysis of this can best be described by reference to Figure 10.2. The stimulus artefact is the response that is detected by the recording electrodes that has been transmitted directly to the electrodes. The stimulus is not transmitted by the normal (but slow) end-plate route and arrives within a few milliseconds. The Relaxograph® quantifies the stimulus artefact by opening a gate from 0.5–1.5 ms after the stimulus and calculating the response as a percentage of the true e.m.g. obtained from 3–13 ms from the stimulus. The value is displayed and recorded. If the value is too high, interference between stimulus artefact and true e.m.g. might occur and the Relaxograph® will not proceed, allowing repositioning of electrodes, especially the ground (black). If, in a particular patient a low artefact cannot be obtained, the Relaxograph® will calculate the artefact after every train-of-four. In normal circumstances it is checked every sixth train.

In clinical use,[37] the Relaxograph® offers the height of the first response to control and the TOF ratio as indices of muscle relaxation. Since it is muscle strength (twitch

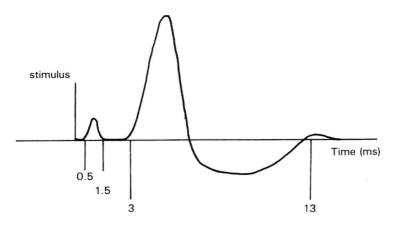

Fig. 10.2 Calculation of the stimulus artefact (see text).

tension) that is of interest to anaesthetists rather than the e.m.g. potential, it is important that correlations are made between the compound e.m.g. and force of contraction. Interpretation of the results from published studies must take into account various factors. Firstly, the earlier published work quantified the e.m.g. in terms of height of the peak deflection, whereas an integrated value is more common now. It appears, however, that the correlation between these two methods is good.[38] Secondly, some studies have recorded the force of contraction of one muscle (adductor pollicis) with the e.m.g. obtained from another muscle or groups of muscles. The Relaxograph® manual advises that the recording electrodes are placed on the hypothenar eminence. This compromises three individual muscles — the opponens, abductor and flexor digiti minimi. This site is recommended because the muscles are more superficial and the signal strength is greater. While it can be argued that if this site is to be used for monitoring then correlations with adductor pollicis should be investigated, it must be realized that the interpretation of the results may only pertain to this combination of monitoring sites, rather than to the correlation of the e.m.g. and the m.m.g. in general. Lastly, it must be remembered that the Relaxograph® is designed as a clinical tool and it must be accepted at this level. The waveform is not displayed and the machine is therefore scientifically unsuitable for research into the e.m.g.

With these points in mind, the following comparative studies have been undertaken. In an early study,[39] using suxamethonium and single stimuli, the mechanical twitch response recovered faster than the thenar e.m.g. While the thenar and hypothenar e.m.g. recovered at different rates within patients, there was no consistent difference in the study group as a whole. With tubocurarine, the thenar and hypothenar e.m.g. responses were less depressed than the mechanical twitch. This study suggests that, upon return of mechanical twitch tension to control values after suxamethonium, a substantial block could still be present as determined by the e.m.g. During recovery from tubocurarine, return of the e.m.g. to control values could be associated with mechanical muscle weakness. The results for suxamethonium have been confirmed in two recent studies. Using a single dose of suxamethonium,[40] mechanical recovery was effected more rapidly than either the peak amplitude or integrated e.m.g. amplitudes. This same pattern of recovery was also seen following discontinuation of a suxamethonium infusion.[41] The more rapid return of m.m.g. over e.m.g. with suxamethonium would be compatible with an alteration in contractile property of the muscle.

Interpretation of studies comparing mechanomyography and electromyography during recovery from non-depolarizing agents have tended to record that, during recovery, the mechanical response lags behind the integrated e.m.g., although the correlation is usually reliable enough for clinical use. Two studies [42,43] which compared the m.m.g. of the thumb with the hypothenar e.m.g., found that e.m.g. TOF ratios of 0.9–1.0 were required for m.m.g. TOF ratios to be reliably greater than 0.6. The correspondence[44] that followed the publication of Kopman's study outlined the criticism of the site for electromyography. A further study by Kopman[45] using the dorsal interosseus muscle e.m.g. and adductor pollicis m.m.g. (with metocurine as relaxant) found a much better correlation. Interestingly, the study found a difference in e.m.g. between patients in whom the thumb was immobilized and those in whom it was preloaded and immobilized. Comparison of the e.m.g. and m.m.g. with two relaxants, alcuronium and atracurium, suggested that a drug specific e.m.g/m.m.g. correlation may exist.[46] Rather confusingly, during recovery from vecuronium, both electrical[47] and mechanical[48] recovery have been found to be more rapid.

Acceleromyography

Acceleromyography quantifies the degree of neuromuscular blockade by measurement of the acceleration of a digit in response to nerve stimulation. Since force is equal to mass multiplied by acceleration, the force of contraction will be directly proportional to the magnitude of acceleration provided that the effective mass of the thumb remains constant. Only one device, the Accelograph (Biometer®)[49] is designed to monitor neuromuscular blockade in this fashion. It consists of an acceleration transducer with stimulating and computing units.

The acceleration transducer is small (0.5×1.0 cm, 20 g) and consists of a piezo-electric ceramic wafer with an electrode on each side. A voltage difference develops between these electrodes when the transducer experiences acceleration. The voltage of the initial positive deflection, approximately 20 mV, is a measure of the maximal acceleration. The stimulator unit is similar to that found in other Biometer® products (Myotest, Myograph). Output currents of 60 mA will be maintained with skin resistances up to 5 kohm. In addition to 1 Hz and TOF patterns of stimulation, post-tetanic counts (PTC) are possible. An Epson compatible printer may be attached for a permanent record. The unit is designed for mains voltage operation, but an inbuilt, rechargeable battery gives 50 hours operation.

Initial set-up of the monitor is straightforward. Stimulating electrodes are placed over the ulnar nerve at the wrist and the electrode is taped to the thumb. The fingers are immobilized on a board, but obviously the thumb is left free to move. No preload is applied. After induction of anaesthesia, but before relaxant administration, the monitor may be switched to automatic mode. The monitor determines supramaximal stimulation and control values of twitch (i.e. acceleration) are adjusted to 100% and displayed. In addition to the values for twitch height, TOF ratio or PTC the display will also show factors such as supramaximal current stimulation, gain factor required to adjust control response to 100%, time to next stimulation, type of stimulation and battery voltage. Fault displays indicate when the electrode circuit is faulty, the skin resistance too high, the supramaximal current is greater than 40 mA or the transducer signals are weak or unstable. In an effort to reduce artefactual recordings from accidental knockings, the recording unit will only operate for a short period after stimulation. Because acceleration is the basis of measurement of the response, it is not possible to calculate tetanic fade.

Comparison between acceleromyography and mechanomyography has been determined by the department that developed the Accelograph. The measurements cannot be determined simultaneously on the same hand and comparisons between two hands in the same patient has been undertaken. In 30 patients,[50] a close linear relationship was found during recovery from vecuronium. Using the TOF ratio, in the range of m.m.g. TOF 0–0.7 the linear relationship was not distinguishable from the line of identity. Taking an m.m.g. TOF ratio of 0.7, the 95% confidence limits for AMG-TOF were approximately 0.55–0.90. Part of this spread of values around the line of identity may be the result of using different hands for each measurement. Above an m.m.g. TOF ratio of 0.7, a.m.g. values tend to be greater. In unparalysed patients it is common for the first response to be of smaller amplitude than the remaining three. This gives a TOF ratio greater than unity. This problem seems to occur when the thumb has been at rest for longer than 2 seconds (personal communication, Biometer®). Unpublished work from our own department accords roughly with the published work from Denmark. Further studies are in progress. The precision of the acceleration transducer was found to be equal to the force-displacement transducer,[51] defining precision as the variation of measurement, given that the true measurement remains unchanged.

REFERENCES

1. Christie T H, Churchill-Davidson H C 1958 The St. Thomas's hospital nerve stimulator. Lancet i: 776
2. Beemer G H, Cass N M 1988 Monitoring the neuromuscular junction. Anaesthesia and Intensive Care 16: 62–66
3. Ali H H 1987 Monitoring of neuromuscular function. International Journal of Clinical Monitoring and Computing 4: 185–189
4. Hudes E, Lee K C 1987 Clinical use of peripheral nerve stimulators in anaesthesia. Canadian Journal of Anaesthesia 34: 525–534
5. Viby-Mogensen J 1982 Clinical assessment of neuromuscular transmission. British Journal of Anaesthesia 54: 209–223
6. Epstein R A, Wyte S R, Jackson S H, Sitter S 1969 The electromechanical response to stimulation by the block-aid monitor. Anesthesiology 30: 43–47
7. Kopman A F, Lawson D 1984 Milliamperage requirements for supramaximal stimulation of the ulnar nerve with surface electrodes. Anesthesiology 61: 83–85
8. Pollmaecher T, Steiert H, Buzello W 1986 A constant current nerve stimulator (neurostim T4). British Journal of Anaesthesia 58: 1443–1446
9. Mylrea K C, Hameroff S R, Calkins J M, Blitt C D, Humphrey L L 1984 Evaluation of peripheral nerve stimulators and relationship to possible errors in assessing neuromuscular blockade. Anesthesiology 60: 464–466
10. Weber S 1984 Observations made in the adductor pollicis may not be applicable to other muscle groups. Anesthesiology 61: 353–354
11 Day N S, Blake G J, Standaert F G, Dretchen K L 1983 Characterization of the train-of-four response in fast and slow muscles: effect of d-tubocurarine, pancuronium, and vecuronium. Anesthesiology 58: 414–417
12. Secher N H, Rube N, Secher O 1982 Effect of tubocurarine on human soleus and gastrocnemius muscles. Acta Anaesthesiologica Scandinavica 26: 231–234
13. Stiffel P, Hameroff S R, Blitt C D, Cork R C 1980 Variability in assessment of neuromuscular blockade. Anesthesiology, 52: 436–437
14. Caffrey R R, Warren M L, Becker K E 1986 Neuromuscular blockade monitoring comparing the orbicularis oculi and adductor pollicis muscles. Anesthesiology 65: 95–97
15. Berger J J, Gravenstein J S, Munsen E S 1982 Electrode polarity and peripheral nerve stimulation. Anesthesiology 56: 402–404
16. Payne J P, Hughes R 1981 Evaluation of atracurium in anaesthetized man. British Journal of Anaesthesia 53: 45–54
17. Ali H H, Savarese J J, Lebowitz P W, Ramsey F M 1981 Twitch, tetanus and train-of-four as indices of recovery from non depolarizing neuromuscular blockade. Anesthesiology 54: 294–297
18. Viby-Mogensen J, Howardy-Hansen P, Chraemmer-Jorgensen B, Ording H, Engbaek J, Nielsen A 1981 Post-tetanic count (ptc): a new method of evaluating an intense non-depolarizing neuromuscular blockade. Anesthesiology 55: 458–461
19. Howardy-Hansen P, Viby-Mogensen J, Gottschau A, Skovgaard L T, Chraemmer-Jorgensen B, Engbaek J 1984. Anesthesiology 60: 372–374
20. Bonsu A K, Viby-Mogensen J, Fernando P U E, Muchhal K, Tamilarasan A, Lambourne A 1987 Relationship of post-tetanic count and train-of-four response during intense neuromuscular blockade caused by atracurium. British Journal of Anaesthesia 59: 1089–1092
21. Fernando P U E, Viby-Mogensen J, Bonsu A K, Tamilarasan A, Muchhal K K, Lambourne A 1987 Relationship between post-tetanic count and response to carinal stimulation during vecuronium-induced neuromuscular blockade. Acta Anaesthesiologica Scandinavica 31: 593–596

22. 1987 Nineteenth Congress of the Scandinavian Society of Anaesthesiologists, Sweden, June 29–July 3
23. Jones R M, Payne J P (eds.) 1988 Recent developments in muscle relaxation. International Congress and Symposium Series, Royal Society of Medicine Services, London
24. O'Hara D A, Fragen R J, Shanks C A 1986 Comparison of visual and measured train-of-four recovery after vecuronium induced neuromuscular blockade using two anaesthetic techniques. British Journal of Anaesthesia 58: 1300–1302
25. Viby-Mogensen J, Jensen N H, Engbaek J, Ording H, Skovgaard L T, Chraemmer-Jorgensen B 1985 Tactile and visual evaluation of the response of the train-of-four nerve stimulation. Anesthesiology 63: 440–443
26. Tammisto T, Wirtavuori K, Linko K 1988 Assessment of neuromuscular block: comparison of three clinical methods and evoked electromyography. European Journal of Anaesthesiology 5: 1–8
27. Nagashima H, Nguyen H D, Conforti M, Duncalf D, Goldiner P L, Foldes F F 1988 A simple method for monitoring muscular relaxation during continuous infusion of vecuronium. Canadian Journal of Anaesthesia 35: 134–138
28. Stanec A, Stanec G 1983 The adductor pollicis monitor-apparatus and method for the quantitative measurement of the isometric contraction of the adductor pollicis muscle. Anesthesia and Analgesia 62: 602–605
29. Viby-Mogensen J, Hansen P H, Jorgensen B C, Ording H, Kann T, Fries B 1980 A new nerve stimulator (myotest). British Journal of Anaesthesia 52: 547–550
30. Weber S 1987 Integrated electromyography: is it the new standard for clinical monitoring of neuromuscular blockade? International Journal of Clinical Monitoring and Computing 4: 53–57
31. Calvey T N 1984 Assessment of neuromuscular blockade by electromyography: a review. Journal of the Royal Society of Medicine 77: 56–59
32. Epstein R M, Epstein R A, Lee A S J 1973 A recording system for continuous evoked electromyography. Anesthesiology 38: 287–289
33. Lee C, Katz R L, Lee A S J, Glaser B 1977 A new instrument for continuous recording of the evoked compound electromyogram in the clinical setting. Anesthesia and Analgesia, 56: 260–270
34. Nightingale D A, Glass A G, Bachman L 1966 Neuromuscular blockade by succinylcholine in children. Anesthesiology 27: 736–741
35. Lam H S, Cass N M, Ng K C 1981 Electromyographic monitoring of neuromuscular blockade. British Journal of Anaesthesia 53: 1351–1356
36. Windsor J P W, Sebel P S, Flynn P J 1985 The neuromuscular transmission monitor. Anaesthesia 40: 146–151
37. Carter J A, Arnold R, Yate P M, Flynn P J 1986 Assessment of the Datex relaxograph during anaesthesia and atracurium-induced neuromuscular blockade. British Journal of Anaesthesia 58: 1447–1452
38. Pugh N D, Kay B, Healy T E J 1984 Electromyography in anaesthesia: a comparison between two methods. Anaesthesia, 39: 574–577
39. Katz R L 1973 Electromyographic and mechanical effects of suxamethonium and tubocurarine on twitch, tetanic and post-tetanic responses. British Journal of Anaesthesia 45: 849–858
40. Shanks C A, Jarvis J E 1980 Electromyographic and mechanical twitch responses following suxamethonium administration. Anaesthesia and Intensive Care 8: 341–344
41. Donati F, Bevan D R 1984 Muscle electromechanical correlations during succinylcholine infusion. Anesthesia and Analgesia 63: 891–894
42. Kopman A F 1985 The relationship of evoked electromyographic and mechanical responses following atracurium in humans. Anesthesiology 63: 208–211
43. Weber S, Muravchick S 1986 Electrical and mechanical train-of-four responses during depolarizing and non depolarizing neuromuscular blockade. Anesthesia and Analgesia 65: 771–776
44. Ali H H 1986 Monitoring neuromuscular function. Anesthesiology, 64: 532
45. Kopman A F 1988 The dose-effect relationship of metocurine: the integrated electromyogram of the first dorsal interosseus muscle and the mechanomyogram of the adductor pollicis compared. Anesthesiology 68: 604–607
46. Harper N J N, Bradshaw E G, Healy T E J 1986 Evoked electromyographic and mechanical responses of the adductor pollicis compared during the onset of meuromuscular blockade by atracurium or alcuronium, and during antagonism by neostigmine. British Journal of Anaesthesia 58: 1278–1284
47. Astley B A, Katz R L, Payne J P 1987 Electrical and mechanical responses after neuromuscular blockade with vecuronium, and subsequent antagonism with neostigmine or edrophonium. British Journal of Anaesthesia 59: 983–988
48. Mortier E, Moulaert P, de Somer A, Rolly G 1988 Comparison of evoked electromyography and mechanical activity during vecuronium-induced neuromuscular blockade. European Journal of

Anaesthesiology 5: 131–141
49. Jensen E, Viby-Mogensen J, Bang, U 1988 The Accelograph: a new neuromuscular transmission monitor. Acta Anaesthesiologica Scandinavica 32: 49–52
50. Viby-Mogensen J, Jensen E, Werner M, Kirkegaard Nielsen H 1988 Measurement of acceleration: a new method of monitoring neuromuscular function. Acta Anaesthesiologica Scandinavica 32: 45–48
51. May O, Kirkegaard Nielsen H, Werne M U 1988 The acceleration transducer — an assessment of its precision in comparison with a force displacement transducer. Acta Anaesthesiologica Scandinavica 32: 239–243

11. Chronic neuropathic pain: aminoglycosides, peripheral somatosensory mechanisms and painful disorders

J. Gallagher and W. Hamann

In their search for an antibiotic against Gram-negative bacteria Waksman and co-workers developed between 1939 and 1943 the first of the clinically useful aminoglycosides, streptomycin.[1,2] Since then the number of aminoglycosides has grown steadily. Although they have maintained therapeutic significance for specific indications, their use is restricted by two main side-effects, oto- and nephrotoxicity. The toxic effects of these substances have attracted the interest of neuroscientists. The resulting work revealed that aminoglycosides are powerful modulators of the normal function of several excitable tissues.[3-9] Where investigated, the actions of aminoglycosides were antagonistic to the physiological effects of Ca^{2+}.[10-12] Recently, streptomycin has been used successfully in the treatment of certain painful disorders.[13] Neomycin is also an antibiotic commonly used in skin ointments. One may speculate that the benefit from these ointments derives not only from the antibiotic, but also from a sensory suppressive effect.

The action of aminoglycosides on nociception is likely to take place at the primary afferent neurone, because the blood-brain barrier does not permit easy passage of these substances.

In what way could aminoglycosides affect nociception in the periphery? Hypothetically, there could be reduction of excitability in peripheral nociceptors, suppression of ectopic or spontaneous activity in primary afferent nociceptor fibres, inhibition of nervous impulses from sympathetic or large to small afferent nerve fibres (ephaptic transmission). There could also be modulation of the pattern of release of excitatory transmitter substance from primary afferent nerve terminals. Finally, exposure to aminoglycosides could produce cell death.

CHEMISTRY

Structurally, all aminoglycosides are polycations consisting of two or more amino-sugars joined in glycosidic linkage to a hexose nucleus. The hexoses or aminocyclitoles found in aminoglycosides are either streptidine or 2-deoxystreptidine. Aminogylcosides containing 2-deoxystreptine are more heat stable and may be autoclaved. The aminocyclitols are usually in a central position of the molecule (Fig. 11.1), streptomycin being an exception from this rule with streptidine in an end position (Fig. 11.2). Commercial products are sold as sulphates, soluble in water, but poorly soluble in alcohol or lipids. They are stable at pH 2–11 with optimal pH in the alkaline range.[2]

Pharmacokinetics

Aminoglycosides are poorly absorbed by the healthy gastrointestinal system. Upon parenteral application, aminoglycosides distribute primarily in the extracellular space with poor distribution into the cerobrospinal fluid. In addition, there appear to be slow trans-membrane transport processes allowing aminoglycosides access to the intracellular space of at least selected cell populations. Peak plasma values are reached within 1 hour following intramuscular injection.[1,2,14] Aminoglycosides are not strongly bound by plasma proteins. In contrast, once attached to pharmacological receptors of a tissue, they are released at a slow rate. Tissue half-lives vary between 40 and 700 hours.[15] It is the combination of low affinity to plasma proteins and high affinity to tissue receptors that make aminoglycosides promising substances for topical or local applications.

The slow release of these substances from the tissue of the inner ear also appears to be the reason for the high aminoglycoside levels persisting in endolymph and perilymph days following cessation of systemic application.[16] Aminoglycosides are not metabolized to any significant degree, and excretion takes place almost exclusively through the kidneys.

Toxicity

Aminoglycosides are toxic drugs and are to be used with caution.[17] The susceptible organs are the vestibulo-cochlear apparatus and the kidney. Toxicity is most com-

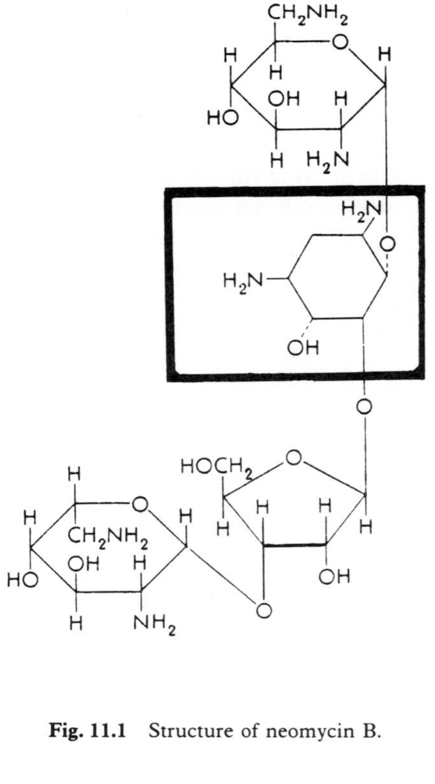

Fig. 11.1   Structure of neomycin B.

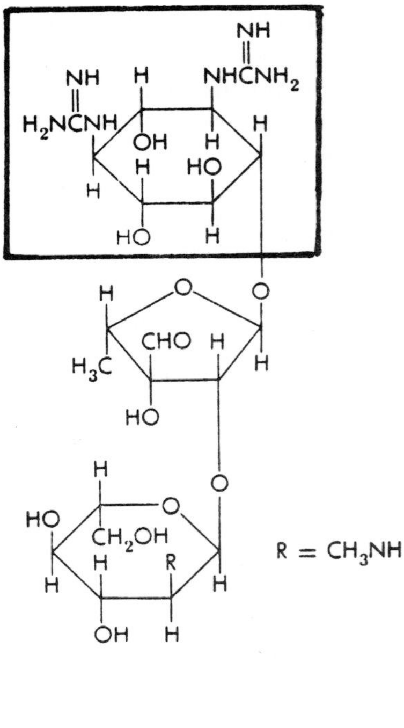

Fig. 11.2   Structure of streptomycin.

monly seen in cases where high doses have been administered frequently and for a long period, and the elderly are most at risk.[1,2] Streptomycin is more likely to affect vestibular function than auditory function, and this is usually heralded by persistent headache and nausea. The incidence of toxicity is difficult to estimate, but 75% of patients treated with 2 g streptomycin a day for more than 60 days have nystagmus or postural imbalance and subclinical damage may occur with smaller doses.[2] Sensitive tests of hearing can detect subclinical changes, which are initially reversible. Nephrotoxicity is less common with streptomycin than with other aminoglycosides such as gentamicin. Renal function impairment is uncommon unless doses of 3–4 g/d are given.[2] Finally, allergy to aminoglycosides is uncommon, but local tender swellings may occur after injection of streptomycin and they may be accompanied by a fever.

MECHANISMS OF ACTION

Cellular function may be affected in a variety of ways by aminoglycosides. To date, no single functional principle has emerged that could explain all known effects. However, most actions of aminoglycosides are antagonized by Ca^{2+}. There would be strong support for the hypothesis that aminoglycosides act either by occupying pharmacological receptor sites for Ca^{2+} or by blockage of Ca^{2+} and other ion channels in cell membranes.

Aminoglycosides distribute primarily in the extracellular space, but some of their cellular actions are clearly intracellular. It is therefore likely that susceptible cells possess transport mechanisms for aminoglycosides.[7] In bacteria such mechanisms have been identified.[18]

Aminoglycosides produce acute suppression of a variety of excitable membranes. To avoid duplication, these are more appropriately discussed in the section about the effects of these drugs on sensory receptors.

Transport processes across cell membranes for aminoglycosides

For a variety of bacteria, the presence of specific transport mechanisms has been established.[19] It appears that damage to the bacterial cell wall may be a facilitating factor, whereas hypoxia causes reduction in transport.[19,20] It would be of interest to know, whether similar principles apply to mammalian tissue. In recent electrophysical and pharmacokinetic studies, it has been shown that aminoglycosides occupy at least two distinct sites (i.e. membrane surface and intracellular space) in the course of their actions. Results from studies of drug uptake in vitro and of drug ototoxicity in cochlear perfusions are suggestive of involvement of an active (energy-requiring) aminoglycoside transport system.[7]

Effect on protein synthesis

The antibiotic action of aminoglycosides has been ascribed to their inhibitory effect on protein synthesis.[2] Aminoglycosides are known to attach to specific fragments of bacterial ribosomes.[21-23] They will thus interfere with transcription during protein synthesis. No experimental data are available for mammalian cells. If similar mechanisms were at work in susceptible mammalian cells, there would be wide-ranging implications regarding survival of a cell. In primary afferent neurones there is likely to be impairment of production and release of peptides and transmitter substances.

It is interesting to note that streptomycin injected close to relevant peripheral nerves may produce pain relief in patients suffering from facial pain or scar pain lasting over periods of weeks or months.[13] One explanation for this unexpectedly long time course may be that streptomycin is transported axonally to the cell bodies in the dorsal root ganglion impairing normal cellular function by interference with protein production.

Mitochondria and cellular respiration

Bacterial, as well as mammalian mitochondria are sensitive to the exposure to aminoglycosides. This is not surprising, as mitochondria are cell organelles with a very high content of calcium. Rat liver mitochondria show an acute and immediate suppression of malate and succinate utilization when exposed to relatively low concentration of neomycin.[24] Renal mitochondria from rats, during progressive decline of renal excretory function induced by gentamicin, showed reduced pyruvate-malate and succinate utilization.[11] This phenomenon could be offset by increased dietary calcium supplementation. In these experiments, the peak renal gentamicin levels were not affected by increased dietary calcium. Thus calcium did not prevent the uptake of gentamicin into the tubular cells. It is more likely that it antagonized the intracellular action of the aminoglycosides. Similar effects of aminoglycosides were observed in bacterial mitochondria. The above results clearly show that, once inside cells, aminoglycosides may suppress cellular respiration.

Another interesting aspect of the results by Humes and colleagues[11] is the time course of the events. Mitochondrial damage became noticeable gradually, over a time course of days. In general, it is unlikely that immediate effects of aminoglycosides on cell function are caused by depression of cellular respiration. It may become an effective mechanism once the slow process of intracellular accumulation has generated sufficiently high intracellular levels.

The phosphoinositide system

Many types of cells, including nerve cells, contain polyphosphoinositide molecules (PIP) in the inner layer of the cell membrane. In response to specific external stimuli, PIP molecules break up into trisphosphoinositol (IP3) and diacylglycerol (DAG). Both substances are released into the cytoplasm and act as so-called second messenger.[25] IP3 raises the intracellular concentration of Ca^{2+} by causing release from stores in the endoplasmatic reticulum, whereas DAG causes activation of protein kinase C, which is believed to facilitate influx of Ca^{2+} through the cell membrane by increasing the transmembrane permeability for Ca^{2+}.[26] For example, application of bradykinin, one of the key mediators in the tissue response to trauma, to neuroblastoma cells in culture will result in the intracellular release of IP3 and DAG. This will cause an increase in the intracellular concentration of Ca^{2+}, in turn resulting in the release of the neurotransmitter acetylcholine.[26] In competition with Ca^{2+}, aminoglycosides bind to PIP thus interfering with the second messenger function of this system.[3]

Phosphoinositide-based second messenger systems seem to be very common. However, the specific actions of DAG and other phosphoinositols are subject to ongoing research.[25,27-29] It is beyond the scope of the chapter to review the rapidly growing literature on this topic.

EFFECT OF SPECIFIC EXCITABLE TISSUES

Action of aminoglycosides on nerve fibres

Sokoll and Diecke[30] measured the conduction velocity and amplitude of the compound action potential of the desheathed frog tibial nerve during exposure to various concentrations of streptomycin. At the relatively high streptomycin concentration of 50 mg/l, the action potential was reduced by 1.1% and at 400 mg/l the conduction velocity was reduced by 10%. Extended periods of exposure (12–18 h) at concentrations of 400 mg/l caused irreversible damage. In man, it is conceivable that such high concentrations of streptomycin may be achieved after injection of 1 g close to a nerve. However, it is unlikely that these concentrations would be sustained for any length of time. The authors did not comment on the effect of streptomycin on non-myelinated nerve fibres.

Action of aminoglycosides on the neuromuscular junction

Since 1956 when Pridgeon noticed a connection between postoperative apnoea and treatment with neomycin, numerous reports have accumulated describing neuromuscular paralysis caused by aminoglycosides.[31,32]

Similarly, neuromuscular paralysis is a well-known complication when treating patients suffering from myasthenia gravis with aminoglycosides. In these patients, respiratory distress may be caused by a single dose within the therapeutic range of streptomycin. Neuromuscular paralysis is mainly caused by a presynaptic mechanism, most probably the inhibition of the release of acetylcholine.[33] Direct excitation of skeletal muscle is little affected by aminoglycosides, whereas indirect excitation is strongly inhibited.

Aminoglycoside-induced neuromuscular paralysis is more effectively antagonized by increased concentration of Ca^{2+} than by neostigmine.[34] Aminoglycosides are likely to occupy Ca^{2+} receptor sites at the presynaptic terminal, thus interfering with the influx of Ca^{2+}, which is a necessary pre-condition for the release of transmitter substance.

Action of aminoglycosides on sensory receptors

Up to this point, the action of aminoglycosides has been considered according to specific cellular functions. To put these actions into perspective they should be considered in their combined effects on peripheral neurones and sensory cells.

In contrast to no information on the effect of aminoglycosides on nociceptors or non-myelinated nerve fibres, there are extensive results on the effect of aminoglycosides on sensory receptors. However, with the exception of work on dermal stretch receptors (Ruffini endings) research has concentrated on secondary receptors. In a seconday receptor, separate sensory cells are attached to the peripheral terminals of primary afferent neurones. If sensory transduction takes place in the sensory cells, it follows that there is an additional site for action of pharmacological substance on these receptors, namely the interface between sensory cell and primary afferent sensory neurone. For receptors in the labyrinth, the lateral line organ of fish and probably for tactile receptor of the Merkel cell type this interface is a chemical synapse.

The effect of Ca^{2+} antagonists and aminoglycosides have been tested in anaesthetized animals from several species. In these experiments, electrophysiological recordings were made from single nerve fibres innervating cutaneous mechanoreceptors.[4,9,35] Repetitive standard mechanical stimuli were applied. Stimuli were within the physiological range of individual receptors under investigation. After the establishment of steady state, a Ca^{2+} antagonist or aminoglycoside were applied, either topically or by close arterial injection; and the extent and time course of action were recorded. In these experiments Ca^{2+} was shown to play a role in stimulus transduction in various cutaneous mechanoreceptors because stimulus transduction was impaired by organic and inorganic calcium-channel blockers. The effect of these substances is reversible within minutes.[9] Manganese concentrations three times higher than for comparable effects in Merkel cell type (secondary) receptors were needed for Ruffini type (primary) mechanoreceptors.

Similar time courses and relative degrees of reduction in sensitivity were observed when these two receptor types were exposed to close arterial infusion of neomycin lasting 10 minutes.[4,35] Also, following chronic daily intraperitoneal injection of very high doses of neomycin into rats over 3 weeks there was only slightly reduced responsiveness of about 20% on the day following the last injection.[5]

The acute action of aminoglycosides is likely to be cell-membrane mediated rather than intracellular in nature because of the extracellular distribution pattern and the relatively slow entry of aminoglycosides into cells.

Aminoglycosides cause reduction or abolition of microphonic responses and afferent nervous activity when applied to receptors of the lateral line system, sacculi, semicircular canals and the cochlea.[6] The binding of a significant number of negatively charged molecules like aminoglycoside to the cell membrane could be expected to interfere with the normal distribution of charge and thus, in a non-specific way, affect the properties of excitable membranes. Since aminoglycosides are strongly cationic, they are expected to bind to the negatively charged phospholipids in biological membranes.[36]

More recently, the specific action of aminoglycosides on hair cells in the inner ear has been discussed by Schacht (7).[7] Present evidence permits the suggestion of three possible ways in which aminoglycosides may block transduction:

1. Owing to the cationic nature of the aminoglycosides, they may compete with Ca^{2+} for binding sites on membranes that activate transduction. By increasing its concentration in the fluid bathing the apices of hair cells, Ca^{2+} was found to counteract the effects of aminoglycoside.[6] Interference of neomycin with Ca^{2+} uptake by neomycin has been demonstrated in vascular smooth muscle and intestinal smooth muscle.

2. By blocking the turnover of polyphosphoinositides in the membrane of hair cells, aminoglycosides might interfere with the transduction of mechanical stimuli. There is a direct correlation between the ototoxicity of various aminoglycosides and their binding strength to lipid films.[37] It is still uncertain, however, whether turnover of phospholipids is central to the transduction process or whether it is related to other cellular activities of receptor cells.

3. The poor ionic selectivity of transduction channels in receptor cells is the basis of a third possible acute mode of action of aminoglycosides on the hair cells. The strong cationic functional groups on the aminoglycosides are thought to enter the transduction channels and block them by plugging. Blockage of the transduction channels should develop rapidly after administration of the drug, and should be dependent upon the transmembrane potential. In a recent study, Ohmori[38] demonstrated in isolated vestibular hair cells of the chick that the mechano-sensitive current was blocked by aminoglycosides. The blockage was clearly voltage dependent.

In conclusion a four-step model about the action of aminoglycosides may be proposed in close agreement with Schacht:[7]

1. An initial, reversible step of electrostatic interaction of aminoglycosides with the plasma membrane, which is antagonized by Ca^{2+}.

2. A possibly energy-dependent uptake process into the intracellular space.

3. Binding to phosphatidylinositol bisphosphates so that further transduction mechanisms and related reactions are affected.

4. Inteference with other cellular functions such as protein synthesis or respiration.

AMINOGLYCOSIDES AND THE TREATMENT OF PAINFUL DISORDERS

Neuropathic pain

Pain of neurological origin (neuropathic pain) follows damage to nervous tissue, which may be traumatic or caused by disease. Pain of this type is characteristically burning in nature. It may have a dysaesthetic component and exhibit allodynia and hyperpathia.* A trigger point may be present and stimulation of this area with a normally innocuous stimulus such as light touch may provoke pain.

The pathophysiological mechanisms that result in post-traumatic pain have not yet been fully elucidated but several hypotheses have been proposed.[39-41] One of these suggests that local tissue damage activates peripheral (unmyelinated) C-fibres, which then initiate sensitization of a group of neurones in the spinal cord, known as wide dynamic-range neurones (WDR). These neurones become sensitized to subsequent afferent impulses. Activity in these neurones correlates well with the perception of pain. In the periphery, axonal damage in some way leads to an increased sensitivity in somatosensory receptors and an exaggerated response to stimulation, which is conducted by Ab fibres. These impulses arrive at the WDR cells and are transmitted to the cortex where they are interpreted as pain. In this way, a normally painless stimulus such as light touch is perceived as painful. In addition, the sensory receptors appear to become more sensitive to efferent sympathetic activity; this accounts for the pain relief that may follow sympathetic blockade.

In general, with the exception of the sympathetically mediated pains, which may respond very well to sympathectomy, neuropathic pain is difficult to treat. It is usually resistant to conventional analgesics, including morphine, but may respond to anticonvulsants and tricyclic antidepressants. These drugs may work by enhancing the

---

*Dysaesthesia: An unpleasant abnormal sensation, whether spontaneous or evoked. Allodynia: pain due to stimulus that does not usually provoke pain. Hyperpathia: a painful syndrome, characterized by increased reaction to a stimulus, as well as an increase in threshold.

descending serotinergic and noradrenergic inhibitory pain pathways and the anti-convulsants may additionly depress activity in irritable nervous tissue as they do in epi-lepsy. Unfortunately, both of these groups of drugs have side-effects and may be poorly tolerated by patients. Less-specific methods of pain relief such as transcutaneous nerve stimulation may also be helpful.

The effects that aminoglycosides may have in modifying stimulus transduction in somatosensory receptors and the function of neurones were discussed in the first part of this chapter. Mechanisms were suggested by which this may occur. It follows that, in conditions where hypersensitivity of peripheral nerves is a predominant feature, the local administration of aminoglycosides may decrease their excitability and thus provide a method of treatment.

To date, there is only one published report describing the successful use of streptomycin in the treatment of pain and this was in the management of trigeminal neuralgia.[13] The department of Pain Relief at Guy's Hospital has used streptomycin in the treatment of various neuropathic pains in a preliminary investigation. These clinical findings will be discussed below, following a brief description of the commonly encountered painful conditions that have their origins in the peripheral nervous system. In each case, the possible applications for aminoglycoside treatment will be discussed.

PAINFUL CONDITIONS WITH PERIPHERAL NERVOUS ORIGIN

So far as possible, the conditions discussed below will be named in accordance with the Descriptions of Chronic Pain Syndromes produced by the International Association for the Study of Pain — Subcommittee on Taxonomy.[42]

Facial pain

Trigeminal neuralgia
Trigeminal neuralgia or Tic Doloureux is an intermittent, but very severe, unilateral pain that is felt in the area of the face that is supplied by one or two of the main branches of the trigeminal nerve. It has several characteristic features that have been well described.[43] It is usually stabbing in nature and the pain is often initiated by stimu-lation of trigger points, with often only the lightest of touch being required. Examination usually reveals no, or minimal, sensory loss.

The aetiology of this condition remains unclear but in approximately 85% of patients microvascular compression of the posterior root of the trigeminal nerve may be demonstrated.[44] The incidence of such compression in the general population is however, unknown. Whatever its aetiology, the pain of 'tic' seems to arise from an irri-table lesion in the trigeminal nerve. Although this rarely produces sensory loss it results in pathological changes in the central and peripheral nervous systems.[45] As with other painful conditions, the pain is triggered by the stimulation of large myelinated Ab fibres and not the classical pain-carrying fibres, C and Ad. The response of the Ab fibres is exaggerated and this is transmitted to the sensitized WDR neurones in the trigeminal ganglion. The activation of these neurones is interpreted by the brain as pain.

Treatment is primarily with carbamezepine, with 70% of patients gaining relief.[43]

Alternative treatments are the partial destruction of the trigeminal ganglion with a radiofrequency lesion, or the surgical decompression of the nerve as it leaves the brain stem. Gangliolysis is successful in 80% of patients at 1 year and 50% will be pain free at 5 years,[43] but some patients find the numbness intolerable and may develop anaesthesia dolorosa (pain in numb areas). Surgical decompression produces an 80% 5-year improvement and does not produce a sensory loss; however, it does involve a posterior fossa craniectomy with its attendant risks. Sectioning of the trigeminal nerve is occasionally necessary and this produces a large area of numbness and consequently a much less satisfactory result.

Injection of trigger spots with local analgesic solution results in brief periods of quiesence, although the pain can be initiated again even before the numbness has completely receded. As stimulation of the trigger spots results in an exaggerated central response and initiates pain, it follows that application of aminoglycosides may attenuate this response and thus reduce or abolish pain. As the branches of the trigeminal nerves lie superficially, in well-described locations, nerve block with aminoglycoside is technically easy. To date, one clinical study reports success using streptomycin.[13]

Secondary trigeminal neuralgia from facial trauma

This painful syndrome follows facial trauma including facial fractures and oral surgery. It is usually a chronic throbbing pain in the distribution of one of the branches of the trigeminal nerve. Unlike primary trigeminal neuralgia, the pain is constant and trigger spots are less commonly found. There may be some associated sensory changes with areas of hypo- and hypersensitive skin. A similar painful condition may occur in patients who have had denervation procedures performed for primary trigeminal neuralgia.

The aetiology of this condition is trauma to branches of the trigeminal nerve. Animal studies have shown that even minor damage to axons may produce cutaneous hypersensitivity in the innervated area, and that the peripheral nerves and dorsal root ganglia show changes in both spontaneous and evoked activity.[46]

Treatment of this condition is more difficult than that of trigeminal neuralgia. Local analgesics and steroid injections often produce only temporary relief and centrally acting drugs, particularly tricyclic anti-depressants, may be more useful. Where patients demonstrate hypersensitivity, injections of aminoglycosides may depress this and afford some relief. The experience in our department is described below.

Facial pain may occur in patients with no history of trauma. In some cases this may have been forgotten but, alternatively the pain may be of psychological origin. These patients may be helped by tricyclic antidepressants and psychiatric help, and are unlikely to respond to local techniques. The diagnosis of psychological pain may be difficult, and is particularly confusing in patients who have already sought dental advice and undergone minor oral surgery in the hope of achieving pain relief.

Localized neuropathic pain

Reflex sympathetic dystrophy

Reflex sympathetic dystrophy (RSD) is a painful syndrome that may complicate sometimes trivial injury to bone and soft tissue. The pain is usually burning in nature and often accompanied by hyperpathia. Initially, the affected area is warm and red but later dystrophic changes may occur in the skin, soft tissue and bone, and the limb may become functionally useless. As the name suggests the syndrome may be accompanied by signs of abnormal sympathetic activity and the role of the sympathetic nervous system is emphasized by the therapeutic effect of sympathetic blockade.

The aetiology of the condition remains uncertain and a recent review discusses the possibilities in detail.[40,41] Initial axonal injury results in changes in the peripheral nerves and sensory receptors. Spontaneous firing may occur and there may be hypersensitivity of the Ad fibres so that normally innocuous stimuli are felt as pain. In addition, the somatosensory receptors appear to be affected by noradrenaline release. Finally, there are thought to be changes in the spinal cord and central nervous system.

The initial treatment of RSD should be sympathetic blockade and the use of the intravenous guanethidine technique described by Hannington-Kiff[47] is particularly useful. Several authors have reported success with this technique.[48,49] It is particularly helpful when hyperpathia is a marked feature of the pain.[49] When this approach fails, centrally acting drugs may be useful and prolonged use of transcutaneous nerve stimulation may also help. Injection of aminoglycosides to the large areas of hypersensitivity usually seen with RSD is rarely feasible. However, as aminoglycosides exert at least part of their action by antagonizing the activity of calcium ions an alternative approach would be the use of calcium antagonist drugs. Prough et al[50] have used nifedipine to treat a group of patients with RSD and have achieved success in 7 out of 11 patients. This is an encouraging result, although a large, controlled study remains to be performed.

Causalgia

Causalgia is the name given to a severe burning pain (the name is derived from the Greek words for burning and pain) that sometimes follows the injury and partial division of peripheral nerves. It was first described by Weir Mitchell after the American Civil war.[51] The pain is more severe but similar in nature to that of RSD and sympathetic hyperactivity is also a feature. It may be considered as a severe variant of RSD and treated accordingly. As with RSD, early and aggressive use of sympathetic blockade should be employed in the hope of avoiding the severe dystrophic changes that may occur.

Post-traumatic localized pain

The following group of conditions all follow injury or damage to peripheral nerves. The aetiology of the pain is changes in neurones in response to trauma, as described previously, and there may also be the development of painful neuromata where nerves have been divided.[52] In some cases, the pain is accompanied by sensory loss.

Stump pain

Stump pain is felt at the extremity of the remaining limb following amputation and should not be confused with phantom limb pain, which is felt in the amputated part of the limb. Stump pain originates from the local neural damage, whereas phantom limb pain has at least some of its origins in the central nervous system. A painful stump is of course common immediately following amputation but, in some patients, it fails to resolve despite apparently satisfactory healing. Reports of its incidence vary but at 6 months post-operation approximately 16% of patients will suffer from it.[53] It is usually a sharp, stabbing pain and often has a well-localized, hypersensitive trigger point on the stump itself. This is probably due to a neuroma being formed at the site of nerve transection. When stump pain occurs after lower limb amputation it often leads to inability to tolerate a prosthesis, with subsequent loss of mobility. Surgical revision of the stump usually leads to reformation of neuroma but, occasionally, it may be possible to reposition a neuroma and make a prosthesis wearable.

Scar pain

Following surgical or other trauma, pain may be experienced in the scar after healing has apparently taken place. It may be due to hypoxia in small nerves being caused by entrapment in scar tissue. The most common scar to cause pain is the thoracotomy scar, in which pain is sufficient to cause the patient to seek medical advice in between 1% and 3% of cases.[54] The pain is usually an extension of the early postoperative ache and also often develops a burning dysaesthetic component with intermittent stabbing pains. Examination usually reveals some sensory changes and hyperpathia and allodynia are common. Occasionally, an exquisitely tender spot is present and represents a neuroma.

Miscellaneous localized pains

Pain may arise of apparently neurological origin where no history of trauma is elicited. Segmental neuralgia is a painful condition characterized by pain in the region of a nerve root, most usually the intercostal nerves. The pain is paroxysmal, burning in nature and the area is often tender. Such conditions are usually the result of local osteoarthritis, or are secondary to infection or metabolic disease. Previous injections of nerves with neurolytics such as phenol may result in this syndrome, and therapeutic radiotherapy is another potent cause. A similar condition giving rise to pain is the abdominal cutaneous nerve entrapment syndrome. Here a cutaneous nerve appears to become trapped in the rectus sheath so that dysaesthetic burning pain is felt; this is exacerbated by contraction of the abdominal muscles.

Many of the localized neuropathic pains described above prove difficult to treat. Local analgesics injections often afford complete but temporary relief, and although steroid is often added, it may not always prolong this. Ablation of the involved nerve, either surgically or chemically should not be performed as it often worsens the pain and also produces numbness, which may be intolerable to the patient. Centrally acting drugs are often used, producing inevitable side-effects. The local injection of aminoglycosides should reduce the hypersensitivity in these nerves without producing numbness and so relieve pain. We have had some success with this technique, although so far only a small number of cases have been treated.

Generalized pain of neurological origin

Peripheral neuropathy

The pain that accompanies a peripheral neuropathy is a widespread, but usually predominantly, distal burning pain. It is often a feature of a general disease such as diabetes mellitus. Frequently, there is an associated sensory loss and autonomic as well as motor function may be disturbed. Because of its generalized distribution it is best treated with centrally acting drugs such as the anticonvulsants and tricyclic antidepressants, but particularly troublesome areas may benefit from local techniques. As with reflex sympathetic dystrophy calcium-channel blockers may prove to be useful in this condition.

CLINICAL EXPERIENCE

Published reports
The only published report concerning the use of an aminoglycoside antibiotics to treat painful conditions in humans is in the treatment of trigeminal neuralgia.[13] In this study, 20 patients with trigeminal neuralgia, who remained in pain despite conventional treatment (including, in some cases, alcohol injection of the trigeminal ganglion) were treated with five local injections of streptomycin. The injections were made subcutaneously and close to the nerves supplying the painful areas and consisted, on each occasion, of 1 g streptomycin dissolved in 2 ml of 2% plain lignocaine. The injections were made at intervals varying between 4 and 7 days. All the patients in this group experienced pain relief usually beginning after the second or third injection and being complete after five. The duration of pain relief experienced ranged from 2–30 months. Of the 20 patients studied, 10 patients had suffered no recurrence at the time of publication with a pain-free interval of 12–30 months (mean 23.3); in patients in whom pain recurred after 18 months retreatment using the same protocol was successful again producing analgesia for a further 6–14 months. Local sensory changes were not seen and so anaesthesia dolorosa was not a problem. The authors of this study reported no local or systemic side-effects.

Experience
In response to the published report and the theoretical and animal evidence outlined above we have used streptomycin to treat a preliminary group of patients. All of our patients were suffering from pain of a neuropathic type with altered sensitivity. The conditions treated are listed in Table 11.1. There were 8 patients with facial pain, most of whom fell into the post-traumatic trigeminal neuralgia category. The other group were also mostly post-traumatic in nature and consisted largely of hypersensitive scar pain. All the patients had proved refractory to conventional methods of treatment including where appropriate the local infiltration of local analgesic solution and steroids. Most patients received two or three injections at weekly intervals.

Table 11.1   Details of patients treated with streptomycin

Condition	Number of patients	Response to streptomycin	
		Relief of Pain	*No Relief*
Secondary trigeminal neuralgia (Post-traumatic)	6	4	2
Secondary trigeminal neuralgia (Post-gangliolysis)	2	1	1
Scar pain	9	7	2
Intercoastal neuralgia	2	2	0

Results

Out of 19 patients, 12 found the streptomycin injections helpful, and in 5 of these complete pain relief was achieved. The results were more impressive in the scar pain group, where 8 out of 11 obtained relief as opposed to the facial pain group in which only 4 out of 8 were helped. In this study, 3 of our patients experienced marked swelling, most commonly after the second injection, and these patients were not treated further. These patients are included in the results and one of them experienced some pain relief once the swelling had subsided. In 2 of these patients the swelling represented tissue reaction but in the 3rd, skin testing suggested true allergy.

These results, which show a success rate of over 50%, are encouraging as these patients are traditionally difficult to help. They are, however, less successful than the previously described paper. This probably results from our use of a lower total dose of streptomycin. The smaller doses were used because of concern about toxicity. It would be worthwhile administering a larger total dose of streptomycin once routine and careful monitoring of renal and auditory function have confirmed its safety.

SUMMARY

In summary, we have found initial results with streptomycin encouraging and worthy of further investigation. The diversity of actions of aminoglycosides on cellular mechanisms make it difficult to predict what will, or will not, happen in specific clinical conditions. Several examples have been given where these substances reduce the level of nervous activity in the peripheral nervous system in laboratory conditions and, so far, these findings have been confirmed in patient studies. It is therefore desirable to conduct more formal and controlled trials of the effect of aminoglycosides in conditions of somatosensory pathology, where changed states of excitability in primary afferent neurones produce pain.

ACKNOWLEDGEMENTS

The authors would like to thank Dr J.R. Wedley, Consultant in Charge, Pain Relief Clinic, Guy's Hospital for his support in this work. Grant support from the Croucher Foundation for W.H., and from The Sir Jules Thorn Charitable Trust for J.G. is gratefully acknowledged.

REFERENCES

1. Aminoglycosides. 1987. In: American hospital formulary drug information. Ed. GK Mc Eroy 50–55, 64–65
2. Sande M A, Mandell G L 1980 The aminoglycosides. In: Goodman L S, Gilman A, Macmillan (eds) The pharmacological basis of therapeutics Macmillan, New York
3. Axelrod J, Burch R M, Jelsman C L 1988 Receptor-mediated activation of phospholipase A2 via GTP-binding proteins: arachidonic acid and its metabolites as second messengers. Trends in Neurosciences 11: 117–122
4. Baumann K I, Cheng-Chew S B, Hamann W C, Leung M S 1984 Tactile responses after neomycin and during vitamin A deficiency in rats. In: Hamann W, Iggo A (eds) Proceedings of the International Symposium on Sensory Receptor Mechanisms. World Scientific Publishing, Singapore, pp. 153–261
5. Baumann K I, Hamann W, Leung M S 1988 Responsiveness of slowly adapting cutaneous mechanoreceptors after close arterial infusion of neomycin in cats. In: Hamann W, Iggo A, (eds) Progress in Brain Research 7: 43–50 Elsevier, Amsterdam

6. Hudspeth A J 1983 Mechano-electrical transduction by hair cells in the acousticolateralis sensory system. Annual review of Neurosciences 6: 187–215
7. Schacht J 1986 Molecular mechanisms of drug-induced hearing loss. Hearing Research 22: 297–304
8. Wilson P, Ramsden R T 1977 Immediate effects of tobramycin on human cochlea and correlation with serum tobramycin levels. British Medical Journal 1: 259–260
9. Yamashita Y, Ogawa H, Taniguchi K 1986 Differential effects of manganese and magnesium on two types of slowly adapting cutaneous mechanoreceptor afferent units in frogs. Pflügers Archives 406: 218–224
10. Bennett W M, Clayton Elliot W, Houghton D C, Gilbert D N, DeFehr J, McCarron D A 1982 Reduction of experimental gentamicin nephrotoxicity by dietary calcium loading. Antimicrobial Agents and Chemotherapy 22: 508–512
11. Humes H D, Sastrasinh M, Weinberg J M 1984 Calcium is a competitive inhibitor of gentamicin-renal membrane binding interactions and dietary calcium supplementation protects against gentamicin nephrotoxicity. Journal of Clinical Investigation 73: 134–147
12. Quarum M L, Houghton D C, Gilbert D N, McCarron D A, Bennett W M 1984 Increasing dietary calcium moderates experimental gentamicin toxicity. Journal of Laboratory and Clinical Medicine 103: 104–114
13. Sokolovic M, Todorovic L, Stajeic Z, Petrovic V 1986 Peripheral streptomycin/lidocaine injections in the treatment of idiopathic trigeminal neuralgia: a preliminary report. Journal of Maxillo-facial Surgery 14: 8–9
14. Reiner N E, Bloxham D D, Thompson W L 1987 Nephrotoxicity of gentamicin and tobramycin given once daily or continuously in dogs. Journal of Antimicrobial Chemotherapy 4: 85–101
15. Schentag J J, Jusko P D, Jusko W J 1977 Renal clearance and tissue accumulation of gentamicin. Clinical Pharmacology and Therapeutics 22(3): 364–370
16. Tran Ba Huy P, Meulemans A, Wassef M, Manuel C, Sterkers O, Amiel C 1983 Gentamicin persistence in rat endolymph and perilymph after a 2-day constant infusion. Antimicrobial Agents and Chemotherapy 23: 344–346
17. Lancet editorial 1986 Aminoglycoside toxicity Lanceti: 670–671
18. Shannon K, Phillips I 1982 Mechanisms of resistance to aminoglycosides in clinical isolates. Journal of Antimicrobial Chemotherapy 9:91–102
19. Bryan L E, Kwan S 1981 Mechanisms of aminoglycoside resistance of anaerobic and facultative bacteria grown anaerobically. Journal of Antimicrobial Chemotherapy 8 (suppl. D) 1–8
20. Mates S M, Patel L, Kaback R, Miller M H 1983 Membrane potential in anaerobically growing *Staphylococcus aureus* and its relationship to gentamicin uptake. Antimicrobial Agents and Chemotherapy 23: 526–530
21. Silverblatt F 1982 Pathogenesis of nephrotoxicity of cephalosporins and aminoglycosides: a review of current concepts . Review of Infectious Diseases 4: S360–S365
22. Le Goffic F, Capmau M L, Tangy F, Baillarge M 1979 Mechanisms of action of aminoglycoside antibiotics: binding studies of tobramycin and its 6-N-acetyl derivative to the bacterial ribosome and its subunits. European Journal of Biochemistry 102: 73–81
23. Luzzatto L. Apirion D, Schelessinger D 1969 Polyribosome depletion of the ribosome cycle by streptomycin in *Escherichia coli.* Journal of Molecular Biology 42: 315–335
24. Cheng-Chew S B, Hamann W, Leung M S, Tsang D 1985 The effect of neomycin on the ultrastructure of touch corpuscles in rats and on cellular respiration. Journal of Physiology 369: 61P
25. Berridge M J 1986 Inositol triphosphate and calcium mobilization. In: Calcium and the cell Eds Evered D Whelan J (Ciba Foundation Symposium 122) Wiley, Chichester, pp. 39–57
26. Miller S 1987 Bradykinin highlights the role of phospholipid metabolism in the control of nerve excitability. Trends in Neurosciences 10: 226–228
27. Kikkawa U, Kitano T, Saito N, Kishimoto A, Tanyyama K, Tanaka C, Nihizuki Y 1986 Role of protein kinase C in calcium-mediated signal transduction. In: Calcium and the cell. Eds Evered D, Whelan J (Ciba Foundation Symposium 122) Wiley, Chichester pp. 197–211
28. Morris A P, Gallacher D V, Irvine R F, Peterson O H 1987 Synergism of inositol triphosphate and tetrakiphosphate in activating Ca^{2+}-dependent K^+ channels. Nature 330: 653–658
29. Simmons B A, Winegard A I, Martin D B 1982 Significance of tissue myo-inositol concentrations in metabolic regulation in nerve. Science 217: 848–851
30. Sokoll M D, Diecke F P J 1969 Some effects of streptomycin on frog nerve in vitro. 177(2): 332–339
31. Pittinger C, Adamson R 1972 Antibiotic blockade of neuromuscular function. Annual review of Pharmacology. 12: 169–184

32. Pittinger C B, Eryasa Y, Adamson R 1970 Antibiotic induced paralysis: Anesthesia and Analgesia. Current Researches 49: 487–501
33. Sokoll M D, Gergis s M 1981 Antibiotics and neuromuscular function. Anesthesiology 55: 148–159
34. Singh Y N, Harvey A L, Marshall I G 1978 Antibiotic-induced paralysis of the mouse phrenic nerve-hemidiaphragm preparation and reversibility by calcium and by neostigmine. Anesthesiology 48: 418–424
35. Baumann K I, Hamann W, Leung M S 1988 Reversible suppression of responsiveness of slowly adapting type 1 mechanoreceptors in the rat following intradermal injection of neomycin. Journal of Physiology, in press
36. Schacht J 1978 Purification of phosphoinositides by chromatography on immobilized neomycin. Journal of Lipid Research 19: 1063–1067
37. Lohdi S, Weiner N D, Schacht J 1979 Interactions of neomycin with monomolecular films of polyphosphoinositides and other lipids. Biochimica et Biophysica Acta 557: 1–8
38. Ohmori H 1985 Mechano-electrical transduction currents in isolated vestibular hair cells of chick. Journal of Physiology 359: 180–217
39. Blumberg H, Janig W 1987 Changes in primary afferent neurones following lesions of their axons. In: Pubols L M (ed.) Effects of injury on trigeminal and spinal somatosensory systems. Alan R. Liss Inc; New York pp. 85–92
40. Payne R 1986 Neuropathic pain syndromes, with special reference to causalgia and reflex sympathetic dystrophy. The Clinical Journal of Pain 2: 59–73
41. Roberts W J 1986 A hypothesis on the physiological basis for causalgia and related pains. Pain 24: 297–311
42. Merskey H. (ed) 1986 Classification of chronic pain. Pain 24: S1–S226
43. Loeser J D 1977 The management of tic douloureux. Pain 3: 155–162
44. Janetta P J 1967 Arterial compression of the trigeminal nerve at the pons in patients with trigeminal neuralgia. Journal of Neurosurgery 26: 159–162
45. Dubner R, Sharav Y, Gracely R H, Price D D 1987 Idiopathic trigeminal neuralgia: sensory features and mechanisms. Pain 31: 23–33
46. Howe J F, Loeser J D, Calvin W H 1977 Mechanosensitivity of dorsal root ganglia and chronically injured axons: a physiological basis for the radicular pain of nerve root compression. Pain 3: 25–41
47. Hannington-Kiff J G 1974 Intravenous regional sympathetic blockade with guanethidine. Lancet i: 1019–1020
48. Hannington-Kiff J G 1977 Relief of Sudeck's atrophy by regional intravenous guanethidine. Lanceti: 1132–1133
49. Loh L, Nathan P W 1978 Painful peripheral states and sympathetic blocks. Journal of Neurology, Neurosurgery and Psychiatry 41: 664–671
50. Prough D S, McLeskey C H, Poehling G G, Koman L A, Weeks D B, Whitworth T, Semble E L 1985 Efficacy of oral nifedipine in the treatment of reflex sympathetic dystrophy. Anesthesiology 62: 796–799
51. Mitchell S W 1872 Injuries to nerves and their consequences. Lippincott, Philadelphia
52. Wall P D, Gutnick M 1974 Ongoing activity in peripheral nerves: the physiology and pharmacology of impulses originating from a neuroma. Experimental Neurology 43: 580–593
53. Jensen T S, Rasmussen P 1984 Amputation pain. In: Wall P D, Melzack R (eds.) Textbook of Pain Churchill Livingstone, Edinburgh
54. Conacher I D 1986 Percutaneous cryotherapy for post – thoracotomy neuralgia. Pain 25: 227–228

Index